MANUAL OF
EMERGENCY AIRWAY
MANAGEMENT

THIRD EDITION

Editor-in-Chief

Ron M. Walls, MD, FRCPC, FACEP, FAAEM

Chairman, Department of Emergency Medicine
Brigham and Women's Hospital
Professor of Medicine
Division of Emergency Medicine
Harvard Medical School, Boston, Massachusetts

Senior Editor

Michael F. Murphy, MD, FRCPC

Professor and Chair
Department of Anesthesiology
Professor Emergency Medicine
Dalhousie University, Halifax, Nova Scotia, Canada

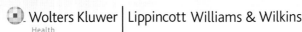
Wolters Kluwer | Lippincott Williams & Wilkins
Health

Philadelphia · Baltimore · New York · London
Buenos Aires · Hong Kong · Sydney · Tokyo

Acquisitions Editor: Frances R. DeStefano
Managing Editor: Chris Potash
Project Manager: Bridgett Dougherty
Senior Marketing Manager: Angela Panetta
Senior Manufacturing Manager: Benjamin Rivera
Creative Director: Doug Smock
Production Services: Aptara, Inc.

530 Walnut Street
Philadelphia, PA 19106
LWW.com

Printed in China

Library of Congress Cataloging-in-Publication Data

Manual of emergency airway management / editor-in-chief, Ron M. Walls;
senior editor, Michael F. Murphy. — 3rd ed.
  p. ; cm.
 Includes bibliographical references and index.
 ISBN-13: 978-0-7817-8494-8 (alk. paper)
 ISBN-10: 0-7817-8494-8 (alk. paper)
 1. Respiratory emergencies—Handbooks, manuals, etc. 2. Respiratory
intensive care—Handbooks, manuals, etc. 3. Airway (Medicine)—
Handbooks, manuals, etc. I. Walls, Ron M. II. Murphy, Michael F.
(Michael Francis), 1954-
 [DNLM: 1. Airway Obstruction—therapy—Handbooks. 2. Emergency
Treatment—Handbooks. 3. Intubation, Intratracheal—Handbooks. WF 39
M2944 2008]
 RC735.R48M36 2008
 616.2'00425—dc22

                                                2007050100

10 9 8 7 6 5 4 3 2 1

Dedication

This edition, like those before it, is dedicated to those intrepid front-line providers who are called on time and again to save a life by rapidly and expertly establishing a definitive airway before a patient's precious intellectual function is lost. They do this quietly and without the expectation of recognition, often while the nation slumbers. They are our true heroes.

PREFACE

In many ways, writing the third edition of this manual was more challenging than either of the previous two. Airway management has progressed dramatically over the four year lifespan of our second edition and, accordingly, so has our way of thinking about it. Through our airway courses, which provide the opportunity to interact with thousands of practicing emergency physicians, intensivists, hospitalists, anesthetists, physician's assistants, nurses, and prehospital providers, we have been struck repeatedly by the demands on the emergency airway manager. There is conflicting and incomplete information, precious little time to perform assessments and make decisions, and even less time to act. This has been reinforced by our own clinical practice on a daily basis, and has driven us to seek simplicity and elegance in airway management, however this might be accomplished.

In producing this edition, we have carefully reviewed the new literature with respect to airway management, evaluated new devices and drugs, and, more important, revisited every principle contained in the previous editions, with a view to ensuring that we present here the very best approach to airway management—the approach we believe is most reliable, most supported by the evidence, and most likely to result in consistent success and good outcomes.

Much has changed. Video laryngoscopy, which was just peeking over the horizon at the time of our second edition, is now mainstream. New optical aids to intubation have come online. Novel drugs, such as suggamadex for the reversal of rocuronium blockade, have emerged; other old favorites, such as etomidate, have come under assault; and certain applications, such as defasciculation, are ready to be retired. Hospitalists and intensivists are increasingly looked to for emergency resuscitation and airway management in the off (and, increasingly, in the "on") hours, as anesthesia departments find their resources too thinly stretched.

In this context, we offer this third edition of the manual. In it, you will find new ways of thinking about old problems, updated algorithms that more accurately reflect practice and technology, and new approaches to both the pharmacology and techniques of airway management. We have expanded our prehospital section, as we have watched the rapid growth of our prehospital airway training programs. Similarly, you will find more information about obesity, pregnancy, and many other conditions. Some old friends, such as the LOAD mnemonic, are departing in favor of a simpler, but equally effective approach. Extraglottic devices are expanding in both indications and availability, and several have been released even since our last edition. Per the previous editions, we have maintained a practical, readable "manual" format in order to be as useful as possible to our readers. However, at the same time, we have expanded and updated our evidence section, so the knowledge basis for our approach is as transparent as possible. We are also fortunate to draw on the collective expertise of experienced, leading academic and clinical emergency physician and anesthesia educators, whose distilled knowledge and experience is a perfect complement to the published literature. At the same time, sadly, we bid adieu to another old friend, Bob Schneider, who has taken his great talents to the arena of homeland security. We thank him for his friendship, collegiality, and constant quest for excellence in our courses and in the previous editions of this book.

The sands of airway management are shifting beneath our feet, and it is hoped that this manual will help the practitioner understand both the actions and the reasons for the actions, and to be better, safer, and more confident airway managers.

We are grateful to our colleagues and teachers, and especially those gifted instructors in The Difficult Airway Course: Emergency, The Difficult Airway Course: Anesthesia, and The Difficult Airway Course: EMS, an increasing number of whom have contributed to this book. Most of all, we are grateful to our students, whose questions continually push us to think critically and to keep exploring.

ACKNOWLEDGMENTS

I have been incredibly fortunate to learn from the giants of our specialty, especially John Marx and Peter Rosen, and to be inspired and challenged daily by my great colleagues, Mike Murphy and Bob Luten. No words could reflect the tremendous influence each has had on me. As I have watched my own family grow and my children have become young adults, I am reminded of the great privilege of being a part of their lives. To my wife, Barb, and my children, Andrew, Blake, and Alexa, thank you for the joy, the inspiration, and the perspective; for always being there for me; and for showing me, by example, what it is all about.

RMW

I wish first to acknowledge my family—Deb, Amanda, Ryan, and Teddy—and to thank them for their tireless support. I am also grateful to my colleagues and close friends, Ron, Bob, and Bob, whose energy and commitment have allowed us to undertake this important mission; the faculty that make it possible to deliver it; and the students who drive us to the cutting edge of emergency airway management.

MFM

CONTRIBUTORS

Aaron E. Bair, MD, MSC
Associate Professor
Emergency Medicine
University of California Davis School
   of Medicine
University of California Davis Medical Center
Sacramento, California

Tobias D. Barker, MD
Instructor in Medicine (Emergency Medicine)
Harvard Medical School
Associate Director,
STRATUS Center for Medical Simulation
Department of Emergency Medicine
Brigham and Women's Hospital
Boston, Massachusetts

Stephen Beed, MD
Associate Professor Anesthesia and Medicine
Dalhousie University
Attending Anesthesiologist and Critical Care
   Physician
Departments of Anesthesia and Critical Care
   Medicine
Queen Elizabeth II Health Sciences Centre
Halifax, Nova Scotia, Canada

Diane M. Birmbaumer, MD
Professor of Clinical Medicine
David Geffen School of Medicine at UCLA
Associate Program Director
Department of Emergency Medicine
Harbor UCLA Medical Center
Torrance, California

Kerry B. Broderick, MD
Assistant Professor
Department of Emergency Medicine
University of Colorado
Staff Physician
Department of Emergency Medicine
Denver Health Medical Center
Denver, Colorado

Calvin A. Brown III, MD
Instructor in Medicine (Emergency
   Medicine)
Harvard Medical School
Associate Director of Student
   Programs
Department of Emergency Medicine
Brigham and Women's Hospital
Boston, Massachusetts

John J. Bruns, Jr., MD
Clinical Assistant Professor
Department of Emergency Medicine
Mount Sinai School of Medicine
Mount Sinai Hospital
New York, New York

**Stephen Bush, MA (OXON), MBBS, FRCS,
   FCEM**
Honorary Senior Lecturer
School of Medicine
University of Leeds
Consultant of Emergency Medicine
Department of Emergency Medicine
St. James University Hospital
Leeds, United Kingdom

David A. Caro, MD
Assistant Professor, Associate Residency
   Director
Department of Emergency Medicine
University of Florida College of Medicine—
   Jacksonville
Jacksonville, Florida

Peter M. C. DeBlieux, MD
LSUHSC Professor of Clinical Medicine
Tulane University Professor of Clinical
   Surgery
Director of Emergency Medicine Services
Department of Emergency Medicine
LSUHSC-MCLNO
New Orleans, Louisianna

Steven A. Godwin, MD, FACEP
Associate Professor
Assistant Dean, Simulation Education
University of Florida College of Medicine,
　Jacksonville
Associated Chair
Department of Emergency Medicine
University of Florida College of Medicine,
　Jacksonville
Jacksonville, Florida

Orlando R. Hung, MD, FRCPC
Professor, Departments of Anesthesia,
　Surgery, and Pharmacology
Dalhousie University
Halifax, Nova Scotia, Canada

Andy S. Jagoda, MD
Professor and Vice Chair
Department of Emergency Medicine
Mount Sinai School of Medicine
Medical Director
Department of Emergency Medicine
Mount Sinai Hospital
New York, New York

**Niranjan Kissoon, MBBS, FRCP(C), FAAP,
　FCCM, FACPE**
Associate Head and Professor
Department of Pediatrics
University of British Columbia
Senior Medical Director
Department of Acute and Critical Care
　Programs
British Columbia's Children's Hospital
Vancouver, British Columbia, Canada

Baruch Krauss, MBBS, EdM, FAAP, FACEP
Assistant Professor of Pediatrics
Harvard Medical School
Faculty, Division of Emergency Medicine
Children's Hospital Boston
Boston, Massachusetts

Eric G. Laurin, MD
Associate Professor of Emergency
　Medicine
Director of Medical Student Education
Department of Emergency Medicine
University of California, Davis
Sacramento, California

Robert C. Luten, MD
Professor, Pediatrics and Emergency
　Medicine
Department of Emergency Medicine
University of Florida
Shands Hospital
Jacksonville, Florida

John D. McAllister, MD
Associate Professor
Departments of Anesthesiology and Pediatrics
Washington University School of Medicine
Clinical Director, Pediatric Anesthesiologist
Department of Anesthesiology
St. Louis Children's Hospital
St. Louis, Missouri

Michael F. Murphy, MD, FRCPC
Professor and Chair Anesthesiology
Professor Emergency Medicine
Dalhousie University
Clinical Chief Anesthesiology
Capital District Health Authority
Halifax, Nova Scotia, Canada

Holly Ann Muir, MD, FRCPC
Vice Chair Clinical Operations
Department of Anesthesiology
Duke University
Chief, Division of Women's Anesthesia
Duke University Medical Center
Durham, North Carolina

Patrick A. Nee, FRCP, FRCS, FCEM
Honorary Lecturer
School of Medical Education
University of Liverpool, United Kingdom
Consultant
Departments of Emergency Medicine and
　Critical Care Medicine
Whiston Hospital
Prescot, Merseyside, United Kingdom

Bret P. Nelson, MD
Assistant Professor
Department of Emergency Medicine
Mount Sinai School of Medicine
Assistant Residency Director
Department of Emergency Medicine
Mount Sinai Hospital
New York, New York

Stephen J. Nelson, NREMTP, CCEMTP
Program Manager, STRATUS Center for
    Medical Simulation
Department of Emergency Medicine
Brigham and Women's Hospital
Boston, Massachusetts

Charles N. Pozner, MD
Assistant Professor of Medicine (Emergency
    Medicine)
Harvard Medical School
Regional Medical Director
Metropolitan Boston EMS Council
Medical Director, STRATUS Center for
    Medical Simulation
Director, of Emergency Medical Services
Brigham and Women's Hospital
Boston, Massachusetts

Ross B. Rodgers, MD
Chief Resident
Department of Emergency Medicine
University of Arizona College of Medicine
Chief Resident
Department of Emergency Medicine
University Medical Center
Tucson, Arizona

John C. Sakles, MD
Associate Professor of Emergency
    Medicine
Department of Emergency Medicine
University of Arizona College of Medicine
Associate Professor
Department of Emergency Medicine
University Medical Center
Tucson, Arizona

Robert E. Schneider, M.D.
Attending Physician
McKay Urology
Charlotte, North Carolina
Senior Medical Advisor for Workforce
    Protection
Office of Health Affairs
Office of the Chief Medical Officer
U.S. Department of Homeland Security
Washington, D.C.

Katren R. Tyler, MD
Assistant Professor
Department of Emergency Medicine
University of California Davis School of
    Medicine
Emergency Physician
Department of Emergency Medicine
University of California Davis Medical
    Center
Sacramento, California

Robert J. Vissers, MD FACEP FRCPC
Chief, Emergency Medicine
Legacy Emanuel Hospital
Adjunct Associate Professor
Oregon Health Sciences University
Portland, Oregon

**Ron M. Walls, MD, FRCPC, FACEP,
    FAAEM**
Professor of Medicine
Division of Emergency Medicine
Harvard Medical School
Chairman, Department of Emergency
    Medicine
Brigham and Women's Hospital
Boston, Massachusetts

Sarah H. Wiser, MD
Clinical Instructor of Anesthesiology
Department of Anesthesiology, Pain and
    Perioperative Medicine
Harvard Medical School
Staff Anesthesiologist
Department of Anesthesiology, Pain and
    Perioperative Medicine
Brigham and Women's Hospital
Boston, Massachusetts

Richard D. Zane, MD
Assistant Professor
Department of Medicine (Emergency
    Medicine)
Harvard Medical School
Vice Chair
Department of Emergency Medicine
Brigham and Women's Hospital
Boston, Massachusetts

CONTENTS

xiii

Section 3. Pharmacology of Airway Management

Section 4. Pediatric Airway Management

Section 5. EMS Airway Management

Section 6. Special Clinical Circumstances

Section 7. Mechanical Ventilation and Monitoring

1

The Decision to Intubate

Ron M. Walls

INTRODUCTION

Loss of the airway, with resultant failure of ventilation and oxygenation, is the terminal pathway for many patients. Timely, effective, and decisive airway management in an emergency can mean the difference between life and death or between ability and disability. In the emergency department (ED), responsibility for airway management resides with the emergency physician. As such, airway management is the single most important skill of the emergency physician, and emergency airway management is one of the defining domains of the specialty of emergency medicine.

> *The emergency physician is responsible for airway management for patients in the emergency department.*

Increasingly, nonanesthesiologists, such as hospitalists or intensivists, are the primary responders to airway emergencies arising on hospital inpatient units. Paramedics and critical care transport personnel are responsible for the out-of-hospital airway. These practitioners must maintain the cognitive base and technical skill set required for swift, decisive airway management, which is often required without warning and in a suboptimal environment.

The emergence of new technology, such as various methods of video and fiberoptic laryngoscopy, is changing the fundamental approach to airway decision making, particularly with respect to difficult intubation. Nevertheless, emergency airway management, whether in the ED or elsewhere in the hospital or prehospital setting, still comprises a definable series of complex actions, each requiring mastery:

- Rapidly assess the patient's need for intubation and the urgency of the situation.
- Determine the best method of airway management.
- Decide whether pharmacological agents are indicated, which to use, in what order, and in what doses.
- Use one of myriad airway devices proficiently to achieve a definitive airway while minimizing the likelihood of hypoxemia, hypercarbia, and aspiration.
- Recognize when the planned airway intervention has failed, and quickly and effectively choose and execute an alternative (rescue) technique.

Physicians responsible for emergency airway management must be proficient with rapid sequence intubation, which requires a thorough knowledge of the pharmacology and effects of neuromuscular blocking agents, sedative or induction agents, and other medications that are used to improve outcome or mitigate adverse effects. The entire repertoire of airway skills must be mastered, ranging from bag-mask ventilation to rapid sequence intubation, techniques for the difficult airway, and rescue maneuvers, including surgical airway techniques, in the event of airway management failure. Emergency airway management requires diligent maintenance of both knowledge and technical bases, continuous learning, sound clinical judgment, and the decisiveness to act when action is indicated. This chapter focuses on the decision to intubate. Subsequent chapters describe the technique of rapid sequence intubation and its place in the new emergency airway algorithms. The airway is rightfully allocated the "A" in the ABC (airway, breathing, circulation) of resuscitation, and in all cases, the airway is paramount and takes precedence over other clinical considerations. Without a secure airway and adequate oxygenation and ventilation, other resuscitative measures are doomed to failure. With the exception of the immediate defibrillation of the cardiac arrest patient, no single resuscitative maneuver takes priority over management of the airway.

Indications for Intubation

The decision to intubate should be based on three fundamental clinical assessments:

1. Is there a failure of airway maintenance or protection?
2. Is there a failure of ventilation or oxygenation?
3. What is the anticipated clinical course?

The results of these three evaluations will lead to a correct decision to intubate or not to intubate in virtually all conceivable cases.

A. **Is there a failure of airway maintenance or protection?**
A patent airway is essential for adequate oxygenation and ventilation, and protection of this airway against aspiration of gastric contents is vital. The conscious, alert patient uses the musculature of the upper airway and various protective reflexes to maintain a patent airway and to protect against the aspiration of foreign substances, gastric contents, or secretions. The ability of the patient to phonate with a clear, unobstructed voice is strong evidence of both airway patency and protection. In the severely ill or injured patient, such airway maintenance and protection mechanisms are often attenuated or lost. If the patient is not able to maintain an adequate airway, an artificial airway may be established by insertion of an oropharyngeal airway or a nasopharyngeal airway. Although such airway devices may restore a patent airway, they do not provide any protection against aspiration. As a general rule, any patient who requires the establishment of an airway also requires protection of that airway, and the use of an oropharyngeal or nasopharyngeal airway should be considered a temporizing measure, pending establishment of a definitive airway.

Any patient who requires the establishment of an airway also requires maintenance and protection of that airway.

A patient who is seemingly able to maintain a patent airway and adequate gas exchange cannot be assumed to be able to protect the airway against the aspiration of gastric contents, which carries a significantly increased risk of morbidity and mortality. It has been widely taught that the gag reflex is a reliable method of evaluating airway protective reflexes. In fact, this concept has never been subjected to adequate scientific scrutiny, and the absence of a gag reflex is neither sensitive nor specific as an indicator of loss of airway protective reflexes. The presence of a gag reflex has similarly not been demonstrated to ensure the presence of airway protection. In addition, testing the gag reflex in a supine, obtunded patient may result in vomiting and possible aspiration. Overall, the gag reflex is not recommended for assessment of airway protection or the need for intubation.

The gag reflex is of no clinical value when assessing the need for intubation.

Evaluation of the ability to swallow spontaneously and to handle normal oropharyngeal secretions is probably a better measure of the patient's ability to protect the airway. Swallowing is a complex reflex that requires the patient to sense the presence of material in the posterior oropharynx, and then to execute a series of intricate and coordinated muscular actions to direct the secretions down past a closed airway into the esophagus. Although this concept also has not been adequately studied, the assessment of spontaneous or volitional swallowing is probably a better tool for assessing the ability to protect the airway than is the presence or absence of a gag reflex. The presence of pooled secretions in the patient's oropharynx should be considered to indicate a potential failure of airway protection. In the absence of an immediately reversible condition, such as opioid overdose or reversible cardiac dysrhythmia, prompt intubation is indicated for any patient who is unable to maintain and protect the airway. A common clinical error is to assume that simply because the patient is "breathing on his or her own," the ability to protect the airway is preserved. Although spontaneous ventilation may be adequate, the patient may be sufficiently obtunded to be at risk for serious aspiration.

B. Is there a failure of ventilation or oxygenation?

If the patient is unable to ventilate adequately, or if adequate oxygenation cannot be achieved despite the use of supplemental oxygen, then intubation is indicated. In such cases, the intubation is being performed to facilitate ventilation and oxygenation rather than to establish or protect the airway. An example is the patient with status asthmaticus, who will generally maintain and protect the airway even when *in extremis.* However, fatigue produces ventilatory failure and, combined with mucous plugging, the resultant hypoxemia will lead to respiratory arrest and death without intervention. Similarly, although the patient with severe adult respiratory distress syndrome may be maintaining and protecting the airway, he or she may have progressive oxygenation failure that can be managed only with endotracheal intubation and positive-pressure ventilation. Unless ventilatory or oxygenation failure is due to a reversible cause, such as opioid overdose, intubation is required.

C. What is the anticipated clinical course?

Most patients who require emergency intubation have one or more of the previously discussed indications: failure of airway maintenance, airway protection, oxygenation, or ventilation. However, there is a large and important group for whom intubation is indicated, even though none of these four fundamental failures is present at the time of evaluation. These are the patients whose conditions, and airways, are predicted to deteriorate, either because of dynamic and progressive changes related to the presenting condition or because the work of breathing will become overwhelming in the face of catastrophic illness or injury. For example, consider the patient who presents with a stab wound to the midzone of the anterior neck and a visible hematoma. At the time of presentation, the patient may have perfectly adequate airway maintenance and protection and be ventilating and oxygenating well. The hematoma, however, provides clear evidence of significant vascular injury. Ongoing bleeding may be clinically occult because the blood often tracks down the tissue planes of the neck (e.g., prevertebral space) rather than causing visible external expansion of the hematoma. Furthermore, the anatomical distortion caused by the enlarging internal hematoma may well thwart a variety of airway management techniques that would have been successful if undertaken earlier. The patient inexorably progresses from awake and alert with a patent airway to a state in which the airway becomes obstructed, often quite suddenly, and the anatomy is so distorted that airway management is difficult or impossible.

> *Acute, progressive anatomical airway distortion is a potential time bomb. Intubate or visualize the airway early, before deterioration occurs!*

Analogous considerations apply to the polytrauma patient who presents with hypotension and multiple severe injuries, including chest trauma. Although this patient initially has adequate airway maintenance and protection, and ventilation and oxygenation may be acceptable, intubation is indicated as part of the management of the constellation of injuries (i.e., as part of the overall management of the patient). The reason for the intubation of such patients becomes clear when one examines the anticipated clinical course of this patient. The hypotension mandates aggressive fluid resuscitation and evaluation for the source of the blood loss, including likely abdominal computed tomography (CT) scan. Pelvic fractures, if unstable, require immobilization and likely embolization of bleeding vessels. Long bone fractures often require operative intervention. Chest tubes may be required to treat hemopneumothorax or in preparation for positive-pressure ventilation during surgery. Combative behavior requires management and evaluation by head

CT scan. Throughout all of this, the patient's shock state causes inadequate tissue perfusion and increasing metabolic debt. This debt significantly affects the muscles of respiration, and progressive respiratory fatigue and failure often supervene. With the patient's ultimate destination certain to be the operating room or the intensive care unit, and the need for complex and potentially painful procedures and diagnostic evaluations, which may require extended periods of time outside the resuscitation suite, this patient is best served by early intubation. In addition, intubation improves tissue oxygenation during shock and helps reduce the increasing metabolic debt burden.

Sometimes, the anticipated clinical course may be such that intubation is mandated because the patient will be exposed to a period of increased risk. For example, the patient with multiple injuries who appears relatively stable might be appropriately managed without intubation while geographically located in the ED. However, if that same patient requires CT scans, angiography, or any other prolonged diagnostic procedure, it may be more appropriate to intubate the patient prior to allowing him or her to leave the ED so that an airway crisis will not ensue in the radiology suite, where recognition may be delayed and response may not be optimal. Similarly, if such a patient is to be transferred from one hospital to another, airway management may be indicated on the basis of the increased risk to the patient during that transfer. Not every trauma patient or every patient with a serious medical disorder requires intubation; however, in general, it is better to err on the side of caution by performing an intubation that might not, in retrospect, have been required, than to delay intubation, thus exposing the patient to a potentially disastrous deterioration. A potentially destructive "fear of intubation" can lead the provider to procrastinate, delaying intubation until the need is indisputable, during which time the patient has deteriorated, and the airway has become more difficult.

If the anticipated clinical course is one of deterioration or if the critically ill or injured patient will be leaving the relatively safe confines of the emergency department, intubate early before deterioration and airway compromise occur.

Approach to the Patient

When evaluating a patient for emergency airway management, the first assessment should be of the patency and adequacy of the airway. In many cases, the adequacy of the airway is confirmed by having the patient speak. Ask questions such as "What is your name?" or "Do you know where you are?" The responses provide information about both the airway and the patient's neurological status. A normal voice, the ability to inhale and exhale in the modulated manner required for speech, and the ability to comprehend the question and follow instructions are strong evidence of adequate upper airway function. Although such an evaluation should not be taken as proof that the upper airway is definitively secure, it is strongly suggestive that the airway is adequate *for the time being*. More important, the inability of the patient to phonate properly, or the presence of stridor or altered mental status precluding responses to the questions mandate an immediate, detailed assessment of the adequacy of the airway and ventilation. After assessing verbal response to questions, conduct a more detailed examination of the mouth and oropharynx. Examine the mouth for bleeding, swelling of the tongue or uvula, abnormalities of the oropharynx (e.g., peritonsillar abscess), or any other abnormalities that might interfere with the unimpeded passage of air through the mouth and oropharynx. Examine the mandible and central face briefly for integrity. A careful examination of the anterior neck requires both visual inspection for deformity, asymmetry, or abnormality and palpation of the anterior neck, including the larynx and trachea. During palpation, assess carefully for the presence of subcutaneous air. This is identified by a crackling feeling on compression of the cutaneous tissues of the neck, much as if a sheet of wrinkled tissue paper were lying immediately beneath the skin. When only a small amount of subcutaneous air is present, this physical finding may be subtle and transient and must be sought carefully. The presence of subcutaneous air indicates disruption of an air-filled passage, often the airway itself, especially in the setting of blunt or penetrating chest or neck trauma. Subcutaneous air in the neck can also be caused by pulmonary injury, esophageal rupture, or, rarely, gas-forming infections. Although these latter two conditions are not immediately threatening to the airway, patients may nevertheless rapidly deteriorate, requiring subsequent airway management.

After inspecting and palpating the upper airway, note the respiratory pattern of the patient. The presence of inspiratory stridor, however slight, indicates some degree of upper airway obstruction. The volume and pitch of stridor on inspiration are related to the velocity of air flow, which in turn depends on the degree to which the patient is conscious and the strength of the inspiratory muscles. Most often, stridor is audible without a stethoscope and should not be confused with "hysterical stridor" or intermittent expiratory moaning, which is often exhibited by patients in pain. Auscultation of the neck with a stethoscope can reveal subauditory stridor that is equally concerning, indicating potential airway compromise. Significant airway compromise may develop before any sign of stridor is evident, particularly in adults. When evaluating the respiratory pattern, observe the chest through several respiratory cycles. Symmetrical, concordant chest movement is the expected finding. In cases where there is significant injury, paradoxical movement of a flail segment of the chest may be observed. If spinal cord injury has impaired intercostal muscle functioning, diaphragmatic breathing may be present. In this form of breathing, there is little movement of the chest wall, and inspiration is evidenced by apparent increase in abdominal volume caused by descent of the diaphragm. Auscultate the chest to assess the adequacy of air exchange. Decreased breath sounds caused by pneumothorax, hemothorax, or other pulmonary pathology may be detected. Acute pneumothorax rarely causes any significant degree of tracheal deviation until the patient is *in extremis,* and tracheal deviation, when found, will likely represent a chronic process.

The assessment of ventilation and oxygenation is a clinical one. Arterial blood gas determinations provide little additional information as to whether intubation is necessary and may be misleading. The clinical impression of the patient's mentation, degree of fatigue, and severity of concomitant injuries or conditions is more important than isolated or even serial determinations of arterial oxygen or carbon dioxide (CO_2) tension. Oxygen saturation is monitored continuously by pulse oximetry, and arterial blood gases are rarely indicated for the purpose of determining arterial oxygen tensions. In certain circumstances, oxygen saturation monitoring is unsuccessful because of poor peripheral perfusion, and arterial blood gases may then be required to assess oxygenation or to provide a correlation with pulse oximetry measurements. Continuous capnography (see Chapter 39) may be used to assess changes in the patient's ability to ventilate adequately, and the measurement of arterial CO_2 tension contributes little additional useful information. In patients with obstructive lung disease, such as asthma or chronic obstructive pulmonary disease, intubation may be required in the face of relatively low CO_2 tensions because of patient fatigue. Other times, extremely high CO_2 tensions may be managed successfully without intubation if the patient is showing clinical signs of improvement (e.g., increased alertness, improving speech, less fatigue).

> *Arterial blood gas values are rarely helpful in the decision to intubate and may be misleading.*

Finally, after assessment of the upper airway and the patient's ventilatory status, including pulse oximetry, capnography, and mentation, consider the patient's anticipated clinical course. If the patient's condition is such that intubation is inevitable and a series of interventions is required, early intubation is preferable. Similarly, if the patient has a condition that is at risk to worsen over time, especially if such worsening is likely to compromise the airway itself, early airway management is indicated. The same consideration applies to patients who require interfacility transfer by air or ground, or a prolonged procedure in an area with diminished resuscitation capability. Intubation before transfer is vastly preferable to a difficult, uncontrolled intubation in an austere environment after the condition has worsened. In all circumstances, the decision to intubate should be given precedence. If doubt exists as to whether the patient requires intubation, err on the side of intubating the patient. It is preferable to intubate the patient and ensure the integrity of the airway than to leave the patient without a secure airway and have an irreversible, preventable catastrophe occur.

EVIDENCE

1. **Is the gag reflex a useful indicator of the need to intubate.** In a study of 111 patients requiring neurological observation in the ED, Moulton et al. (1) found no correlation between the Glasgow Coma Scale (GCS) and the presence or absence of a gag reflex. The gag reflex was noted to be variably present across the range of GCS from 6 to 15, independent of the patient's perceived need for intubation (1). The gag reflex is not involved in laryngeal closure or protection of the airway. Bleach (2) found an absent gag reflex in 27% of fully conscious patients who had undergone speech therapy and videofluoroscopy to assess for possible aspiration after neurological events. There was no correlation between aspiration and the presence (or absence) of the gag reflex (2). Davies et al. (3) studied 140 healthy adults, half of whom were elderly, and found that 37% lacked any gag reflex. Chan et al. (4) studied 414 patients with acute poisoning and noted absence of the gag reflex to be only 70% sensitive in identifying patients who required intubation. Contrary to those studies that find the gag reflex frequently absent in the normal population, absence of a gag reflex was 100% specific in identifying patients requiring intubation; however, the use of a GCS score of 8 or less outperformed the gag reflex, and evaluation of the gag reflex added nothing to the assessment of the GCS score alone (4).

REFERENCES

1. Moulton C, Pennycook A, Makower A. Relation between the Glasgow Coma Scale and the gag reflex. *BMJ* 1991;303:1240–1241.
2. Bleach N. The gag reflex and aspiration: a retrospective analysis of 120 patients assessed by videofluoroscopy. *Clin Otolaryngol* 1993;18:303–307.
3. Davies AE, Kidd D, Stone SP, et al. Pharyngeal sensation and gag reflex in healthy subjects. *Lancet* 1995;345:487–488.
4. Chan B, Gaudry P, Grattan-Smith TE, et al. The use of Glasgow Coma Score in poisoning. *J Emerg Med* 1993;11:579–582.

2

The Emergency Airway Algorithms

Ron M. Walls

APPROACH TO THE AIRWAY

This chapter presents and discusses the emergency airway algorithms, which the authors have developed, used, taught, and refined for more than 12 years. When we first set out to try to codify the cognitive aspects of emergency airway management, we were both liberated and impaired by the complete lack of any such algorithms to guide us. In developing The Airway Course, then The Difficult Airway Course: Emergency, The Difficult Airway Course: Anesthesia, and The Difficult Airway Course: EMS, and in applying successively each iteration of the emergency airway algorithms to tens of thousands of real and simulated cases involving thousands of providers, we felt guided by both our continuous learning about optimal airway management and the empirical application of these principles on a large scale. These algorithms, or adaptations of them, now appear in many of the major emergency medicine textbooks and online references. They are used in airway courses, for residency training, and in didactic teaching sessions, both for in-hospital and out-of-hospital providers. They have stood the test of time and have benefited from constant updating. This current iteration reflects broader application of flexible fiberoptic (FO) methods, new options with extraglottic devices (EGDs), and a near revolution in video and rigid FO laryngoscopy, causing us to rethink concepts related to the definition and management of the "difficult airway" (see Chapter 7). Together, as before, these algorithms comprise a fundamental, reproducible approach to the emergency airway. The purpose is not to provide a "cookbook," which one could universally and mindlessly apply, but rather to describe a reproducible set of decisions and actions to enhance performance and maximize the opportunities for success, even in difficult or challenging cases. The specialized algorithms all build from concepts found in the main emergency airway algorithm, which details the evaluation of the patient for the presence of a crash airway, a difficult airway, or a failed airway. The algorithms do not attempt to deal with the decision to intubate. This is covered in Chapter 1. Therefore, the entry point for the emergency airway algorithm is immediately after the decision to intubate has been made.

The algorithms are intended as guidelines for management of the emergency airway. Although they are not meant to be interpreted as strict rules, covering every possible eventuality, they are designed to present distinct, recognizable patterns and to guide the actions to be taken for each pattern. The goal is to simplify some of the complexities of emergency airway management by defining distinct classes of airway problems. For example, we single out those patients who are essentially dead or near death (i.e., unresponsive, agonal) and manage them using a distinct pathway, the crash airway algorithm. Similarly, a patient with a difficult airway must be identified and managed according to sound principles. Serious problems can ensue if a neuromuscular blocking agent is given to a patient with a difficult airway, unless the difficulty was identified and planned for, and the neuromuscular blocking agent is part of that planned approach.

By grouping patients with certain characteristics together, the algorithms assist the clinician in applying basic notions of pattern recognition so that each patient can be identified as a member of one of a small number of groups, and each group has a defined series of actions. For example, in the case of a difficult airway, the difficult airway algorithm facilitates formulation of a distinct, but reproducible plan, which is individualized for that particular patient, yet lies within the overall approach that is predefined for difficult airways.

In human factors analysis, failure to recognize a pattern is often a precursor to medical error.

Algorithms are best thought of as a series of *key questions* and *critical actions*, with the answer to each question guiding the next critical action. Figures 2-1 and 2-2 provide an overview of the algorithms, and how they work together. When a patient requires intubation, the first question is "Is this a crash airway?" (i.e., is the patient unconscious, near death, with agonal or no respirations, expected to be unresponsive to the stimulation of direct laryngoscopy?). If the answer is "yes," the patient is managed as a crash airway

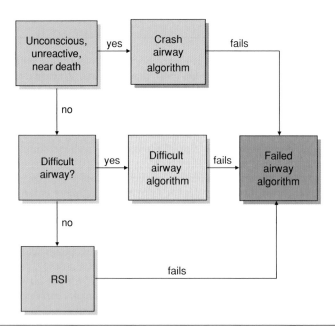

Figure 2-1 ● Universal Emergency Airway Algorithm. This algorithm demonstrates how the emergency airway algorithms work together. For all algorithms, green represents the main algorithm, yellow is the difficult airway algorithm, blue is the crash airway algorithm, red is the failed airway algorithm, and orange represents an end point. © 2008 The Difficult Airway Course: Emergency.

using the crash airway algorithm (Fig. 2-3). If the answer is "no," the next question is "Is this a difficult airway?" (see Chapter 7). If the answer is "yes," the patient is managed as a difficult airway (Fig. 2-4). If the answer is "no," then neither a crash airway nor a difficult airway is present, and rapid sequence intubation (RSI) is recommended, as described on the main algorithm (Fig. 2-2). Regardless of the algorithm used initially (main, crash, or difficult), if airway failure occurs, the failed airway algorithm (Fig. 2-5) is immediately invoked. The working definition of the failed airway is crucial and is explained in much more detail in the following sections. It has been our experience that airway management errors occur much more often because the provider does not recognize the situation (e.g., failed airway), as opposed to recognizing the situation, but not knowing what actions to take.

The Emergency Airway Algorithm (Main Algorithm)

The main emergency airway algorithm is shown in Fig. 2-2. It begins after the decision to intubate and ends when the airway is secured, whether intubation is achieved directly or via one of the other algorithms. The algorithm is navigated by following defined steps with decisions driven by the answers to a series of key questions:

- **Key question 1: Is this a crash airway?** If the patient presents in an essentially unresponsive state and is deemed to be unlikely to respond in any way to direct laryngoscopy, then the patient is defined as a crash airway. Here, we are identifying patients who are in full cardiac or respiratory arrest, or patients with agonal cardiorespiratory activity (e.g., agonal, ineffective respirations, pulseless idioventricular rhythm). These patients, who have been referred to as the "nearly dead or the newly dead," are managed in a manner appropriate for their extremis condition. If a crash

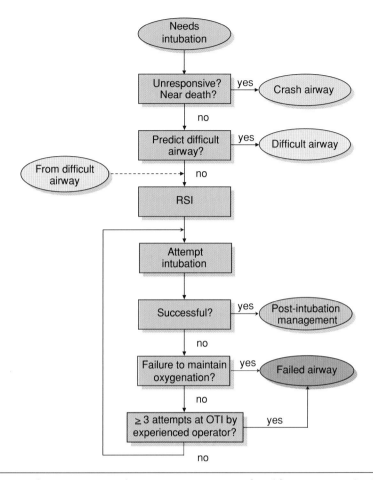

Figure 2-2 ● Main Emergency Airway Management Algorithm. See text for details. © 2008 The Difficult Airway Course: Emergency.

airway is identified, exit this main algorithm and begin the crash airway algorithm (Fig. 2-3). Otherwise, continue on the main algorithm.

- **Key question 2: Is this a difficult airway?** If the airway is not identified as a crash airway, the next task is to determine whether it is a difficult airway, which encompasses difficult laryngoscopy and intubation, difficult bag-mask ventilation (BMV), difficult cricothyrotomy, and difficult extra-glottic device (EGD) use. Chapter 7 outlines the assessment of the patient for a potentially difficult airway using the various mnemonics (LEMON, MOANS, SHORT, and RODS) corresponding to these dimensions of difficulty. It is understood that virtually all emergency intubations are difficult to some extent. However, the evaluation of the patient for attributes that predict difficult airway management is extremely important. If the patient represents a particularly difficult airway situation, then he or she is managed as a difficult airway, using the difficult airway algorithm (Fig. 2-4), and one would exit the main algorithm. Although it is the LEMON assessment for difficult laryngoscopy and intubation that may be the main driver, evaluation for the other difficulties (BMV, cricothyrotomy, EGD) is also critical at this point. If the airway is not identified as particularly difficult, continue on the main algorithm to the next step, which is to perform RSI.
- **Critical action: Perform RSI.** In the absence of an identified crash or difficult airway, RSI is the method of choice for managing the emergency airway. RSI is described in

detail in Chapter 3 and affords the best opportunity for success with the least likelihood of adverse outcome of any possible airway method, when applied to appropriately selected patients. This step assumes that the appropriate sequence of RSI (the seven Ps) will be followed as described in Chapter 3. If the patient is in extreme respiratory distress, or if haste is indicated for any reason, an accelerated or immediate RSI protocol can be used (see Chapter 3).

> *In the absence of difficult airway predictors, rapid sequence intubation is the most rapid, most effective, and safest method of emergency airway management.*

During RSI, intubation is attempted. According to the standard nomenclature of the National Emergency Airway Registry, a multicenter study of emergency intubation, *an attempt is defined as activities occurring during a single continuous laryngoscopy maneuver, beginning when the laryngoscope is inserted into the patient's mouth, and ending when the laryngoscope is removed, regardless of whether an endotracheal tube is actually inserted into the patient.* In other words, if several attempts are made to pass an endotracheal tube through the glottis during the course of a single laryngoscopy, these aggregate efforts count as one attempt. If the glottis is not visualized and no attempt is made to insert a tube, the laryngoscopy is still counted as one attempt. These distinctions are important because of the definition of the failed airway that follows.

- **Key question 3: Was intubation successful?** If the first oral intubation attempt is successful, the patient is intubated, postintubation management is initiated, and the algorithm terminates. If the intubation attempt is not successful, continue on the main pathway.
- **Key question 4: Can the patient's oxygenation be maintained?** When the first attempt at intubation is unsuccessful, it is often possible and appropriate to attempt a second laryngoscopy without interposed BMV because oxygen saturations often remain acceptable for an extended period of time due to proper preoxygenation. In general, supplemental oxygenation with a bag and mask is not necessary until the oxygen saturation falls into the low 90% range. When the oxygen saturation reaches this level, the appropriate first maneuver is BMV of the patient. This approach underscores the importance of assessing the likelihood of successful BMV (MOANS, see Chapter 7) before beginning the intubation sequence. In the vast majority of cases, especially when neuromuscular blockade has been used, BMV will provide adequate ventilation and oxygenation for the patient, defined as maintenance of the oxygen saturation at 90% or higher. If BMV is not capable of maintaining the oxygen saturation above 90%, better technique, including oral and nasal airways, two-person two-handed technique, and optimal positioning of the patient will usually result in effective ventilation (see Chapter 5). If BMV fails despite optimal technique, the airway is considered a failed airway, and one must exit the main algorithm immediately and initiate the failed airway algorithm (Fig. 2-5). Recognition of the failed airway is crucial because delays caused by persistent, futile attempts at intubation will waste critical seconds or minutes and may sharply reduce the time remaining for a rescue technique to be successful before brain injury ensues.
- **Key question 5: Have three attempts at orotracheal intubation been made by an experienced operator?** There are two essential definitions of the failed airway: (a) "can't intubate, can't oxygenate" (CICO) (described previously); and (b) "three failed attempts by an experienced operator." If three separate attempts at orotracheal intubation by an experienced operator have been unsuccessful, then the airway is again defined as a failed airway, despite the ability to adequately oxygenate the patient using a bag and mask. If an experienced operator has used a particular method of laryngoscopy, such as direct laryngoscopy or video laryngoscopy, for three attempts without success, the likelihood of success with further attempts is minimal. The airway must be recognized as a failed airway and managed as such using the failed

airway algorithm. If there have been fewer than three unsuccessful attempts at intubation, but BMV is successful, then it is appropriate to attempt orotracheal intubation again, provided the oxygen saturation is maintained and the operator can identify an element of the laryngoscopy that can be improved (e.g., patient positioning, longer blade). Similarly, if the initial attempts were made by an inexperienced operator, such as a trainee, and the patient is adequately oxygenated, then it is appropriate to reattempt oral intubation until three attempts by an *experienced* operator have been unsuccessful. Rarely, a fourth attempt at laryngoscopy may be appropriate before declaring a failed airway. This most often occurs when the operator identifies a particular strategy for success (e.g., using a smaller diameter endotracheal tube or switching to a greatly oversized blade) during the third unsuccessful attempt. Similarly, it is possible that an *experienced* operator will recognize on the *very first attempt* that further attempts at orotracheal intubation will not be successful. In such cases, provided that the patient has been optimally positioned for intubation, good relaxation has been achieved, the BURP (see Chapter 6) or other external laryngeal maneuvers have been used, and the operator is convinced that further attempts at laryngoscopy would be futile, the airway should be immediately regarded as a failed airway and the failed airway algorithm initiated.

> *It is not essential to make three laryngoscopic attempts before labeling an airway as failed, but three failed attempts by an experienced operator should always be considered a failed airway, unless the laryngoscopist identifies a particular opportunity for success during the last attempt.*

The Crash Airway Algorithm

Entering the crash airway algorithm (Fig. 2-3) indicates that one has identified an unconscious, unresponsive patient with immediate need for airway management. It is assumed throughout that BMV with high flow oxygen is occurring as preparations are made to intubate.

- **Critical action: Intubate immediately:** The first step in the crash algorithm is to attempt oral intubation immediately by direct, video, or FO laryngoscopy without pharmacological assist. In these patient circumstances, direct oral intubation has success rates comparable to RSI, presumably because the patients have flaccid musculature and are unresponsive in a manner similar to that achieved by RSI.
- **Key question 1: Was intubation successful?** If yes, carry on with postintubation management and general resuscitation. If intubation was not successful, resume BMV and proceed to the next step.
- **Key question 2: Is bag-mask oxygenation adequate?** If oxygenation using a bag and mask is judged to be successful, then further attempts at oral intubation are possible. *If BMV is unsuccessful in the context of a single failed oral intubation attempt with a crash airway, then a failed airway is present.* One further attempt at intubation may be rapidly tried, but no more than one, because intubation has failed, and the failure of BMV places the patient in serious and immediate jeopardy. This is a CICO failed airway, analogous to that described previously. Exit here and proceed directly to the failed airway algorithm (Fig. 2-5).

  > *Adequacy of bag-mask oxygenation with a crash airway is usually not determined by pulse oximetry, but by assessment of chest rise and the feel of the bag (as it reflects patency of the airway, delivered tidal volume, airway resistance, and pulmonary compliance).*

- **Critical action: Administer succinylcholine 2 mg/kg intravenous push:** If intubation is not successful, it is reasonable to assume that the patient has residual muscle tone and is not optimally relaxed. The dose of succinylcholine is increased here because these patients often have severe circulatory compromise, impairing the distribution and

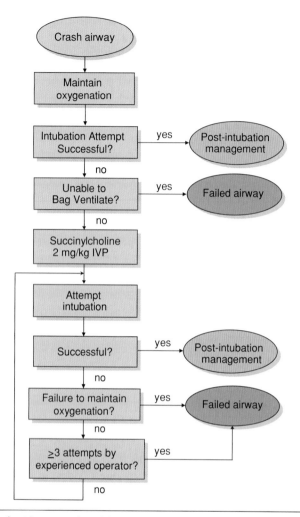

Figure 2-3 ● Crash Airway Algorithm. The portion at the bottom is essentially identical to the corresponding portion of the main emergency airway algorithm. © 2008 The Difficult Airway Course: Emergency.

rapidity of the onset of succinylcholine. BMV is continued for 60 seconds to allow the succinylcholine to distribute. Remember, it is oxygen the patient requires most, not the endotracheal tube. From this point onward, the crash airway algorithm is virtually identical to the corresponding portion of the main airway algorithm, with the exception that the patient has not been adequately preoxygenated, and pulse oximetry is generally incapable of accurately reflecting the state of oxygenation in the crash airway patient. The sequence and rationale, however, are identical from this point on.

- **Critical action: Attempt intubation:** After allowing time for the succinylcholine to circulate, another attempt is made at oral intubation.
- **Key question 3: Was the intubation successful?** If intubation is achieved, then proceed to postintubation management. If not, another attempt is indicated if oxygenation is maintained.
- **Key question 4: Is oxygenation adequate?** If oxygenation cannot be maintained at any time, the airway becomes a CICO failed airway, requiring implementation of the failed airway algorithm.

- **Key question 5: Have there been three or more attempts at intubation by an experienced operator?** If the answer to this question is "yes," then consistent with the previous definition, the situation represents a failed airway. If fewer than three attempts have been made by an experienced operator, then a repeated attempt at oral intubation is justified and one cycles through another intubation attempt. Crash airway patients can be anticipated to experience rapid desaturation, so after each unsuccessful intubation attempt, as defined previously, the patient should receive BMV, and this ventilation must be effective.

   If succinylcholine is administered to a crash patient, count the subsequent intubation attempt as attempt 1.

The Difficult Airway Algorithm

Assessment and management of the difficult airway is discussed in detail in Chapter 7. This algorithm (Fig. 2-4) represents the clinical approach that should be used in the event of an anticipated difficult airway.

- **Critical action: Call for assistance:** The "call for assistance" box is linked as a dotted line because this is an optional step, dependent on the particular clinical circumstances, skill of the airway manager, available equipment and resources, and availability of additional personnel. Assistance might include personnel, special airway equipment, or both.
- **Key question 1: Is there adequate time?** In the context of the difficult airway, *oxygen is time*. If ventilation and oxygenation are adequate and oxygen saturation can be

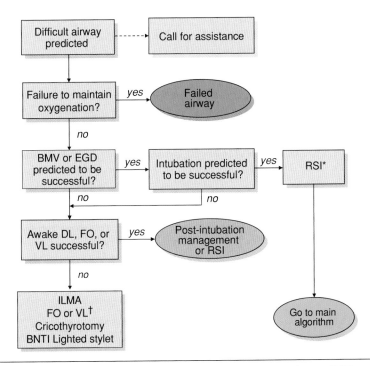

Figure 2-4 ● Difficult Airway Algorithm. BMV, bag-mask ventilation; EGD, extra-glottic device; DL, direct laryngoscopy; FO, fiberoptic method; VL, video laryngoscopy; ILMA, intubating laryngeal mask; BNTI, blind nasotracheal intubation.
*RSI may require a double set-up. See text for details.
†If not used for awake laryngoscopy. © 2008 The Difficult Airway Course: Emergency.

maintained over 90%, then a careful assessment and a methodical, planned approach can be undertaken, even if significant preparation time is required. However, if oxygenation is inadequate, then additional oxygenation or BMV is initiated. If oxygenation cannot be maintained, the situation is equivalent to a "can't intubate (the identified difficult airway is a surrogate for can't intubate), can't oxygenate (adequate oxygenation saturation cannot be achieved)" failed airway. Move immediately to the failed airway algorithm. Certain difficult airway patients will have chronic pulmonary disease, for example, and may not be able to reach oxygen saturation of 90%, but can be kept stable and viable at, say, 86%. Whether to call this case a failed airway is a matter of judgment, but if a decision is made to proceed down the difficult airway algorithm rather than switching to the failed airway algorithm, it is essential to be aware that in cases such as this desaturation will occur rapidly during intubation attempts (see Chapter 3) and to be vigilant with respect to hypoxemia.

- **Key question 2: Despite the presence of the difficult airway, is RSI indicated?** Because we have identified that the patient is adequately oxygenated, the next step is to consider RSI. This decision hinges on two key factors.

  The first, and most important, factor is whether one predicts with confidence that gas exchange can be maintained by BMV or the use of some other adjunct (e.g., an EGD [see Chapter 10]) if a neuromuscular blocking drug is administered rendering the patient paralyzed and apneic. This answer may already be known if BMV has been required to maintain the patient's oxygenation. If the patient has been breathing spontaneously and oxygenating adequately to this point, BMV may have not been attempted. Nonetheless, it is crucial that one performs an evaluation as to whether BMV or an EGD is likely to be successful because this is a virtually essential prerequisite for RSI. The assessment of a patient with respect to predicting difficult BMV and EGD use is described in Chapter 7. In some cases, it may be desirable to attempt a trial of BMV, but this approach does not reliably predict the ability to bag-mask ventilate the patient after paralysis.

  Second, if BMV or EGD is predicted to be successful, then the next consideration is whether intubation is reasonably likely to be successful, despite the difficult airway attributes. In reality, many patients with identified difficult airways undergo successful emergency intubation employing RSI, so if there is a reasonable likelihood of success with oral intubation, *despite the difficult airway*, then RSI may be undertaken. Remember, this is predicated on the fact that one has already judged that gas exchange (BMV or EGD) will be successful following neuromuscular blockade. In some cases, the RSI may be done using a "double setup," in which the patient is evaluated for difficult cricothyrotomy (see Chapter 7) and prepared (i.e., landmarks identified, skin prepped) for cricothyrotomy, and the surgical instruments are open and ready before the RSI is initiated. In most cases, however, when RSI is undertaken despite identification of difficult airway attributes, appropriate care during the technique and planning related to the particular difficulties present will result in success.

  To reiterate these two fundamental principles, if gas exchange employing BMV or EGD is not confidently assured of success in the context of difficult intubation, *or* if the chance of successful oral intubation is felt to be poor, then RSI is not recommended.

  Rapid sequence intubation is often both safe and effective even in a patient with an identified difficult airway, but identifying the difficult airway in advance permits careful planning and use of a double setup when indicated.

- **Critical action: Perform "awake" laryngoscopy:** Just as RSI is the cornerstone of emergency airway management overall, "awake" laryngoscopy is the cornerstone of difficult airway management. The goal of this maneuver is to gain a high degree of confidence that should one induce and paralyze a patient, the airway can be secured. Or, alternatively, the airway can be secured during the "awake look." This technique, which is discussed in detail in Chapter 8, requires moderate to deep sedation of the patient, similar to that used for painful procedures, and the liberal use of local anesthesia (usually topical) to permit laryngoscopy without inducing and paralyzing the patient. The principle here is that the patient is awake enough to maintain the airway and effective spontaneous ventilation, but sufficiently obtunded to tolerate the awake look procedure. Thus, strictly speaking, "awake" is somewhat of a misnomer. The laryngoscopy can be done with a standard laryngoscope, flexible FO scope, video laryngoscope (e.g., the Glidescope or the Storz Videolaryngoscope) or a semirigid FO intubating stylet, such as the Bonfils or the Shikani Optical Stylet. These devices are discussed in detail in Chapters 12 to 14. Two possible outcomes are possible from this awake examination. First, the glottis may be adequately visualized, informing the operator that oral intubation using that device will succeed. If the difficult airway is static (i.e., chronic, such as with ankylosing spondylitis), then the best approach might be to proceed with RSI, now that it is known that the trachea can be intubated, using that same device. If, however, the difficult airway is dynamic (i.e., acute, as in smoke inhalation or angioedema), then it is likely better to proceed directly with intubation during this awake laryngoscopy, rather than to back out and perform RSI. This decision is predicated on the possibility that the airway might deteriorate further in the intervening time, arguing in favor of immediate intubation during the awake examination, rather than assuming that the glottis will be visualized with equal ease a few minutes later during an RSI. Intervening deterioration, possibly contributed to by the laryngoscopy itself, might make a subsequent laryngoscopy more difficult or even impossible (see Chapter 8). The second possible outcome during the awake laryngoscopic examination is that the glottis is not adequately visualized to permit intubation. In this case, the examination has confirmed the suspected difficult intubation and reinforced the decision to avoid neuromuscular paralysis. A failed airway has been avoided and several options remain. Oxygenation should be maintained as necessary at this point.

> *Awake laryngoscopy is the cornerstone of difficult airway management when rapid sequence intubation is not believed to be sufficiently likely to result in successful intubation.*

Although the awake look is the crucial step in management of the difficult airway, it is not infallible. In a very small number of patients, an awake look may provide a better view of the glottic structures than is visible after the administration of a neuromuscular blocking drug. Thus, although the likelihood that the glottis will be less well seen after paralysis than during the awake look is remote, it is not unheard of, and the airway manager must always be prepared for this rare eventuality.

- **Critical action: Select an alternative airway approach:** At this point, we have clarified that we have a patient with difficult airway attributes, who has proven to be a poor candidate for laryngoscopy, and thus is inappropriate for RSI. There are a number of options available here. If the awake laryngoscopy was done using a direct laryngoscope, a video or FO laryngoscopy is likely to provide a superior view of the glottis. The main fallback method for the difficult airway is cricothyrotomy (open or Seldinger technique), but the patient may be amenable to an extraglottic airway that facilitates intubation, i.e. one of the intubating laryngeal mask airways (ILMAs). In highly select cases, blind nasotracheal intubation may be possible, but requires an anatomically intact and normal upper airway. The lighted stylet can be used, either with or without an ILMA for some patients, but is limited by obesity and dark skin pigmentation, and the fact that profound topical anesthesia is needed. The choice of which of these to use will depend on the operator's experience, available equipment, the particular difficult airway attributes the patient possesses, and the urgency of the intubation. The devices and techniques are described in Section 2 of this book. Whichever technique is used, the goal is to place a cuffed endotracheal tube in the trachea, so any device that does not result in an intubated, protected airway should not be used.

The Failed Airway Algorithm

At several points in the preceding algorithms, it may be determined that airway management has failed. The definition of the failed airway (see previous discussion in this chapter and in Chapter 7) is based on one of two criteria being satisfied: (a) a failure of an intubation attempt in a patient for whom oxygenation cannot be adequately maintained with a bag and mask, or (b) three unsuccessful intubation attempts by an experienced operator and adequate oxygenation. Unlike the difficult airway, where the standard of care dictates the placement of a cuffed endotracheal tube in the trachea providing a definitive, protected airway, the failed airway calls for action to provide emergency oxygenation sufficient to prevent patient morbidity (especially hypoxic brain injury) by whatever means possible, until a definitive airway can be secured (Fig. 2-5). Thus, the devices considered for the failed airway are somewhat different from, but inclusive of, the devices used for the difficult airway (see Chapter 7). When a failed airway has been determined to occur, the response is guided by whether bag-mask oxygenation is adequate.

- **Critical action: Call for assistance:** As is the case with the difficult airway, it is best to call for any available and necessary assistance as soon as a failed airway is identified. Again, this action may be a stat consult to emergency medicine; anesthesia; surgery; or an ear, nose, and throat specialist, or it may require a call for special equipment or a respiratory therapist. In the prehospital setting, the consult may be with a second paramedic or other available skilled personnel.

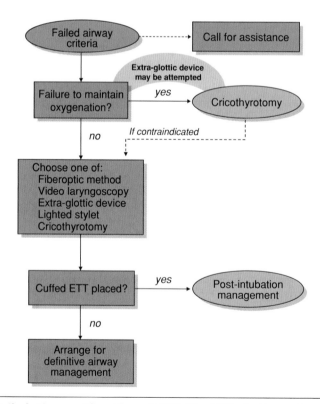

Figure 2-5 ● **Failed Airway Algorithm.** © 2008 The Difficult Airway Course: Emergency.

- **Key question 1: Is oxygenation adequate?** As is the case for the difficult airway, this question addresses the time available for a rescue airway. If the patient is a failed airway because of three failed attempts by an experienced operator, in most cases, oxygen saturation will be adequate, and there is time to consider various approaches. If, however, the failed airway is because of a CICO situation, then there is little time left before cerebral hypoxia will result in permanent deficit, and immediate cricothyrotomy is indicated. There may be rare circumstances when cricothyrotomy is contraindicated, for example, by a large hematoma across the anterior neck. Even in such cases, however, the contraindications are relative, and cricothyrotomy remains the first consideration, unless it is the opinion of the operator that cricothyrotomy would not be possible in the particular circumstance at hand. The only partial exception to the rule that a CICO situation mandates immediate cricothyrotomy as the first rescue step is when the operator makes a single attempt to insert a rapidly placed extraglottic airway device, *simultaneously with the preparation for a cricothyrotomy.* In other words, when the attempt with this alternative device is in parallel with, and not instead of, preparation for immediate cricothyrotomy, it may be prudent and reasonable to attempt a single placement of a rapid, reliable rescue device, which, if successful, converts the CICO situation into a *can't* intubate, *can* oxygenate situation, allowing time for consideration of a number of different approaches to securing the airway.

    Can't intubate, can't oxygenate = cricothyrotomy in the vast majority of circumstances!

- **Critical action:** Achieve an airway using an FO method, video laryngoscopy, an extraglottic device, a lighted stylet, or cricothyrotomy. In the can't intubate, but can oxygenate situation, various devices are available to provide an airway, and most also provide some degree of airway protection. In addition to FO intubation and the lighted stylet, both of which establish a cuffed endotracheal in the trachea, the ILMAs have a high likelihood of providing effective ventilation and will usually permit intubation through the device. Other extraglottic airways vary in their ability to facilitate endotracheal intubation (see Chapter 10). In practical terms, if the patient is able to be successfully ventilated and oxygenated with a bag and mask, the preference is to use a device that places a cuffed endotracheal tube in the trachea (e.g., FO or video method, lighted stylet, ILMA) rather than a nondefinitive temporizing device (e.g., Combitube). Cricothyrotomy always remains the final common pathway if other measures are not successful, or if the patient's oxygenation becomes compromised.

- **Key question 3: Does the device used result in a definitive airway?** If the device used results in a definitive airway (i.e., a cuffed endotracheal tube in the trachea), then one can move on to postintubation management. If an EGD has been used, such as a Combitube or an ILMA, without successful intubation, then arrangements must still be made to provide a definitive airway. A definitive airway may be provided in the operating room, intensive care unit, or emergency department (ED), once the necessary personnel and equipment are available. Until then, constant surveillance is required to ensure that the airway, as placed, continues to provide adequate oxygenation, with cricothyrotomy always available as a backup.

Conclusions

These algorithms are significantly updated and simplified from those in the previous editions of this book. They represent our best thinking regarding a recommended approach to emergency airway management. The algorithms are intended as guidelines only. Individual decision making, clinical circumstances, skill of the physician, and available resources will determine the final, best approach to airway management in any individual case. Understanding the fundamental concepts of the difficult and failed airway; identification, in advance, of the difficult airway; recognition of the crash airway; and the use of RSI as the airway management method of choice for most emergency intubations, however, will result in successful airway management with minimal morbidity.

EVIDENCE

1. **Is RSI superior to sedation alone for intubation?** Blinded anesthesia studies comparing intubating conditions and success under conditions of deep general anesthesia with various neuromuscular blocking agents have included a control group that received no neuromuscular blocking agent. Despite the deep level of anesthesia, much deeper than that existing in the ED during conditions of RSI, the intubating conditions in the no neuromuscular blockade group were so inferior that both authors subsequently advised against including such a control group in the future (1,2). Recently, 70% of patients undergoing general anesthesia with fentanyl 2 μg/kg and propofol 2 mg/kg, but without succinylcholine, demonstrated unacceptable intubating conditions with vocal cords either adducted or closing, excessive patient movement, or sustained coughing, compared to only 2% of patients receiving 1.0 mg/kg of succinylcholine (3). Increasing the dose of succinylcholine from 0.5 to 1.5 mg/kg increases the incidence of excellent intubating conditions from 56% to 85% (4). In two other studies, 19 of 20 and 10 of 10 patients had poor intubating conditions or impossible intubation when neuromuscular blocking agents were not used, despite appropriate doses of anesthetic agents (5,6). In a study of 49 patients in an air medical service, Bozeman et al. (7) compared intubations done with etomidate alone to those done after introduction of an RSI protocol and reported good or acceptable intubating conditions in 79% of RSI patients versus 13% intubated using etomidate alone. Glottic views and intubation difficult scoring were both significantly superior in the RSI group. Intubation success rates were 92% for RSI versus 25% for etomidate alone (7).

2. **What is the success rate of RSI for emergency intubations?** Sakles et al. (8) prospectively studied 610 ED intubations from one high-volume center. In this series, RSI was used in 515 (84%), with a success rate of 98.9%; 7 patients underwent cricothyrotomy. The overall complication rate was 8.0%; 95% confidence interval, 6% to 11% (8). Tayal et al. (9) reported on RSI in 417 of 596 (70%) critically ill patients requiring emergent intubation. Intubations by residents and attendings were successfully completed within two attempts in 97% of the patients. Major immediate adverse events (hypotension, hypoxemia, dysrhythmia) were uncommon (1.4%), and there was no death attributable to RSI. Initial reports from the National Emergency Airway Registry project, a multicenter study of ED intubations that has now gathered data on more than 15,000 ED intubations, show very high success rates with a low incidence of adverse events. Sivilotti et al. (10) reported on 3,407 ED intubations, of which 2,380 (70%) were intubated using RSI. Ninety-five percent of the patients were intubated in the first two laryngoscopic attempts, and 98.5% were successfully intubated without requiring a second (rescue) method. Emergency medicine physicians performed the initial intubation in 2,118 (89%) cases (10). Similar success is reported for pediatric intubations in the NEAR I project (11). RSI is the method of choice for most intubations and is also the most common rescue maneuver when another intubation method fails (12). Sagarin et al. (13) reported on 7,498 intubations at 31 centers in the NEAR project. The first intubator was successful in 90% of intubations, and intubation success improved with year of residency training in emergency medicine. Cricothyrotomy was required in less than 1% of cases (13). Graham et al. (14) studied RSIs in seven hospitals in Scotland, and reported Cormack-Lehane grades 1 or 2 in 92% of cases. Zukerbraun et al. (15) reported 100% success in 77 consecutive pediatric patients undergoing RSI at a single center. In a comparison of etomidate

and midazolam for prehospital RSI, Swanson et al. (16) found success rates of more than 98%, regardless of which sedative agent was used.

3. **What is the evidence supporting the alternate airway devices as rescue devices?** Parr et al. (17) reported on the use of the ILMA for two anesthesia patients with failed oral intubation due to impossible laryngoscopic visualization of the glottis. Both patients were successfully ventilated with a bag and mask, had the ILMA placed, then were intubated through the ILMA. One hundred percent of 254 patients with identified difficult airways were successfully ventilated with the ILMA, and 96.5% of those on whom intubation was attempted ($n = 200$) were successfully intubated within five attempts through the ILMA (18). One hundred patients with identified difficult airways were randomized to undergo intubation either using an ILMA or with an FO scope. Success required intubation within three attempts, and success rates were 45/49 (92%) for FO and 48/51 (94%) for ILMA. When the first method of intubation failed (seven patients total), all patients were successfully intubated within two attempts using the other method (19). Both the Combitube and the LMA appear to be easy to place and ventilate with, even by inexperienced personnel (20). These devices are discussed in more detail in the relevant chapters.

4. **Evidence for the algorithms.** Unfortunately, there are no systematized data supporting the algorithmic approach presented in this chapter. The algorithms are the result of careful review of the American Society of Anesthesiologists difficult airway algorithm and composite knowledge and experience of the editors, who functioned as an expert panel in this regard. There has not been, and likely never will be, a study comparing, for example, the outcomes of cricothyrotomy versus alternate airway devices in the CICO situation, and clearly randomization of such patients is not ethical. Thus, the algorithms are derived from a rational body of knowledge (described previously) and represent a recommended approach, but cannot be considered to be scientifically proven as the only or even necessarily the best way to approach any one clinical problem or patient. Rather, they are designed to help guide a consistent approach to both common and uncommon airway management situations.

REFERENCES

1. Cicala R, Westbrook L. An alternative method of paralysis for rapid-sequence induction. *Anesthesiology* 1988;69:983–986.

2. Baumgarten RK, Carter CE, Reynolds WJ, et al. Priming with nondepolarizing relaxants for rapid tracheal intubation: a double-blind evaluation. *Can J Anaesth* 1988;35:5–11.

3. Naguib M, Samarkandi A, Riad W, et al. Optimal dose of succinylcholine revisited. *Anesthesiology* 2003;99:1045–1049.

4. Stewart KG, Hopkins PM, Dean SG. Comparison of high and low doses of suxamethonium. *Anaesthesia* 1991;46:833–836.

5. Kahwaji R, Bevan DR, Bikhazi G, et al. Dose-ranging study in younger adult and elderly patients of ORG 9487, a new rapid-onset, short duration muscle relaxant. *Anesth Analg* 1997;84:1011–1018.

6. Pino RM, Ali HH, Denman WT, et al. A comparison of the intubation conditions between mivacurium and rocuronium during balanced anesthesia. *Anesthesiology* 1998;88:673–678.

7. Bozeman WP, Kleiner DM, Huggett V. A comparison of rapid sequence intubation and etomidate-only intubation in the prehospital air medical setting. *Prehosp Emerg Care* 2006;10:8–13.

8. Sakles JC, Laurin EG, Rantapaa AA, et al. Airway management in the emergency department: a one-year study of 610 tracheal intubations. *Ann Emerg Med* 1998;31:325–332.

9. Tayal VS, Riggs RW, Marx JA, et al. Rapid-sequence intubation at an emergency medicine residency: success rate and adverse events during a two-year period. *Acad Emerg Med* 1999;6:31–37.

10. Sivilotti MA, Filbin MR, Murray HE, et al., on behalf of the NEAR investigators. Does the sedative agent facilitate emergency rapid-sequence intubation? *Acad Emerg Med* 2003; 10:612–620.

11. Sagarin MJ, Chiang V, Sakles JC, et al., on behalf of the NEAR investigators. Rapid sequence intubation for pediatric emergency airway management. *Pediatr Emerg Care* 2002;18:417–423.

12. Bair AE, Filbin MR, Kulkami R, et al., on behalf of the NEAR investigators. Failed intubation in the emergency department: analysis of prevalence, rescue techniques, and personnel. *J Emerg Med* 2002;23:131–140.

13. Sagarin MS, Barton ED, Chng YM, et al. Airway management by U.S. and Canadian emergency medicine residents: a multicenter analysis of more than 6,000 endotracheal intubation attempts. *Ann Emerg Med* 2005;46:328–336.

14. Graham CA, Oglesby AJ, Beard D, et al. Laryngoscopic views during rapid sequence intubation in the emergency department. *Can J Emerg Med* 2004;6:416–420.

15. Zuckerbraun NS, Pitetti RD, Herr SM, et al. Use of etomidate as an induction agent for rapid sequence intubation in a pediatric emergency department. *Acad Emerg Med* 2006;13: 602–609.

16. Swanson ER, Fosnocht DE, Jensen SC. Comparison of etomidate and midazolam for prehospital rapid-sequence intubation. *Prehosp Emerg Care* 2004;8:273–279.

17. Parr MJA, Gregory M, Baskett PJ, et al. The intubating laryngeal mask: use in failed and difficult intubations. *Anaesthesia* 1998;53:343–348.

18. Ferson DZ, Rosenblatt WH, Johansen MJ, et al. Use of the intubating LMA-Fastrach in 254 patients with difficult airways. *Anesthesiology* 2001;95:1175–1181.

19. Langeron O, Semjen F, Bourgain JL, et al. Comparison of the intubating laryngeal mask airway with the fiberoptic intubation in anticipated difficult airway management. *Anesthesiology* 2001;94:968–972.

20. Yardy N. A comparison of two airway aids for emergency use by unskilled personnel. The Combitube and laryngeal mask. *Anaesthesia* 1999;54:179–183.

3

Rapid Sequence Intubation

Ron M. Walls

INTRODUCTION

Definition

Rapid sequence intubation (RSI) is the administration, after preoxygenation, of a potent induction agent followed immediately by a rapidly acting neuromuscular blocking agent to induce unconsciousness and motor paralysis for tracheal intubation. The technique is predicated on the fact that the patient has not fasted before intubation and, therefore, is at risk for aspiration of gastric contents. The preoxygenation phase before drug administration permits a period of apnea to occur safely between the administration of the drugs and intubation of the trachea, therefore obviating the need for positive-pressure ventilation. In other words, the purpose of RSI is to render the patient unconscious and paralyzed and then to intubate the trachea without the use of bag-mask ventilation, which may cause gastric distention and increase the risk of aspiration. Sellick's maneuver (posterior pressure on the cricoid cartilage) has been widely recommended and used to occlude the esophagus and supposedly prevent passive regurgitation, but it has been shown to impair glottic visualization in some cases, and the evidence supporting its use is tenuous. In this edition of the manual, we have demoted Sellick's maneuver to "optional" status.

> *Rapid sequence intubation is the virtually simultaneous administration, after preoxygenation, of a potent sedative agent and a rapidly acting neuromuscular blocking agent to facilitate rapid tracheal intubation without interposed positive-pressure ventilation.*

Indications and Contraindications

RSI is the cornerstone of emergency airway management. Other techniques, such as blind nasotracheal intubation or intubation using sedation with or without topical anesthesia, may be useful in certain patients presenting with a difficult airway (see Chapter 2). However, the superiority of RSI in terms of success rates, complication rates, and control of adverse effects makes it the procedure of choice for the majority of emergency department intubations. Contraindications to RSI are relative. Difficult intubation per se is not a contraindication to RSI; rather, it indicates to the physician that a careful preintubation assessment and plan are required (see Chapter 2 and Figs. 2-2 and 2-4). Other relative contraindications pertain more to the choice of individual agents for the intubation rather than to the use of a rapid sequence technique. These relative contraindications are discussed in various places throughout this text and within the discussions of the pharmacology of each agent.

TECHNIQUE

RSI can be thought of as a series of discrete steps, referred to as the seven Ps. These are shown in Box 3-1.

BOX 3-1 The Seven Ps of Rapid Sequence Intubation

1. Preparation
2. Preoxygenation
3. Pretreatment
4. Paralysis with induction
5. Positioning
6. Placement with proof
7. Postintubation management

A. *Preparation*

Before initiating the sequence, the patient is thoroughly assessed for difficulty of intubation (see Chapters 2 and 7). Fallback plans in the event of failed intubation are established, and the necessary equipment is located. The patient is in an area of the emergency department that is organized and equipped for resuscitation. Cardiac monitoring, blood pressure monitoring, and pulse oximetry should be used in all cases. Continuous capnography provides additional valuable monitoring information, particularly after intubation. The patient has at least one, and preferably two, secure, well-functioning intravenous lines. Pharmacological agents are drawn up in properly labeled syringes. Vital equipment is tested. If a direct laryngoscope is to be used, the blade of choice is affixed to the laryngoscope handle and clicked into the "on" position to ensure that the light functions and is bright. If a video or fiberoptic laryngoscope is to be used, it is turned on, image quality is verified, and any necessary antifog solution is applied. The endotracheal tube (ETT) of the desired size is prepared, and the cuff tested for leaks. If difficult intubation is anticipated, a smaller tube (6.0 or 6.5 mm) should also be prepared. Selection and preparation of the tube, as well as the use of the intubating stylet and bougie, are discussed in Chapter 6. Throughout this preparatory phase, the patient should be receiving preoxygenation as described in the next section.

B. *Preoxygenation*

Preoxygenation is essential to the "no bagging" principle of RSI. Preoxygenation is the establishment of an oxygen reservoir within the lungs, blood, and body tissue to permit several minutes of apnea to occur without arterial oxygen desaturation. The principle reservoir is the functional residual capacity in the lungs, which is approximately 30 mL/kg. Administration of 100% oxygen for 3 minutes replaces this predominantly nitrogenous mixture of room air with oxygen, allowing several minutes of apnea time before hemoglobin saturation decreases to less than 90% (Fig. 3-1). Similar preoxygenation can be achieved much more rapidly by having the patient take eight vital capacity breaths (the greatest volume breaths the patient can take) while receiving 100% oxygen.

Time to desaturation varies, depending on particular patient attributes, with children, morbidly obese patients, and late-term pregnant women desaturating much more rapidly than an average healthy adult.

Note the bars indicating recovery from succinylcholine paralysis on the bottom right of Fig. 3-1. This demonstrates the fallacy of the oft-cited belief that a patient will quite likely recover sufficiently from succinylcholine-induced paralysis to breathe on his or her own before sustaining injury from hypoxemia, even if intubation and mechanical ventilation are both impossible. Although many patients will recover adequate neuromuscular function to breathe on their own before catastrophic desaturation, many others, including almost all children, will not, and even those who do are dependent on optimal preoxygenation before paralysis.

A healthy, fully preoxygenated 70-kg adult will maintain oxygen saturation over 90% for 8 minutes, whereas an obese (127-kg) adult will desaturate to 90% in less than 3 minutes. A 10-kg child will desaturate to 90% in less than 4 minutes. The time for desaturation from 90% to 0% is even more important and is much shorter. The healthy 70-kg adult desaturates from 90% to 0% in less than 120 seconds, and the small child does so in 45 seconds. A late-term pregnant woman is a high oxygen user and has an increased body mass, so she desaturates quickly in a manner analogous to that of the obese patient. Particular caution is required in this circumstance because both the obese patient and the pregnant woman are also difficult to intubate and to bag-mask ventilate.

The time to desaturate from 90% to 0% is dramatically less than the time to desaturate from 100% to 90%.

Most emergency departments do not use systems that are capable of delivering 100% oxygen. Typically, emergency department patients are preoxygenated using the

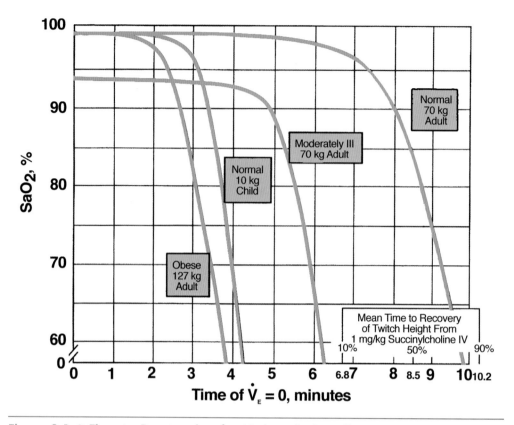

Figure 3-1 ● **Time to Desaturation for Various Patient Circumstances.** *Source:* From Benumof J, Dagg R, Benumof R. Critical hemoglobin desaturation will occur before return to an unparalyzed state following 1 mg/kg intravenous succinylcholine. *Anesthesiology* 1997;87:979.

"100% nonrebreather mask," which delivers approximately 65% to 70% oxygen (see Chapter 5). In physiologically well patients in whom difficult intubation is not anticipated, this percentage is often sufficient and adequate preoxygenation is achieved. However, higher inspired fractions of oxygen are often desirable and can be delivered by active breathing through the demand valve of bag-mask systems equipped with a one-way exhalation valve, or by specially designed high-concentration oxygen delivery devices. Oxygen delivery is discussed in detail in Chapter 5. The use of pulse oximetry throughout intubation enables the physician to monitor the level of oxygen saturation, thus eliminating guesswork.

The old recommendation that an intubator should hold his or her breath during the laryngoscopy to determine the maximal time that the patient should be without ventilation predated pulse oximetry and has no place in modern airway management.

C. *Pretreatment*
Pretreatment is the administration of drugs to mitigate adverse effects associated with the intubation or the patient's underlying comorbidities. These adverse effects include bronchospastic reactivity of the airways to the ETT in patients with reactive airways disease, the intracranial pressure (ICP) response to airway manipulation in patients with elevated ICP, and systemic release of sympathetic adrenergic amines (the reflex sympathetic response to laryngoscopy [RSRL]). We have revisited our former recommendation regarding use of a defasciculating dose of a competitive

---

BOX 3-2 Pretreatment Drugs for Rapid Sequence Intubation

Fentanyl   When sympathetic responses should be blunted (increased intracranial pressure (ICP), aortic dissection, intracranial hemorrhage, ischemic heart disease)

Lidocaine   For reactive airways disease or increased ICP

neuromuscular blocking agent in patients with elevated ICP who are receiving succinylcholine and, on the basis of available evidence, can no longer recommend this practice. Similarly, we no longer recommend the routine use of atropine before succinylcholine in small children. The pretreatment drugs are shown in Box 3-2 and discussed in detail in Chapter 17. Because there are three classes of patients for whom pretreatment is indicated, the mnemonic "ABC" can be used (Fig. 3-2): **A**sthma (representing reactive airways disease), **B**rain (representing elevated ICP), and **C**ardiovascular (representing those at risk from RSRL; i.e., patients with ischemic heart disease, vascular disease [especially cerebrovascular disease], hypertension, and vascular events, such as aortic dissection, intracranial hemorrhage, etc.). The two drugs, fentanyl and lidocaine, and their relationship to the ABC conditions can be represented in a Venn diagram (Fig. 3-2). The pretreatment agents, when indicated, are administered 3 minutes before the induction agents and succinylcholine.

D. *Paralysis with induction*

In this phase, a rapidly acting induction agent is given in a dose adequate to produce prompt loss of consciousness (see Chapter 18). Administration of the induction agent is immediately followed by the neuromuscular blocking agent, usually succinylcholine (see Chapter 19). Both medications are given by intravenous push. The concept of RSI does not involve the slow administration of the induction agent, nor does it involve a titration-to-end point approach. The sedative agent and dose should

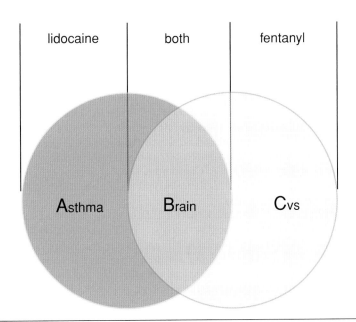

Figure 3-2 ● Pretreatment Agents for Rapid Sequence Intubation—the ABC Approach.
CVS, cardiovascular system.

be selected with the intention of rapid intravenous administration of the drug. Although rapid administration of these induction agents can increase the likelihood and severity of side effects, especially hypotension, the entire technique is predicated on rapid loss of consciousness, rapid neuromuscular blockade, and a brief period of apnea without interposed assisted ventilation before intubation. Therefore, the induction agent is given as a rapid push followed immediately by a rapid push of the succinylcholine. Within a few seconds of the administration of the induction agent and succinylcholine, the patient will begin to lose consciousness and respirations will decline, and then cease.

E. *Positioning*

After 20 to 30 seconds, apnea virtually universally will be present. If succinylcholine has been used as the neuromuscular blocking agent, fasciculations will be observed during this time. The patient will become increasingly flaccid. The oxygen mask used for pre-oxygenation remains in place to prevent the patient from acquiring even a partial breath of room air. At this point, the patient is positioned optimally for intubation (see Chapter 6), with consideration for cervical spine immobilization in trauma. Sellick's maneuver, the application of firm pressure (see Chapter 6) on the cricoid cartilage to prevent passive regurgitation of gastric contents, was formerly widely recommended, but there is little evidence to support its use, and emerging evidence demonstrates that it can worsen laryngoscopic view and impair tube insertion over a bougie. Thus, it is considered optional. If used, Sellick's maneuver is initiated immediately on the observation that the patient is losing consciousness and maintained throughout the entire intubation sequence until the ETT has been correctly placed, the position verified, and the cuff inflated. If there is difficulty visualizing the glottis or inserting the ETT, Sellick's maneuver, if used, is discontinued, and external laryngeal manipulation or other maneuvers are used as indicated. Some patients, as discussed in Section 6 of this manual, will be sufficiently compromised that they require assisted ventilation to maintain oxygen saturations over 90% before, during, and after the intubation. Such patients, especially those with profound hypoxemia, should be bag-mask ventilated throughout the sequence to prevent worsening hypoxemia. In such cases, the application of Sellick's maneuver may minimize the volume of gases passed down the esophagus to the stomach, possibly decreasing the likelihood of regurgitation.

F. *Placement with proof*

Approximately 45 seconds after the administration of the succinylcholine, or 60 seconds if rocuronium is used, test the patient's jaw for flaccidity and intubate. Because of the *minutes* of safe apnea time permitted by the preoxygenation, the intubation can be performed gently and carefully with due attention to the patient's dentition and proper attention to technique to minimize the potential for trauma to the airway. The glottic aperture is visualized, and the ETT is placed. The stylet is removed, and the ETT cuff is inflated. Tube placement is confirmed as described in Chapter 6 to prove that the tube is correctly placed within the trachea. End-tidal carbon dioxide (CO_2) detection is mandatory. A capnometer, such as a colorimetric end-tidal CO_2 detector, is sufficient for this purpose. Continuous capnography is recommended, however. Sellick's maneuver, if used, is then discontinued on the order of the intubator.

G. *Postintubation management*

After placement is confirmed, the ETT must be taped or tied in place. Mechanical ventilation should be initiated as described in Chapter 37. A chest radiograph should be obtained to assess pulmonary status and ensure that mainstem intubation has not occurred. Hypotension is common in the postintubation period and is often caused by diminished venous blood return as a result of the increased intrathoracic pressure that attends mechanical ventilation, exacerbated by the hemodynamic effects of the induction agent. Although this form of hypotension is often self-limited and responds to intravenous fluids, more ominous causes should be sought. Blood pressure should be measured, and if significant hypotension is present, the management steps in Table 3-1 should be undertaken.

TABLE 3-1

Hypotension in the Postintubation Period

Cause	Detection	Action
Pneumothorax	Increased peak inspiratory pressure (PIP), difficulty bagging, decreased breath sounds	Immediate thoracostomy
Decreased venous return	Worst in patients with high PIPs secondary to high intrathoracic pressure or those with marginal hemodynamic status before intubation	Fluid bolus, treatment of airway resistance (bronchodilators); increase inspiratory flow rate to allow increased expiratory time; try $\downarrow V_T$, respiratory rate, or both if S_pO_2 is adequate
Induction agents	Other causes excluded	Fluid bolus, expectant
Cardiogenic	Usually in compromised patient; ECG; exclude other causes	Fluid bolus (caution), pressors

Long-term sedation is usually indicated. Recently, there is an increased focus on avoidance of paralysis, except when necessary, and use of a sedation scale, such as the Richmond Agitation Sedation Scale, to optimize patient comfort (Box 3-3). Sedation is administered to reach the desired sedation goal, and neuromuscular blockade is used only if the patient then requires it for management. This avoids the use of neuromuscular blockade to eliminate (and obscure) patient response, when the cause of the patient's agitation is inadequate sedation. A sample sedation protocol is shown in Fig. 3-3. Maintenance of intubation and mechanical ventilation require both sedation and analgesia, and these can be titrated to patient response (Fig. 3-3). A reasonable sedation starting point is lorazepam 0.05 mg/kg or midazolam 0.2 mg/kg, combined with an analgesic such as fentanyl 2 to 3 μg/kg, morphine 0.2 mg/kg, or hydromorphone (Dilaudid) 0.03 mg/kg. Fentanyl may be preferable because of its superior hemodynamic stability. When a neuromuscular blocking agent is required, a full paralytic dose should be used (e.g., vecuronium 0.1 mg/kg). Sedation and analgesia are difficult to titrate when the patient is paralyzed, and "topping up" doses should be administered regularly, before physiological stress (hypertension, tachycardia) is evident. For patients requiring serial examination, principally patients with neurological conditions, propofol by infusion is preferable, because it can be discontinued or decreased with rapid recovery of consciousness. Propofol infusion can be started at 25 to 50 mcg/kg/min and titrated. An initial bolus of 0.5 to 1 mg/kg may be given if rapid sedation is desired.

Timing the Steps of RSI

Successful RSI requires a detailed knowledge of the precise steps to be taken and also of the time required for each step to achieve its purpose. Preoxygenation requires at least 3 minutes for maximal effect. In hurried circumstances, eight vital capacity breaths (if possible) can accomplish equivalent preoxygenation in less than 30 seconds. It is recommended that pretreatment drugs be given 3 minutes before the administration of the sedative and neuromuscular blocking agent. The pharmacokinetics of the sedatives and

BOX 3-3 Richmond Agitation Sedation Scale

Score	Term	Description	
+4	Combative	Overtly combative, violent, immediate danger to staff	
+3	Very agitated	Pulls or removes tube(s) or catheter(s), aggressive	
+2	Agitated	Frequent nonpurposeful movement, fights ventilator	
+1	Restless	Anxious but movements not aggressive, vigorous	
0	Alert and calm		
−1	Drowsy	Not fully alert, but has sustained awakening (eye opening/eye contact) to *voice* (>10 seconds)	Verbal stimulation
−2	Light sedation	Briefly awakens with eye contact to *voice* (<10 seconds)	
−3	Moderate sedation	Movement or eye opening to *voice* (but no eye contact)	
−4	Deep sedation	No response to voice, but movement or eye opening to *physical* stimulation	Physical stimulation
−5	Unarousable	No response to *voice* or *physical* stimulation	

Procedure for Richmond Agitation Sedation Scale Assessment
1. Observe patient.
   a. Patient is alert, restless, or agitated.   (score 0 to +4)
2. If not alert, state patient's name and *say* to open eyes and look at speaker.
   b. Patient awakens with sustained eye opening and eye contact.   (score −1)
   c. Patient awakens with eye opening and eye contact, but not sustained.   (score −2)
   d. Patient has any movement in response to voice but no eye contact.   (score −3)
3. When no response to verbal stimulation, physically stimulate patient by shaking shoulder and/or rubbing sternum.
   e. Patient has any movement to physical stimulation.   (score −4)
   f. Patient has no response to any stimulation.   (score −5)

Adapted from Sessler CN, Gosnell M, Grap MJ, et al. The Richmond Agitation-Sedation Scale: validity and reliability in adult intensive care patients. *Am J Respir Crit Care Med* 2002;166:1338–1344; Ely EW, Truman B, Shintani A, et al. Monitoring sedation status over time in ICU patients: the reliability and validity of the Richmond Agitation Sedation Scale (RASS). *JAMA* 2003;289:2983–2991.

neuromuscular blockers would suggest that a 45-second interval between administration of these agents and initiation of endotracheal intubation is optimal, extending to 60 seconds if rocuronium is used. Thus, the entire sequence of RSI can be described as a series of timed steps. For the purposes of discussion, time zero is the time at which the sedative agent and succinylcholine are pushed. The recommended sequence is shown in Table 3-2.

An example of RSI performed for a generally healthy 40-year-old, 80-kg patient is shown in Table 3-3. Other examples of RSI for particular patient conditions are in the corresponding sections throughout the text.

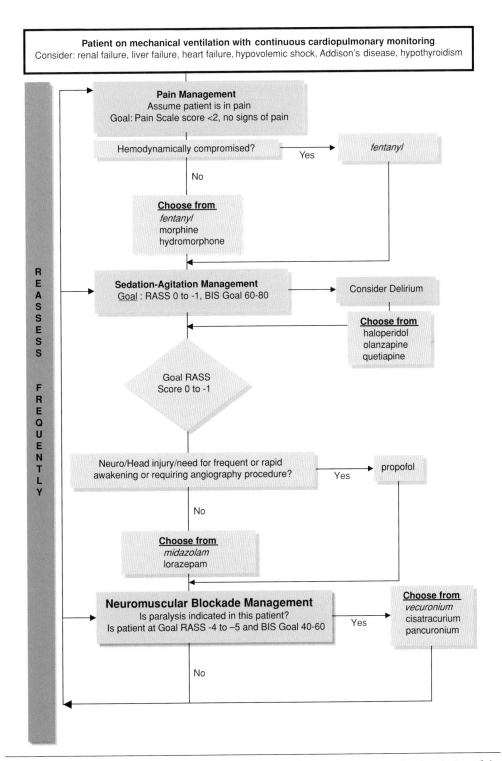

Figure 3-3 ● **Postintubation Management Protocol.** See also Box 3-3 for description of the Richmond Agitation Sedation Scale. *Source:* The protocol, reproduced with permission, was developed for use at Brigham and Women's Hospital, Boston.

TABLE 3-2
Rapid Sequence Intubation

Time	Action (seven Ps)
Zero minus 10 minutes	Preparation: *Assemble all necessary equipment, drugs, etc.*
Zero minus 5 minutes	Preoxygenation
Zero minus 3 minutes	Pretreatment
Zero	Paralysis with induction: *Administer induction agent by intravenous (IV) push, followed immediately by paralytic agent by IV push*
Zero plus 20–30 seconds	Positioning: *Position patient for optimal laryngoscopy; Sellick's maneuver, if desired, is applied now*
Zero plus 45 seconds	Placement with proof: *Assess mandible for flaccidity; perform intubation; confirm placement*
Zero plus 1 minute	Postintubation management: *Long-term sedation/paralysis as indicated*

Success Rates and Adverse Events

RSI has a very high success rate in the emergency department, approximately 99% in most modern series. The National Emergency Airway Registry (NEAR), an international multicenter study of more than 10,000 emergency department intubations, reported greater than 99% success for RSI when used on patients with medical emergencies and greather than 97% for trauma patients. RSI success rates are higher than those for other emergency airway management methods, and RSI is the main rescue technique when other methods, such as

TABLE 3-3
Rapid Sequence Intubation for Healthy 80-kg Patient

Time	Action (seven Ps)
Zero minus 10 minutes	Preparation
Zero minus 5 minutes	Preoxygenation
Zero minus 3 minutes	Pretreatment: *None indicated*
Zero	Paralysis with induction: *Etomidate 24 mg intravenous (IV) push; succinylcholine 120 mg IV push*
Zero plus 20–30 seconds	Positioning: *Position patient for optimal laryngoscopy; Sellick's maneuver, if desired, is applied now*
Zero plus 45 seconds	Placement with proof: *Confirm with $ETCO_2$, Physical Examination*
Zero plus 1 minute	Postintubation management: *Long-term sedation/paralysis as indicated*

$ETCO_2$, end-tidal CO_2 detection.

blind nasotracheal intubation, fail. The NEAR investigators classify events related to intubation as follows:

- Immediate complications, such as witnessed aspiration, broken teeth, airway trauma, undetected esophageal intubation
- Technical problems, such as mainstem intubation, cuff leak, recognized esophageal intubation
- Physiological alterations, such as pneumothorax, pneumomediastinum, cardiac arrest, dysrhythmia

This system allows witnessed complications to be identified and all adverse events to be captured, but avoids the incorrect attribution of various technical problems (e.g., recognized esophageal intubation or tube cuff failure) or physiological alterations (e.g., cardiac arrest in a patient who was *in extremis* before intubation was undertaken and which may or may not be attributable to the intubation) as complications. Overall, event rates are low in the NEAR studies; immediate complications are seen in approximately 3% of RSI patients. Hypotension and alterations in heart rate can result from the pharmacological agents used or from stimulation of the larynx with resultant reflexes. Other studies have reported consistent results. The most catastrophic complication of RSI is unrecognized esophageal intubation, which is rare in the emergency department, but occurs with alarming frequency in some prehospital studies. This situation underscores the importance of the confirmation of tube placement described in Chapter 6. It is incumbent on the person who administers neuromuscular blocking agents and potent sedatives to the patient to be able to establish an airway and maintain mechanical ventilation. This process may require a surgical airway as a final rescue for a failed oral intubation attempt (see Chapter 2 and Fig. 2-5). Aspiration of gastric contents can occur but is uncommon. Overall, the true complication rate of RSI in the emergency department is low and the success rate is exceedingly high, especially when one considers the serious nature of the illnesses for which patients are intubated, as well as the limited time and information available to the clinician performing the intubation.

"Accelerated" and "Immediate" RSI

When time is of the essence, the RSI sequence can be compressed so the steps are conducted much more rapidly than the standard RSI outlined previously.

1. Accelerated RSI
   - Shorten preoxygenation to 30 seconds by using eight vital capacity breaths
   - Shorten the pretreatment interval to 1 or 2 minutes from 3 minutes
2. Immediate RSI
   - Preoxygenate with eight vital capacity breaths
   - Eliminate pretreatment

EVIDENCE

1. **What is the optimal method for preoxygenation?:** Standard preoxygenation has traditionally been achieved by 3 minutes of normal tidal volume breathing of 100% oxygen. Panditt et al. (1) showed that eight vital capacity breaths achieves similar preoxygenation to that of 3 minutes of normal tidal volume breathing and that both of these methods are superior to four vital capacity breaths. The time to desaturation of oxyhemoglobin to 95% is 5.2 minutes after eight vital capacity breaths versus 3.7 minutes after 3 minutes of tidal volume breathing versus 2.8 minutes after four vital capacity breaths (2,3). Preoxygenation of normal healthy patients can produce an average of 8 minutes of apnea time before desaturation to 90% occurs, but the times are much less (as little as 3 minutes) in patients with cardiovascular disease, obese patients, and small

children (4). Sufficient recovery from succinylcholine paralysis cannot be relied on before desaturation occurs, even in properly preoxygenated healthy patients (4,5). Term pregnant women also desaturate more rapidly than nonpregnant women and desaturate to 95% in less than 3 minutes, compared with 4 minutes for nonpregnant controls. Preoxygenating in the upright position prolongs desaturation time in nonpregnant women to 5.5 minutes, but does not favorably affect term pregnant patients (6,7).

2. **Evidence:** Evidence regarding the use of pretreatment drugs, induction agents, and neuromuscular blocking agents are discussed in the *Evidence* sections of the relevant chapters.

3. **Sellick's maneuver:** A meta-analysis of the studies of Sellick's maneuver by Brimacombe and Berry (8) concluded that there is no hard evidence supporting its routine use during RSI, but the practice remains firmly entrenched. Sellick's maneuver may be applied improperly or not at all during a significant proportion of emergency department RSIs (9). Even when applied by experienced practitioners, Sellick's maneuver can increase peak inspiratory pressure and decrease tidal volume or even cause complete obstruction during bag-mask ventilation (10). Cricoid pressure appears to enhance the success rate of fiberoptic intubation, increasing rapid insertion success from 33% to more than 60% in one series (11). Properly applied, cricoid pressure tends to improve laryngoscopic view during conventional direct laryngoscopy, but it may interfere with both insertion of and ventilation through the laryngeal mask airway (12,13). Cricoid pressure is capable of moving the cervical spine approximately 5 mm in normal subjects, which suggests that it might present a hazard in patients with unstable cervical spine injuries; however, its use in patients with cervical spine injuries has never been assessed (14). A two-handed technique has been advocated, but it has never been shown to be superior to the one-handed technique in terms of prevention of aspiration and results in a worse laryngoscopic view (15).

4. **Is RSI superior to intubation with sedation alone?:** This is also discussed in the evidence sections for Chapters 2 and 19. Bozeman et al. (16) compared the use of etomidate alone to etomidate plus succinylcholine in a prehospital flight paramedic program and found that RSI outperformed etomidate-alone intubations by all measures of ease of intubation. An analysis of 200 prehospital intubations performed before and after institution of an RSI protocol found that intubation success increased from 73% before RSI was used to 96% with RSI (17). Li et al. (18) found similar improvement when RSI was introduced in the emergency department. The only direct comparison between RSI and blind nasotracheal intubation showed that higher success rates and more rapid intubation are achieved by RSI in poisoned patients (19). Dufour et al. (20) reported very high success and low complication rates in 219 patients undergoing RSI in a community hospital in Canada. Pediatric RSI has also been studied. A multicenter report of pediatric intubation by the NEAR investigators identified 156 pediatric intubations from among 1,288 total intubations, with 81% of pediatric intubations having been done using RSI (21). A study of 105 children younger than 10 years (average age, 3 years) who underwent RSI with etomidate as the induction agent showed stable hemodynamics and high success and safety profiles (22). Bair et al. (23) analyzed 207 (2.7%) failed intubations among 7,712 intubations in the NEAR project and found that the greatest proportion of rescue procedures (49%) involved the use of RSI to achieve intubation after failure of oral or nasotracheal intubation by non-RSI methods.

REFERENCES

1. Pandit JJ, Duncan T, Robbins PA. Total oxygen uptake with two maximal breathing techniques and the tidal volume breathing technique: a physiologic study of preoxygenation. *Anesthesiology* 2003;99:841–846.

2. Baraka AS, Taha SK, Aouad MT, et al. Preoxygenation: comparison of maximal breathing and tidal volume breathing techniques. *Anesthesiology* 1999;91:612–616.

3. Ramez Salem M, Joseph NJ, Crystal GJ, et al. Preoxygenation: comparison of maximal breathing and tidal volume techniques. *Anesthesiology* 2000;92:1845–1847.

4. Benumof JL, Dagg R, Benumof R. Critical hemoglobin desaturation will occur before return to an unparalyzed state following 1 mg/kg intravenous succinylcholine. *Anesthesiology* 1997;87:979–982.

5. Hayes AH, Breslin DS, Mirakhur RK, et al. Frequency of haemoglobin desaturation with the use of succinylcholine during rapid sequence induction of anaesthesia. *Acta Anaesthesiol Scand* 2001;45:746–749.

6. Heier T, Feiner JR, Lin J, et al. Hemoglobin desaturation after succinylcholine-induced apnea: a study of the recovery of spontaneous ventilation in healthy volunteers. *Anesthesiology* 2001;94:754–759.

7. Baraka AS, Hanna MT, Jabbour SI, et al. Preoxygenation of pregnant and nonpregnant women in the head-up versus supine position. *Anesth Analg* 1992;75:757–759.

8. Brimacombe JR, Berry AM. Cricoid pressure. *Can J Anaesth* 1997;44:414–425.

9. Olsen JC, Gurr DE, Hughes M. Video analysis of emergency medicine residents performing rapid-sequence intubations. *J Emerg Med* 2000;18:469–472.

10. Allman KG. The effect of cricoid pressure application on airway patency. *J Clin Anesth* 1995;7:197–199.

11. Asai T, Murao K, Johmura S, et al. Effect of cricoid pressure on the ease of fibrescope-aided tracheal intubation. *Anaesthesia* 2002;57:909–913.

12. Vanner RG, Clarke P, Moore WJ, et al. The effect of cricoid pressure and neck support on the view at laryngoscopy. *Anaesthesia* 1997;52:896–900.

13. Aoyama K, Takenaka I, Sata T, et al. Cricoid pressure impedes positioning and ventilation through the laryngeal mask airway. *Can J Anaesth* 1996;43:1035–1040.

14. Gabbott DA. The effect of single-handed cricoid pressure on neck movement after applying manual in-line stabilization. *Anaesthesia* 1997;52:586–588.

15. Cook TM. Cricoid pressure: are two hands better than one? [comment]. *Anaesthesia* 1996;51:365–368.

16. Bozeman WP, Kleiner DM, Huggett V. Intubating conditions produced by etomidate alone vs. rapid sequence intubation in the prehospital aeromedical setting. *Acad Emerg Med* 2003;10:445–456.

17. Rose WD, Anderson LD, Edmond SA. Analysis of intubations: before and after establishment of a rapid sequence intubation protocol for air medical use. *Air Med J* 1994;13:475–478.

18. Li J, Murphy-Lavoie H, Bugas C, et al. Complications of emergency intubation with and without paralysis. *Am J Emerg Med* 1999;17:141–143.

19. Dronen SC, Merigian KS, Hedges JR, et al. A comparison of blind nasotracheal and succinylcholine-assisted intubation in the poisoned patient. *Ann Emerg Med* 1987;16:650–652.

20. Dufour DG, Larose DL, Clement SC. Rapid sequence intubation in the emergency department. *J Emerg Med* 1995;13:705–710.

21. Sagarin MJ, Chiang V, Sakles JC, et al. National Emergency Airway Registry (NEAR) investigators. Rapid sequence intubation for pediatric emergency airway management. *Pediatr Emerg Care* 2002;18:417–423.

22. Guldner G, Schultz J, Sexton P, et al. Etomidate for rapid-sequence intubation in young children: hemodynamic effects and adverse events. *Acad Emerg Med* 2003;10:134–139.

23. Bair AE, Filbin MR, Kulkarni RG, et al. The failed intubation attempt in the emergency department: analysis of prevalence, rescue techniques, and personnel. *J Emerg Med* 2002;23:131–140.

4

Applied Functional Anatomy of the Airway

Michael F. Murphy

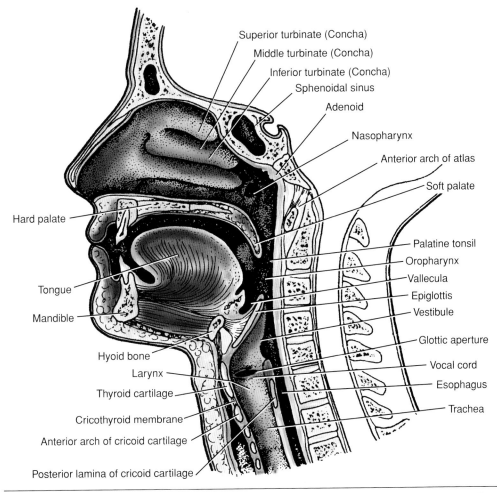

Superior turbinate (Concha)
Middle turbinate (Concha)
Inferior turbinate (Concha)
Sphenoidal sinus
Adenoid
Nasopharynx
Anterior arch of atlas
Soft palate
Hard palate
Palatine tonsil
Oropharynx
Vallecula
Epiglottis
Tongue
Vestibule
Mandible
Glottic aperture
Hyoid bone
Vocal cord
Larynx
Esophagus
Thyroid cartilage
Trachea
Cricothyroid membrane
Anterior arch of cricoid cartilage
Posterior lamina of cricoid cartilage

Figure 4-1 ● Sagittal View of the Upper Airway. Note the subtle inferior tilt of the floor of the nose from front to back, the location of the adenoid, the location of the vallecula between the base of the tongue and the epiglottis, and the location of the hyoid bone in relation to the posterior limit of the tongue. *Source:* From Kastendieck JG. Airway management. In: Rosen P, ed. *Emergency medicine: concepts and clinical practice*, 2nd ed. St. Louis, MO: Mosby; 1988, with permission.

There are many salient features of the anatomy and physiology of the airway to consider with respect to airway management maneuvers. This chapter discusses the anatomical features most involved in the act of intubation, the important vascular structures, and the innervation of the upper airway. Chapter 7 builds on these anatomical and functional relationships to describe anesthesia techniques for the airway. Chapter 20 addresses developmental and pediatric anatomical features of the airway.

We consider each anatomical structure in the order in which it appears as we enter the airway: the nose, the mouth, the pharynx, the larynx, and the trachea (Fig. 4-1).

THE NOSE

The external nose consists of a bony vault, a cartilaginous vault, and a lobule. The bony vault comprises the nasal bones, the frontal processes of the maxillae, and the nasal spine of the frontal bone. The nasal bones are buttressed in the midline by the perpendicular plate of the ethmoid bone that forms part of the bony septum. The cartilaginous vault is formed by the upper lateral cartilages that meet the cartilaginous portion of the septum in the midline. The nasal lobule consists of the tip of the nose, the lower lateral cartilages, the fibrofatty alae that form the lateral margins of the nostril, and the columella. The cavities of each nostril are continuous with the nasopharynx posteriorly.

Important Anatomical Considerations

- Kiesselbach's plexus (Little's area) is a very vascular area located on the anterior aspect of the septum in each nostril. Epistaxis most often originates from this area. During the act of inserting a nasal trumpet or a nasotracheal tube, it is generally recommended that the device be inserted in the nostril such that the leading edge of the bevel (the pointed tip) is away from the septum. The goal is to minimize the chances of trauma and bleeding from this very vascular area. This means that the device is inserted "upside down" in the left nostril and rotated 180 degrees after the tip has proceeded beyond the cartilaginous septum. Although some authors have recommended the opposite (i.e., that the bevel tip approximate the nasal septum to minimize the risk of damage and bleeding from the turbinates), the bevel away from the septum approach makes more sense and is the recommended method.
- The major nasal airway is between the laterally placed inferior turbinate, the septum, and the floor of the nose. The floor of the nose is tilted slightly downward front to back, approximately 10 to 15 degrees. Thus, when a nasal tube, trumpet, or fiberscope is inserted through the nose, it should not be directed upward or even straight back. Instead, it should be directed slightly inferiorly to follow this major channel. Before nasal intubation of an unconscious adult patient, some authorities recommend gently but *fully* inserting one's gloved and lubricated little finger to ensure patency and to maximally dilate this channel before the insertion of the nasal tube. In addition, placing the endotracheal tube (ETT; preferably an Endotrol tube) in a warm bottle of saline or water softens the tube and attenuates its damaging properties.
- The nasal mucosa is exquisitely sensitive to topically applied vasoconstricting medications such as phenylephrine, epinephrine, oxymetazoline, or cocaine. Cocaine has the added advantage of providing profound topical anesthesia and is the only local anesthetic agent that produces vasoconstriction; the others cause vasodilatation. Shrinking the nasal mucosa with a vasoconstricting agent can increase the caliber of the nasal airway by as much as 50% to 75% and may reduce epistaxis incited by nasotracheal intubation, although there is little evidence to support this claim. Cocaine has been implicated in coronary vasoconstriction when applied to the nasal mucosa, so it should be used with caution in patients with coronary artery disease (see *Evidence* section at the end of this chapter).
- The nasal cavities are bounded posteriorly by the nasopharynx. The adenoids are located posteriorly in the nasopharynx just above the nasal surface of the soft palate and partially surround a depression in the mucosal membrane where the eustachian tube enters the nasopharynx. During insertion, the nasotracheal tube often enters this depression and resistance is encountered. Continued aggressive insertion can cause the nasotracheal tube to penetrate the mucosa and pass submucosally deep to the naso- and oropharyngeal mucous membrane (Fig. 4-2). Although alarming when one recognizes that this has occurred, no specific treatment is advised, except that withdrawing the tube and trying the opposite nostril is advised. Despite the theoretical risk of infection, there is no literature to suggest that this occurs. Documentation of the complication and communication to the accepting team on admission is mandatory.
- The soft palate rests on the base of the tongue during quiet nasal respiration, sealing the oral cavity anteriorly.

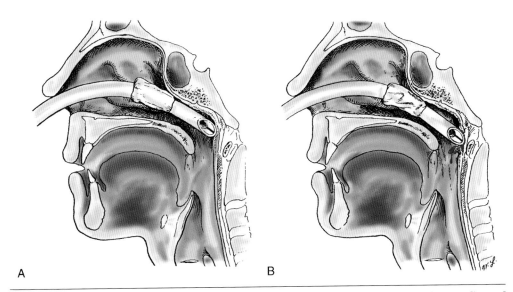

Figure 4-2 ● Mechanism of Nasopharyngeal Perforation and Submucosal Tunneling of the Nasotracheal Tube (NTT). A: The NTT entering the pit of the adenoid where the eustachian tube enters the nasopharynx. **B:** The tube perforating the mucous membrane. *Source:* From Tintinalli JE, Claffey J. Complications of nasotracheal intubation. *Ann Emerg Med* 1981;10:142–144, with permission.

- The contiguity of the paranasal sinuses with the nasal cavity is believed to be responsible for the infections of the paranasal sinuses that may be associated with prolonged nasotracheal intubation. Although this fact has led some physicians to condemn nasotracheal intubation, fear of infection should not deter the emergency physician from considering nasotracheal intubation when indicated. Securing the airway in an emergency takes precedence over possible later infective complications, and in any case, the intubation can always be changed to an oral tube or tracheostomy, if necessary.
- A nasotracheal intubation is relatively contraindicated in patients with basal skull fractures (i.e., when the maxilla is fractured away from its attachment to the base of the skull) because of the risk of penetration into the cranial vault (usually through the cribriform plate) with the ETT. Careful technique avoids this complication: the cribriform plate is located cephalad of the nares, and tube insertion should be directed slightly caudad (see previous discussion). Maxillary fractures (e.g., LeFort fractures) may disrupt the continuity of the nasal cavities and are a relative contraindication to blind nasal intubation. Again, cautious insertion, especially if guided by a fiberscope, can mitigate the risk.

THE MOUTH

The mouth, or oral cavity, is bounded externally by the lips and is contiguous with the oropharynx posteriorly (Fig. 4-3).

- The tongue is attached to the symphysis of the mandible anteriorly and anterolaterally and the stylohyoid process and hyoid bone posterolaterally and posteriorly, respectively. The posterior limit of the tongue corresponds to the position of the hyoid bone (Fig. 4-1). The clinical relevance of this relationship will become apparent when the 3-3-2 rule is described in Chapter 7.

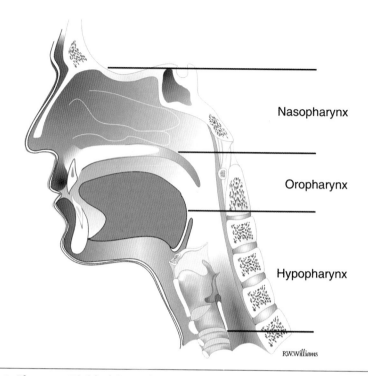

Nasopharynx

Oropharynx

Hypopharynx

R.W.Williams

Figure 4-3 ● Pharynx Divided into Three Segments: Nasopharynx, Oropharynx, and Hypopharynx. *Source:* From Redden RJ. Anatomic considerations in anesthesia. In: Hagberg CA, ed. *Handbook of difficult airway management.* Philadelphia: Churchill Livingstone; 2000:7, with permission.

- The potential spaces in the hollow of the mandible are collectively called the mandibular space, which is subdivided into three potential spaces on either side of the midline sublingual raphe: the submental, submandibular, and sublingual spaces. The tongue is a fluid-filled noncompressible structure. During conventional laryngoscopy, the tongue is ordinarily displaced to the left and into the mandibular space, permitting one to expose the larynx for intubation under direct vision. If the mandibular space is small relative to the size of the tongue (e.g., hypoplastic mandible, lingual edema in angioedema, lingual hematoma), the ability to visualize the larynx may be compromised. Infiltration of the mandibular space by infection (e.g., Ludwig's angina), hematoma, or other lesions may limit the ability to displace the tongue into this space and render orotracheal intubation difficult or impossible.
- Subtle geometric distortions of the oral cavity that limit one's working and viewing space, such as a high arched palate with a narrow oral cavity or buck teeth with an elongated oral cavity, may render orotracheal intubation difficult. Chapter 6 elaborates on these issues.
- Salivary glands continuously secrete saliva, which can defeat attempts at achieving sufficient topical anesthesia of the airway to undertake awake laryngoscopy or other active airway intervention maneuvers in the awake or lightly sedated patient—for example, laryngeal mask airway insertion, lighted stylet intubation, and so on.
- The condyles of the mandible articulate within the temporomandibular joint (TMJ) for the first 30 degrees of mouth opening. Beyond 30 degrees, the condyles *translate* out of the TMJ anteriorly onto the zygomatic arches. Once translation has occurred, it is possible to employ a jaw thrust maneuver to pull the mandible and tongue

forward. This is the most effective method of opening the airway to alleviate obstruction or permit bag-mask ventilation. A jaw thrust to open the airway is not possible unless this translation has occurred (see Chapter 5).

THE PHARYNX

The pharynx is a U-shaped fibromuscular tube extending from the base of the skull to the lower border of the cricoid cartilage where, at the level of the sixth cervical vertebra, it is continuous with the esophagus. Posteriorly, it rests against the fascia covering the prevertebral muscles and the cervical spine. Anteriorly, it opens into the nasal cavity (the nasopharynx), the mouth (the oropharynx), and the larynx (the laryngo- or hypopharynx).

- The oropharyngeal musculature has a normal tone, like any other skeletal musculature, and this tone serves to keep the upper airway open during quiet respiration. Respiratory distress is associated with pharyngeal muscular activity that attempts to open the airway further. Benzodiazepines and other sedative hypnotic agents may attenuate some of this tone. This explains why even small doses of sedative hypnotic medications (e.g., midazolam) may precipitate total airway obstruction in patients presenting with partial airway obstruction.
- An "awake look" is advocated during the difficult airway algorithm (see Chapter 2). Being able to see the epiglottis or posterior glottic structures employing topical anesthesia and sedation reassures one that at least this much, and probably more, of the airway will be visualized during an intubation attempt following the administration of a neuromuscular blocking drug. In practice, the glottic view is usually improved following neuromuscular blockade. Rarely, however, the loss of pharyngeal muscle tone caused by the neuromuscular blocking agent leads to the cephalad and anterior migration of the larynx worsening the view at direct laryngoscopy. Although uncommon, this tends to occur more often in morbidly obese or late-term pregnancy patients, in whom there may be submucosal edema.
- The glossopharyngeal nerve supplies sensation to the posterior one-third of the tongue, the valleculae, the superior surface of the epiglottis, and most of the posterior pharynx. This nerve is accessible to blockade (topically or by injection) because it runs just deep to the inferior portion of the palatopharyngeus muscle (the posterior tonsillar pillar) (Fig. 4-4).

THE LARYNX

The larynx extends from its oblique entrance formed by the aryepiglottic folds, the tip of the epiglottis, and the posterior commissure between the arytenoid cartilages (interarytenoid folds) through the vocal cords to the cricoid ring (Fig. 4-5).

- The superior laryngeal branch of the vagus nerve supplies sensation to the undersurface of the epiglottis, all of the larynx to the level of the false vocal cords, and the pyriform recesses posterolateral to either side of the larynx (Fig. 4-5). The nerve enters the region by passing through the thyrohyoid membrane just below the inferior cornu of the hyoid bone (Fig. 4-6). It then divides into a superior and an inferior branch; the superior branch passes submucously through the vallecula, where it is visible to the naked eye, on its way to the larynx; and the inferior branch runs along the medial aspects of the pyriform recesses.
- The larynx is the most heavily innervated sensory structure in the body, followed closely by the carina. Stimulation of the unanesthetized larynx during intubation

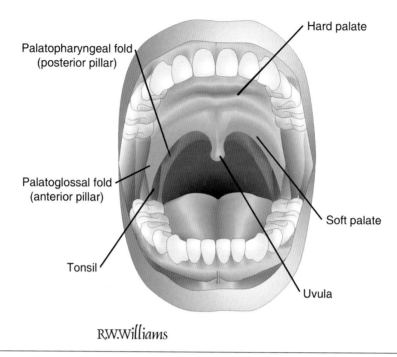

R.W.Williams

Figure 4-4 ● The Oral Cavity. Note the position of the posterior pillar. The glossopharyngeal nerve runs at the base of this structure. *Source:* From Redden RJ. Anatomic considerations in anesthesia. In: Hagberg CA, ed. *Handbook of difficult airway management.* Philadelphia: Churchill Livingstone; 2000:8 with permission.

causes tremendous reflex sympathetic activation. Blood pressure and heart rate may as much as double. This may lead to the elevation of intracranial pressure, particularly in patients with imperfect autoregulation; aggravate or incite myocardial ischemia in patients with underlying coronary artery disease; or incite or aggravate large vessel dissection or rupture (e.g., penetrating injury to a carotid, thoracic aortic dissection, or abdominal aortic rupture).

- The pyramidal arytenoid cartilages sit on the posterior aspect of the larynx (Fig. 4-5). The intrinsic laryngeal muscles cause them to swivel, opening and closing the vocal cords. An ETT that is too large may, over time, compress these structures, causing mucosal and cartilaginous ischemia and resultant permanent laryngeal damage. A traumatic intubation may dislocate these cartilages posteriorly (more often a traumatic curved blade–related complication) or anteriorly (more often a straight blade traumatic complication), which, unless diagnosed early and relocated, may lead to permanent hoarseness.
- The larynx bulges posteriorly into the hypopharynx, leaving deep recesses on either side called the pyriform recesses or sinuses. Foreign bodies (e.g., fish bones) occasionally become lodged there. During active swallowing, the larynx is elevated and moves anteriorly, the epiglottis folds down over the glottis to prevent aspiration, and the bolus of food passes midline into the esophagus. When not actively swallowing (e.g., the unconscious patient), the larynx rests against the posterior hypopharynx such that a nasogastric (NG) tube must traverse the pyriform recess to gain access to the esophagus and stomach. Ordinarily, an NG tube introduced through the right nostril passes to the left at the level of the hypopharynx and enters the esophagus through the left pyriform recess. Similarly, with a left nostril insertion, the NG tube gains access to the esophagus through the right pyriform recess.

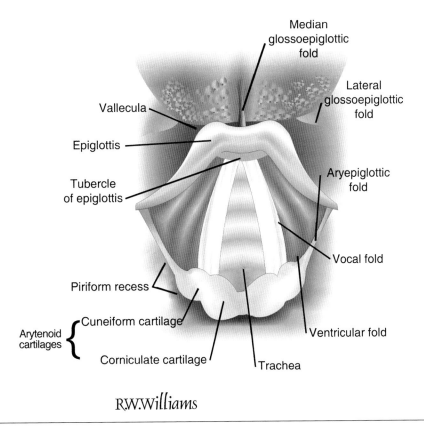

Median
glossoepiglottic
fold

Lateral
glossoepiglottic
fold

Vallecula

Epiglottis

Tubercle
of epiglottis

Aryepiglottic
fold

Vocal fold

Piriform recess

Cuneiform cartilage

Arytenoid
cartilages {

Ventricular fold

Corniculate cartilage

Trachea

R.W.Williams

Figure 4-5 ● Larynx Visualized From the Oropharynx. Note the median glossoepiglottic fold. It is pressure on this structure by the tip of a curved blade that flips the epiglottis forward, exposing the glottis during laryngoscopy. Note that the valleculae and the pyriform recesses are different structures, a fact often confused in the anesthesia literature. The cuneiform and corniculate cartilages are called the arytenoid cartilages. The ridge between them posteriorly is called the posterior commissure. *Source:* From Redden RJ. Anatomic considerations in anesthesia. In: Hagberg CA, ed. *Handbook of difficult airway management.* Philadelphia: Churchill Livingstone; 2000:9 with permission.

- The cricothyroid membrane extends between the upper anterior surface of the cricoid cartilage to the inferior anterior border of the thyroid cartilage. Its height tends to be about the size of the tip of the index finger externally in both male and female adults. Locating the cricoid cartilage and the cricothyroid membrane quickly in an airway emergency is crucial. It is usually easily done in men because of the obvious laryngeal prominence (Adam's apple). Locate the laryngeal prominence, and then note the anterior surface of the thyroid cartilage immediately caudad, usually about one index finger's breadth in height. There is an obvious soft indentation caudad to this anterior surface with a very hard ridge immediately caudad to it. The soft indentation is the cricothyroid membrane, and the ridge is the cricoid cartilage. Because of the lack of a distinct laryngeal prominence in women, locating the membrane can be much more difficult. In women, place your index finger in the sternal notch. Then drag it cephalad in the midline until the first, and ordinarily the biggest, transverse ridge is felt. This is the cricoid ring. Superior to the cricoid cartilage is the cricothyroid membrane, and superior to that, the anterior surface of the thyroid cartilage, then the thyrohyoid space and thyroid cartilage. The cricothyroid membrane is higher in the neck in a woman than a man because the woman's thyroid cartilage is relatively smaller than the man's.

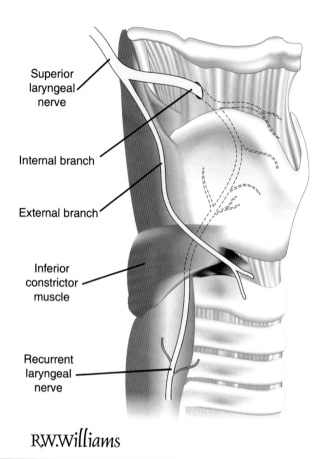

R.W.Williams

Figure 4.6 ● Oblique View of the Larynx. Note how the internal branch of the superior laryngeal nerve pierces the thyrohyoid membrane midway between the hyoid bone and the superior border of the thyroid cartilage. *Source:* From Redden RJ. Anatomic considerations in anesthesia. In: Hagberg CA, ed. *Handbook of difficult airway management.* Philadelphia: Churchill Livingstone; 2000:11 with permission.

- The cricothyroid membrane measures 6 to 8 mm from top to bottom. If one pierces the membrane in its midportion to perform a retrograde intubation, the puncture point is a mere 3 to 5 mm below the vocal cords, which may not be far enough into the airway to retain the ETT when the wire is cut at the skin. The technique of passing the wire from the outside to the inside of the distal end of the ETT through the Murphy eye enables an additional 4 to 5 mm of insertion, reducing this risk. The proximity of the cricothyroid membrane to the vocal cords is also the driving factor in using small tracheal hooks during surgical cricothyroidotomy to minimize any risk to the cords (see Chapter 15).

TRACHEA

The trachea begins at the inferior border of the cricoid ring. The sensory supply to the tracheal mucosa is derived from the recurrent laryngeal branch of the vagus nerve. The trachea is between 9 and 15 mm in diameter in the adult and is 12 to 15 cm long. It may be somewhat larger in the elderly. The adult male trachea will generally easily accept an 8.5-mm inner diameter (ID) ETT; a 7.5-mm ID ETT may be preferable in women. If the patient being intubated might require bronchoscopic pulmonary toilette after admission (e.g., chronic obstructive pulmonary disease, airway burns), consider increasing to a 9.0-mm ID tube for men and an 8.0-mm ID tube for women.

SUMMARY

Functional anatomy is important to expert airway management. Attention to the nuances and subtleties of anatomy in relation to technique will often mean the difference between success and failure in managing airways, particularly difficult airways. A clear understanding of the relevant anatomical structures, their blood supply, and their innervation will guide the choice of intubation and anesthesia techniques and will enhance understanding regarding the best approach to each patient. It also provides a basis for understanding how complications are best avoided, or if they occur, how they may be detected.

EVIDENCE

1. **General:** The reviews by Morris (1) and Redden (2) provide excellent descriptions of the functional anatomy of the upper airway.
2. **Nasotracheal intubation:** Nasotracheal intubation has largely been supplanted by other methods of emergency airway management that have a higher success rate and fewer complications. Several authors have addressed the complications of nasotracheal intubation (3–10). Some are serious, such as severe epistaxis (1%–10%), intracranial intubation (3), and bronchial obstruction (4). Others are potentially serious, such as retropharyngeal dissection (5,6) and sinusitis, particularly if the nasotracheal tube is left in place longer than 3 to 7 days (7,8). Most immediate complications of nasotracheal intubation are mild and self-limited (e.g., mild to moderate epistaxis) (2,11). Softening the ETT in warm water or saline has been demonstrated to reduce the complication rate, particularly epistaxis (12).
3. **Cocaine and coronary vasoconstriction:** It is well known that recreational cocaine use is associated with coronary spasm, leading to myocardial ischemia and infarction as well as sudden death (13). It is important to realize that medically administered cocaine to produce nasal vasoconstriction has produced similar complications (14–16).

REFERENCES

1. Morris IR. Functional anatomy of the upper airway. *Emerg Med Clin North Am* 1988;6: 639–669.
2. Redden RJ. Anatomic considerations in anesthesia. In: Hagberg CA, ed. *Handbook of difficult airway management*. Philadelphia: Churchill Livingstone; 2000:1–13.
3. Marlow TJ, Goltra DD Jr, Schabel SI. Intracranial placement of a nasotracheal tube after facial fracture: a rare complication. *J Emerg Med* 1997;15:187–191.
4. Skouteris CA, Mylonas AI, Galanaki EJ, et al. Acute bronchial obstruction after nasotracheal intubation: report of a case. *J Oral Maxillofac Surg* 2002;60:1188–1192.
5. Tintinalli JE, Claffey J. Complications of nasotracheal intubation. *Ann Emerg Med* 1981;10: 142–144.

6. Landess WW. Retropharyngeal dissection: a rare complication of nasotracheal intubation revisited—a case report. *AANA J* 1994;62:273–277.

7. Holdgaard HO, Pedersen J, Schurizek BA, et al. Complications and late sequelae following nasotracheal intubation. *Acta Anaesthesiol Scand* 1993;37:475–480.

8. Bach A, Boehrer H, Schmidt H, et al. Nosocomial sinusitis in ventilated patients: nasotracheal versus orotracheal intubation. *Anaesthesia* 1992;47:335–339.

9. Conetta R, Nierman DM. Pneumocephalus following nasotracheal intubation. *Ann Emerg Med* 1992;21:100–102.

10. Rhee KJ, Muntz CB, Donald PJ, et al. Does nasotracheal intubation increase complications in patients with skull base fractures? *Ann Emerg Med* 1993;22:1145–1147.

11. Rosen CL, Wolfe RE, Chew SE, et al. Blind nasotracheal intubation in the presence of facial trauma. *J Emerg Med* 1997;15:141–145.

12. Lu PP, Liu HP, Shyr MH, et al. Softened endotracheal tube reduces the incidence and severity of epistaxis following nasotracheal intubation. *Acta Anaesthesiol Sin* 1998;36:193–197.

13. Minor RL Jr, Scott BD, Brown DD, et al. Cocaine induced myocardial infarction in patients with normal coronary arteries. *Ann Intern Med* 1992;115:797–806.

14. Lange RA, Cigarroa RG, Yancy CW Jr, et al. Cocaine induced coronary artery vasoconstriction. *N Engl J Med* 1989;321:1557–1562.

15. Ross GS, Bell J. Myocardial infarction associated with inappropriate use of topical cocaine as treatment for epistaxis. *Am J Emerg Med* 1992;10:219–222.

16. Laffey JG, Neligan P, Ormonde G. Prolonged perioperative myocardial ischemia in a young male: due to topical intranasal cocaine? *J Clin Anesth* 1999;11:419–424.

5

Supplemental Oxygenation and Bag-Mask Ventilation

Tobias D. Barker and Robert E. Schneider

Bag-mask ventilation is the cornerstone of airway management.

Although all airway skills are important, perhaps the most important skill, and one of the most difficult to perform correctly, is the ability to use a bag and mask to effectively oxygenate and ventilate a patient. Once mastered, however, confident bag-mask ventilation (BMV) reduces both the urgency to intubate and the anxiety that universally accompanies a failed attempt at laryngoscopy and intubation, especially if muscle relaxants have been used to facilitate intubation. In fact, competence with BMV is a prerequisite to using paralytic agents to secure the airway. A well-designed sequential approach to basic airway management is essential to the practice of emergency medicine physicians, critical care physicians, hospitalists, emergency medical services providers, and anesthesia practitioners.

SUPPLEMENTAL OXYGENATION

There is a stepwise progression that must be understood and followed in administering oxygen to nonintubated, spontaneously breathing patients who cannot maintain acceptable oxygen saturation on room air. Many patients arrive to the emergency department with a nasal cannula connected to oxygen at 2 to 3 L/minute flow rate. If ineffective at maintaining adequate oxygen saturations, the nasal cannula should immediately be replaced with a nonrebreathing mask at 15 L of flow, so named because of the one-way valves incorporated into the mask to prevent the patient from entraining room air. There has been tremendous confusion in the past regarding the actual percentage of oxygen that can be successfully delivered through a nonrebreathing mask. For years, most physicians believed that a nonrebreather was capable of delivering upward of 95% oxygen. This belief was fueled by the original name of the mask, 100% nonrebreather mask, which is clearly misleading. Many well-conducted studies have subsequently shown that the *maximum* percentage of oxygen that can be delivered effectively is actually 70% to 75% because the mask does not effectively seal and prevent the entrainment of room air, and the reservoir is too small to provide a sufficient volume of oxygen to meet the large demand that occurs during inspiration. In common use, the nonrebreather probably provides oxygen at about 65%. Replacing the nasal cannula with a nonrebreathing mask and then observing changes in pulse oximetry readings over a 2 to 3 minute period allows one to quickly assess the efficacy of the nonrebreathing mask.

If the expected improvement in oxygenation does not occur, the nonrebreather should be removed and replaced with any one of several specific resuscitation bags and masks. Initially, the patient must be reassured that a tight-fitting mask will be placed on his or her face and encouraged to continue breathing spontaneously without any assistance from the care provider. Utmost attention must be directed to ensuring a tight mask seal. After 3 or 4 minutes, the patient's oxygenation should be reassessed, and if not improving, synchronous augmentation of the patient's inspiratory effort (500–700 cc tidal volume of oxygen with each spontaneous inspiration) should be undertaken. In a nontachypneic patient (less than 20 breaths/minute), this procedure is simply done. In a tachypneic patient (greater than 20 breaths/minute), synchronous augmentation will be quite difficult. Continued attempts at augmenting each inspiratory effort may result in asynchronous bagging, leading to insufflation of the patient's stomach and increased risk of vomiting or regurgitation of gastric contents. To combat this, an appropriate cadence of bagging must be selected to allow effective enhancement of every third or fourth inspiratory effort. This is fairly easy to do and allows the care provider time to be certain a good seal is achieved and maintained. If synchronous assist fails, continuous positive airway pressure or bilevel positive airway pressure may be helpful (see Chapter 38), or endotracheal intubation will be required.

BAG-MASK VENTILATION

There is a paucity of literature that adequately describes effective BMV. It is not glamorous, most health care providers mistakenly think that they are proficient at it, and it is given little attention in most airway textbooks and courses. This makes BMV appear mundane as an airway management maneuver. However, one quickly realizes its importance, given the fact that effective bag-mask oxygenation and ventilation buys time as one works through the array of potential solutions in managing a difficult or failed airway. Simply stated, the ability to effectively oxygenate and ventilate a patient with a bag and mask leaves three failed attempts at laryngoscopy and intubation as the only pathway to a failed airway.

Successful BMV depends on a patent airway, an adequate mask seal, and proper ventilation. Creating an adequate mask seal requires an understanding of the design features of the mask, the anatomy of the patient's face, and the interrelationship between the two. A patent airway permits the delivery of appropriate tidal volumes without insufflating the stomach. Techniques used in producing a patent airway often include head extension, chin lift, and jaw thrust maneuvers. Proper ventilation must take into account not only giving the appropriate volume, but also giving it at the correct rate and with the appropriate amount of force.

The specific type of bag used in BMV is also important. Bags that minimize dead space, incorporate unidirectional airflow valves (e.g., duckbill inspiratory valves), and use one-way expiratory valves to prevent the entrainment of room air during inspiration will deliver 90% to 97% oxygen to spontaneously breathing or ventilated patients. This is in sharp distinction to improperly configured bags that provide high oxygen concentration during active bagging, but deliver only 30% oxygen during spontaneous patient breathing. This suboptimal oxygenation is due to the lack of a one-way expiratory valve on the bag, leading to entrainment of room air.

A typical mask consists of three main parts:

- A round 15-mm orifice that fits a standard 22-mm female connector on the bag portion of the assembly
- A hard shell, or body of the mask; this is often clear, to allow continuous visualization of the patient's mouth and nose so immediate intervention can be employed if the patient visibly regurgitates
- A circumferential cushion, or inflatable collar, which, when properly inflated, evenly distributes downward pressure onto the patient's face, promoting an effective mask seal

It is easier to establish an adequate mask seal if the mask is too large than if it is too small. In masks with inflatable collars, the collar must be inflated to the extent that it forms an adequate seal. An inadequate seal may indicate that air should be added to or removed from the mask empirically according to the operator's best judgment to maximize a facial seal.

Opening the Airway

The airway should be opened before placing the mask on the face. There are two maneuvers commonly used to open the airway. The head tilt, chin lift is the primary maneuver used in any patient in whom cervical spine injury is not a concern. In this technique, the clinician uses two hands to extend the patient's neck and open the airway. While one hand applies downward pressure to the patient's forehead, the tips of the index and middle finger of the second hand lift the mandible at the mentum, which lifts the tongue from the posterior pharynx. The jaw thrust maneuver also moves the tongue anteriorly with the mandible, minimizing its obstructing potential. An effective jaw thrust is achieved by

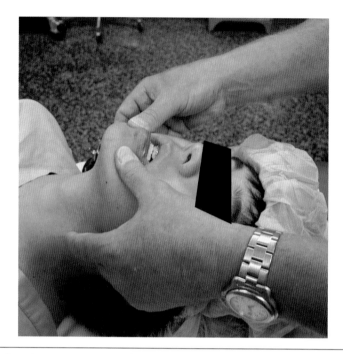

Figure 5-1 ● Jaw thrust maneuver employing a two-hand technique.

forcibly and fully opening the mouth to "translate" the condyles of the mandible out of the temporomandibular joint, then pushing the mandible forward and maintaining a forward position with the help of the oral airway (Fig. 5-1). The jaw thrust is the safest first approach to opening the airway of a patient with a potential cervical spine injury because, properly performed, it can generally be accomplished without moving the neck. The reduced emphasis on the jaw thrust technique in the current advanced cardiac life support (ACLS) guidelines has to do with reducing the complexity of cardiopulmonary resuscitation for lay persons, rather than opposition to its use. Both the jaw thrust and head tilt, chin lift techniques have been shown in multiple studies to improve airway patency, and skilled airway managers should feel comfortable with either.

Airway Adjuncts

Once an open airway has been established, it must be maintained. Oropharyngeal and nasopharyngeal airways (Fig. 5-2A and B) devices are important adjuncts in achieving this goal. Both will prevent the tongue from occluding the airway and provide an open conduit for air to pass. Unless BMV is expected to be needed only transiently (e.g., while naloxone takes effect), an oropharyngeal airway (OPA) should be placed whenever BMV is required. The OPA may be supplemented by one, or even two, nasopharyngeal airways. Neither of these airway devices will protect the trachea from aspiration of secretions or gastric contents.

Positioning the Mask

With the mandible pulled forward, the mask is placed on the face and sealed. The mask should be placed on the patient's face *detached* from the bag. This is a simple, but often neglected, point. Leaving the bag and mask connected during initial placement makes the procedure awkward and clumsy. The nasal part of the mask should be opened and placed on

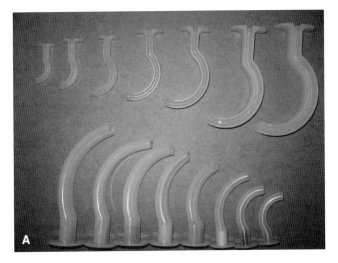

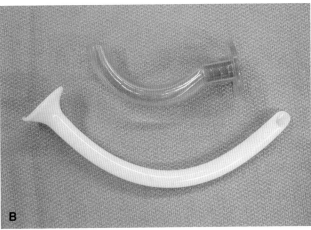

Figure 5-2 ● **A:** The family of Guedel (*bottom row*) and Berman (*top row*) oropharyngeal airways. **B:** A Guedel oropharyngeal airway and a nasopharyngeal airway (also called a nasal trumpet).

the bridge of the nose. The body of the mask is then levered down onto the patient's face (Fig. 5-3), covering the nose and mouth, and is adjusted cephalad (superior) or caudad (inferior) to allow optimum positioning.

One must be cognizant at all times of the patient's orbits and resist any temptation to rest the ulnar surfaces of either wrist or the mask cushion on the orbits during BMV. This inadvertent compression may produce a profound vagal response and significantly reduce retinal blood flow.

Single-Hand Mask Hold

Ordinarily, the operator's nondominant hand is placed on the mask with the distal pads of the thumb and the index finger used to hold the mask in place, rocking it gently from side to side to achieve the best seal. The remaining fingers are used to pull the mandible up into the mask to keep the airway open. A common tendency, especially if any difficulty

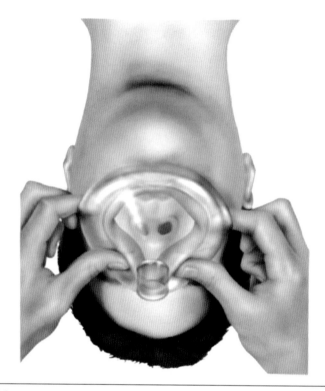

Figure 5-3 ● After opening the nasal portion of the mask, it is positioned on the face to incorporate the nares and mouth inside the body of the mask.

is encountered, is to pinch the body of the mask with the thumb and index finger pads. If this occurs, a mask leak may be produced or worsened if already present. If the operator's hand is large enough, the web space between the thumb and index finger may appose the mask connector, allowing the rest of the hand to fall comfortably onto the body of the mask at a 45-degree angle (Fig. 5-4); however, most people do not have hands this large, meaning that the index finger and thumb web space is a variable distance from the collar of the mask (Fig. 5-5). This hand position allows even distribution of downward pressure as the mask is gently sealed onto the patient's face. The long, ring, and little fingers should lie comfortably on the body of the mask, although their respective finger pads contact the mentum of the chin and body of the mandible and must be ready to pull the mandible into the mask (chin lift), if necessary (Fig. 5-6). Ordinarily, the tip of the long finger placed beneath the mentum is used to keep the mandible in a "thrusted position." Several authors recommend placing the volar pad of the little finger posterior to the angle of the mandible to attempt a jaw thrust maneuver (Fig. 5-5). This method of producing a jaw thrust maneuver is extremely difficult to perform and maintain for any length of time, especially with small hands. Alternatively, the mandible can be kept forward by "hooking" the long finger under the mentum while the remaining fingers lie comfortably along the undersurface of the mandibular body (Fig. 5-7). It is important to be certain the volar pads elevate only on the bony parts of the mandible; pressure to the soft tissues of the neck may occlude the airway. When holding the mask with one's left hand, it may be necessary to gather the left cheek with the hypothenar eminence of the hand and compress it into the mask cushion while rocking the mask to the right to establish a more efficient mask seal.

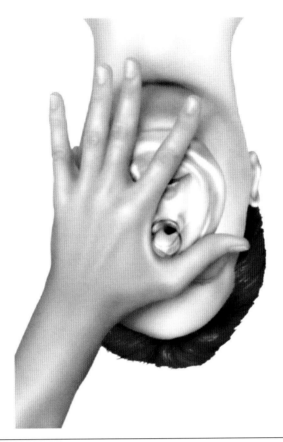

Figure 5-4 ● An effective single-handed mask seal can be achieved by placing the thumb/index finger web space against the mask connector at 45 degrees and gently pushing the mask onto the face with the web space, not the palm of the hand. This single-hand mask hold is best suited to individuals with large hands.

Two-Hand Mask Hold

The two-hand mask hold is the most effective method of opening the airway while achieving and maintaining an adequate mask seal. It is the method of choice in an emergency situation when a one-handed mask hold is not producing adequate ventilation. The two-handed, two-person technique mandates that one operator's sole responsibility is to ensure proper mask placement on the patient's face by simultaneously using both hands to open the airway and achieve an effective mask seal. An assistant is needed to squeeze the bag, but the most experienced airway manager should be handling the mask seal.

Initially, the operator opens the airway and translates the mandible forward. Standing at the head of the patient, the long fingers of both hands are placed behind the angle of the mandible (Fig. 5-8). The mouth is then opened with the thumbs (Fig. 5-9) and the mandible pulled to a "thrusted" position (Fig. 5-1) in which the bottom teeth are now in front of the top teeth. The long fingers maintain the thrusted position while the mask is applied to the face as discussed previously.

The operator's hands may be placed on the mask in one of two ways. In the first method, the index finger and thumb distal phalanges of both hands are placed in apposition to one another along the inferior and superior ridges of the mask, respectively (Fig. 5-10). The volar

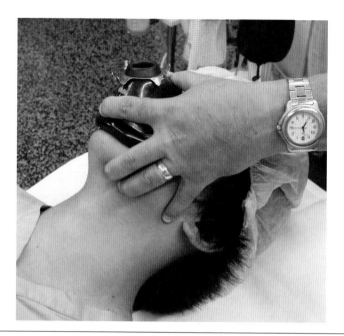

Figure 5-5 ● Single-hand mask hold for individuals with medium-size hands.

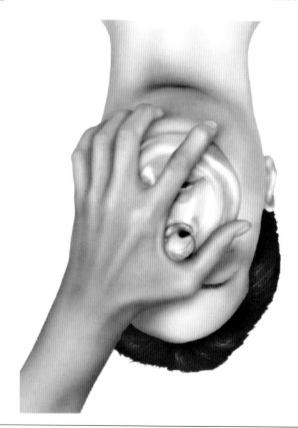

Figure 5-6 ● **The Thumb and Index Finger Lie Passively on The Mask.** The long, ring, and little finger volar pads capture the body of the mandible and mentum and perform a chin lift maneuver.

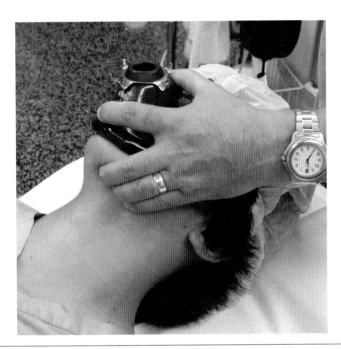

Figure 5-7 ● Single-hand mask hold for individuals with small hands.

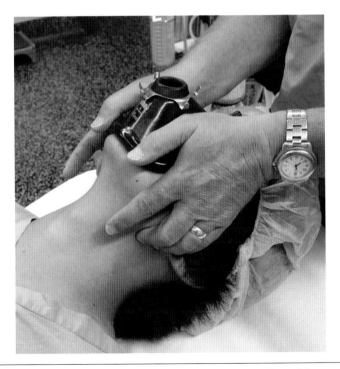

Figure 5-8 ● Initial Position of Hands for a Two-hand Mask Hold. Note the tips of the long fingers behind the angle of the mandible. For this to occur, the wrists must be in an ulnar deviated position.

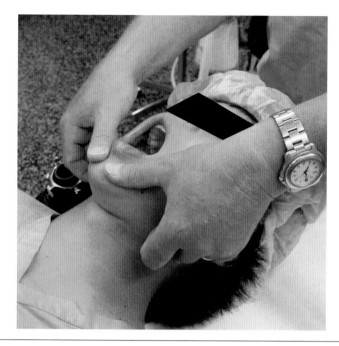

Figure 5-9 ● Mouth opening employing thumbs to depress the mandibular mentum with a rocking motion to open the mouth.

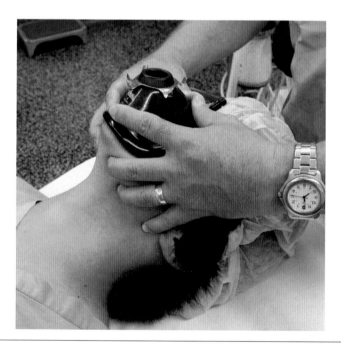

Figure 5-10 ● **Conventionally Taught Position of Fingers for a Two-hand Mask Hold.** Thumbs are cephalad (superiorly) and index fingers are caudad (inferiorly), leaving only three fingers to create and maintain jaw thrust and chin lift maneuver. This is not a comfortable position to maintain for any length of time.

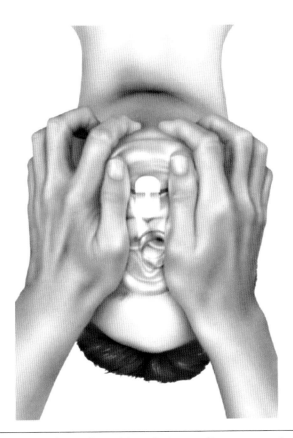

Figure 5-11 ● Two-handed Mask Hold Technique: Emergency technique two-hand mask hold position: metacarpophalangeal joints of both thumbs appose the mask connector and thenar eminences to compress the mask into the face, allowing the other four fingers to create and maintain the jaw thrust position. This is a much more comfortable position for prolonged ventilation.

pads of the remaining three fingers of each hand (long, ring, and little fingers) are fully abducted and used to capture the mandible and perform a simultaneous jaw thrust and chin lift maneuver, opening the airway and creating an optimum mask seal. In the second method, both thenar eminences can be positioned parallel to one another with the thumbs pointing caudad (inferior), executing gentle downward pressure to push the mask into the face to effect a seal (Fig. 5-11), while the long fingers, positioned behind the angles of the mandible, perform a jaw thrust maneuver (Fig. 5-8). This mask hold position is more comfortable and less prone to fatigue compared to that described previously.

In desperate situations, a single care provider employing a two-hand mask hold can achieve oxygenation and ventilation by squeezing the bag between his or her elbow and chest/lateral abdomen, or between his or her knees if on the floor while using both hands to optimize the mask seal until help can be recruited.

Ventilating the Patient

Once the airway is opened and an optimal mask seal obtained, the resuscitation bag is connected to the mask, and the patient is ventilated. When fully inflated, the standard adult resuscitation bag contains 1,500 cc of oxygen. This entire volume should not and cannot be delivered repeatedly without insufflating the stomach. The goal of effective oxygenation and

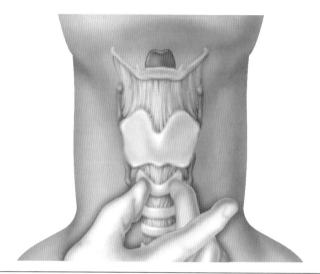

Figure 5-12 ● Proper application of Sellick's maneuver (cricoid pressure) involves the thumb and long finger properly positioned on the cricoid (not the thyroid) cartilage and applying posterior pressure to occlude the esophagus against the anterior surface of the C-6 vertebral body. Note that the index finger is free to apply external laryngeal manipulation.

ventilation is to deliver 10 to 12 reduced tidal volume breaths (500 cc) per minute without exceeding the proximal and distal esophageal sphincter opening pressures of approximately 25 cm of water. High upper airway peak inspiratory pressures result from short inspiratory times, large tidal volumes, incomplete airway opening, increased airway resistance, and decreased compliance. Several things can be done to minimize the potential for gastric inflation and its complications. Deliver each breath over 1 second, and deliver a tidal volume that is sufficient to produce a visible chest rise (500–600 mL). Do not, however, deliver more volume or use more force than is needed to produce visible chest rise. This goal of delivering smaller tidal volumes with each breath while avoiding rapid or forceful breaths is also reflected in the new ACLS guidelines.

Sellick's Maneuver

While ventilating, performing a Sellick's maneuver correctly may reduce gastric insufflation. Until more definitive literature is published, we suggest it be applied if resources permit. Sellick's maneuver is performed by pressing the cricoid cartilage posteriorly, causing it to occlude the esophagus against the spinal column (Fig. 5-12). This requires an additional health care provider and should only be used if the patient is unresponsive. A common error is to apply pressure to the thyroid cartilage instead of the cricoid cartilage, causing airway occlusion.

SUMMARY

BMV is a dynamic process. One must continually assess the adequacy of gas exchange that one is providing. Listening and feeling for areas of mask leak and observing the rise and fall of the chest are crucial to success. With the nondominant hand placed appropriately on the mask, a left-sided mask leak will be felt by the care provider's hypothenar eminence. An assistant may be required to evaluate the integrity of the seal on the right side of the mask and compress the right cheek into the mask cushion as needed. It may be necessary to rock the mask up or down or from side to side (pronation or supination) to achieve a better mask seal. It may also be necessary to frequently reperform the jaw thrust maneuver to re-establish airway patency because it is common for the mandible to slip back to its normal position during BMV. When squeezing the bag and delivering effective tidal volumes, the care provider should simultaneously feel resistance in the bag and observe rise and fall of the patient's chest. Other signs of adequate ventilation are improvement in oxygen saturation, the appearance of an appropriate waveform on a capnograph, and color change from purple to yellow on an end-tidal carbon dioxide (CO_2) detector, provided the patient is generating CO_2.

Occasionally, one may be able to deliver an inspiratory breath, but passive expiration fails to occur. This ordinarily occurs when the degree of jaw thrust is inadequate. Removal of the bag-mask unit from the face and re-creation of a jaw thrust will ordinarily permit expiration.

When initial BMV fails to establish or maintain adequate oxygen saturation, better bag and mask techniques must be used. If a single-hand mask hold is being used, one should immediately employ a two-handed, two-person technique and focus on the following options:

1. Is the mask seal optimal? If not, how can this be improved (e.g., applying KY jelly to a beard; placing unfolded gauze 4 × 4s fluffed and compressed inside the mouth along the buccal pouches [cheeks] to create a better mask seal; reinserting the patient's false teeth; gathering both cheeks inside the body of the mask; ensuring that the entire mouth and all airway adjuncts are within the body of the mask, not disrupting the seal) (Fig. 5-13)?

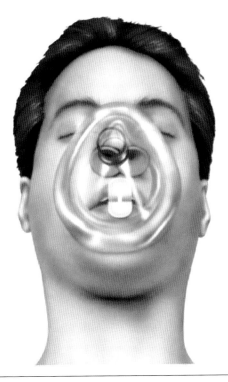

Figure 5-13 ● Two nasal airways and an oral airway inserted and placed inside the body of the mask to ensure an effective mask seal.

2. Are all upper airway adjuncts being properly used? The most common error is the failure to use oral and/or nasal airways. Oral or nasal airways should always be used when an unresponsive patient is being ventilated with a bag and mask; two nasal airways and an oral airway should be used in cases where persistent difficulty is encountered in delivering adequate ventilation and oxygenation (Fig. 5-13).

3. Does the jaw thrust maneuver need to be redone to more effectively open the airway?

4. Does a more experienced person need to be recruited to help optimize bag-mask technique?

EVIDENCE

1. **How much oxygen is the patient actually receiving with different oxygen delivery systems?** Standard textbooks in respiratory therapy (1,2) and anesthesiology (3) describe oxygen delivery systems and the concentrations of oxygen that they characteristically deliver.

2. **How can I determine whether a superior resuscitation bag is being used?** Not all self-inflating ventilation bags deliver high concentrations of oxygen. Only those bags with duckbill inhalation valves, one-way exhalation valves, and small dead space can be expected to deliver inhaled concentrations of oxygen greater than 90% (4,5). Duckbill valve bags without one-way exhalation valves have been shown to deliver less than 40% oxygen (5).

3. **What is the optimal technique to ventilate the patient during BMV?** The primary goal is oxygenation without gastric inflation. This is best accomplished by focusing on avoiding high airway pressures during BMV (e.g., longer inspiratory times, smaller tidal volume, optimal airway opening) (6–9). The recommended tidal volume of 500 cc is best achieved by squeezing the bag with one hand rather than squeezing the bag against one's body (10).

4. **Should Sellick's maneuver be performed during BMV?** If the necessary personnel are available, it is possibly helpful to use this technique during BMV. Note that literature exists both supporting and questioning the utility of Sellick's maneuver. Proper application of cricoid pressure does appear to reduce the volume of air entering the stomach when BMV is performed with low to moderate pressures (11). There is also literature, however, indicating that this technique may not occlude the esophagus at all (12) or may impair ventilation by partially obstructing the upper airway (13). In addition, although not developed to be used as an adjunct to improve visualization during laryngoscopy, there are studies both supporting its ability to improve (14) and worsen (15) visualization of the airway during direct laryngoscopy.

REFERENCES

1. Shapiro BA, Kacmarek RM, Cane RD, et al. *Clinical application of respiratory care*, 4th ed. St. Louis, MO: Mosby; 1991.

2. Kacmarek RM, Stoller JK, eds. *Current respiratory care*. Toronto, Ontario, Canada: BC Decker; 1988.

3. Vender JS, Clemency MV. Oxygen delivery systems, inhalation therapy and respiratory therapy. In: Benumof JL, ed. *Airway management: principles and practice*. St. Louis, MO: Mosby; 1996.

4. Cullen P. Self-inflating ventilation bags. *Anaesth Intensive Care* 2001;29:203.

5. Nimmagadda U, Salem MR, Joseph NJ, et al. Efficacy of preoxygenation with tidal volume breathing: comparison of breathing systems. *Anesthesiology* 2000;93:693–698.

6. American Heart Association. 2005 American Heart Association Guidelines for Cardiopulmonary Resuscitation and Emergency Cardiovascular Care. *Circulation* 2005;112(Suppl I):IV.

7. Uzun L, Ugur MB, Altunkaya H, et al. Effectiveness of the jaw-thrust maneuver in opening the airway: a flexible fiberoptic endoscopic study. *ORL J Otorhinolaryngol Relat Spec* 2005;67:39.

8. Guildner CW. Resuscitation—opening the airway. A comparative study of techniques for opening an airway obstructed by the tongue. *JACEP* 1976;5:588.

9. Davis K Jr, Johannigman JA, Johnson RC Jr, Branson RD. Lung compliance following cardiac arrest [published correction appears in *Acad Emerg Med* 1995;2:1115]. *Acad Emerg Med* 1995;2:874–878.

10. Wolcke B, Schneider T, Mauer D, et al. Ventilation volumes with different self-inflating bags with reference to the ERC guidelines for airway management: comparison of two compression techniques. *Resuscitation* 2000;47:175–178.

11. Petito SP, Russell WJ. The prevention of gastric inflation—a neglected benefit of cricoid pressure. *Anaesth Intensive Care* 1988;16:139.

12. Smith KJ, Dobranowski JD, Yip Gietal, et al. Cricoid pressure displaces the esophagus: an observational study using magnetic resonance imaging. *Anesthesiology* 2003;99:60–64.

13. Hartsilver EL, Vanner RG. Airway obstruction with cricoid pressure. *Anaesthesia* 2000;55:208.

14. Levitan RM, Kinkle WC, Levin WJ, et al. Laryngeal view during laryngoscopy: a randomized trial comparing cricoid pressure, backward-upward-rightward pressure, and bimanual laryngoscopy. *Ann Emerg Med* 2006;47:548–555.

15. Snider DD, Clarke D, Finucane BT. The "BURP" maneuver worsens the glottic view when applied in combination with cricoid pressure. *Can J Anaesth* 2005;52:100–104.

6

Endotracheal Intubation

Michael F. Murphy, Tobias D. Barker, and Robert E. Schneider

LARYNGOSCOPY AND OROTRACHEAL INTUBATION

Direct laryngoscopy is the centerpiece of orotracheal intubation. Laryngoscopy is a learned skill, and when it is performed properly, it provides optimal exposure of the glottic opening, facilitating endotracheal intubation. Laryngoscopy is a multifaceted procedure that requires both dexterity and creativity to align the oral, pharyngeal, and laryngeal axes of the airway so that the laryngoscopist is provided the best possible view of the glottis.

Although there are many different types of laryngoscopic blades, they are essentially either straight or curved. Typically, the straight blades are intended to pick up the epiglottis to optimize visualization of the glottic opening. The curved blades are used to negotiate around the base of the tongue to make contact with the hyoepiglottic ligament. Depressing this ligament with the blunt (and usually beaded tip) of a curved blade produces elevation of the epiglottis and exposure of the glottis. Both types of blades can be used either way, although the best success rates are achieved when they are used as intended. Airway managers need to be familiar with both techniques so if one fails the other can be used.

A *best attempt* at laryngoscopy has six components: (a) performance by a reasonably experienced laryngoscopist, (b) no significant muscle tone (paralysis), (c) optimal positioning of the airway (e.g., sniff position), (d) the use of external laryngeal manipulation, (e) appropriate length of blade, and (f) type of blade. With this definition and no other confounding considerations, the optimal attempt at laryngoscopy and intubation may be achieved on the first attempt and should take no more than three attempts. Because there are different techniques of laryngoscopy, the laryngoscopist needs to choose one method that works best, and use or practice it often, although not to the exclusion of the others.

Anatomy of Intubation

To appreciate the intricacies of laryngoscopy, one must first understand the anatomy of the upper airway. The anatomy of the upper airway, including the larynx, is described in Chapter 4. In the larynx, the vocal cords, which define the glottic opening, lie at the midportion of the thyroid cartilage, and are inferior and posterior to the flexible epiglottis. During laryngoscopy, these constant relationships serve as important anatomical landmarks. When in trouble, one *must* find the epiglottis because it leads to the cords. There will be occasions during routine or difficult laryngoscopy when the esophagus is exposed and mistaken for the vocal cords. Unless one has a landmark or consistent reference point to confirm the airway anatomically, esophageal intubation may result, or intubation may be unsuccessful. Whenever one is uncertain whether the visualized opening is the glottis or the esophagus, the epiglottis must be found. Once identified, the tip of the epiglottis can usually be elevated with either the straight or the curved blade exposing the cords and the arytenoid cartilages, allowing confident placement of the endotracheal tube (ETT) into the airway.

The single greatest obstacle to successful laryngoscopy is the tongue. To the laryngoscopist, the tongue is the enemy, and the epiglottis is a friend. Anatomically, the base of the tongue may block access to the glottic opening. When the tongue is large in relation to the oral cavity (Mallampati Class III or IV), it can inhibit adequate exposure of the glottic aperture. For this reason, preintubation assessment of the patient's airway is essential. In the mnemonic LEMON, discussed in Chapter 7, the *M* stands for Mallampati, serving as a reminder to examine the oral cavity to assess the relative size of the tongue in relationship to the oropharynx and the mandibular space. The laryngoscope blade is the tool that controls and maneuvers the tongue. In general, the larger the tongue, the wider the blade (i.e., no. 3 or 4) that should be selected. Fundamental to successful laryngoscopy is the selection of a blade, curved or straight, that will be wide and long enough to capture the tongue at the initiation of laryngoscopy, sweep it leftward out of the visual field, and permit direct visualization of the airway.

Laryngoscope Blades: History and Application

There are two fundamental laryngoscope blade designs, and practitioners typically have preferences for one or the other, even though it is essential that airway managers have facility with both.

Although orotracheal intubation employing a laryngoscope blade was initially described in the late 19th century, it became popularized in the early 20th century by Sir Ivan Magill, who used a semicircular straight blade modified from the ear, nose, and throat surgeon's anterior commissure laryngoscope. This "Magill blade" was inserted at the right corner of the mouth, taking advantage of the fact that the distance from the molars to the glottis was less than the distance from the incisors to the glottis, a factor that improved the airway manager's view of the vocal cords. The tip of the blade picked up the epiglottis, enhancing the view of the glottis. An uncuffed, blunt-tipped, gum elastic ETT was then inserted down the semicircular flange of the blade through the vocal cords and into the trachea. Most of these patients were breathing spontaneously (usually on ether anesthesia), although if positive-pressure ventilation was needed, as it commonly was after the introduction of curare and succinylcholine in the 1940s, oil-soaked gauze was packed around the ETT. This technique became known as the "paraglossal" or "retromolar" technique and remained the standard technique until the 1940s when balloons were applied to ETTs to permit positive-pressure ventilation with the use of neuromuscular blockade. Even today, moving the blade from the midline to the paraglossal position may rapidly convert an intubation failure to a success, particularly if an endotracheal tube introducer, such as an Eschmann introducer (EI), is used. It is a maneuver that may improve the laryngeal view so substantially that every airway manager ought to be aware of it.

Modifications of the Magill blade include other straight blade variants, such as the Miller, Wisconsin, Phillips, Henderson, Guedel, and others. A common feature to most of these blades is that the tip is fairly sharp, as opposed to the curved blade where the tip is squared off and blunt to minimize trauma in the vallecula as it is advanced to depress the hyoepiglottic ligament to flip the epiglottis up to enhance glottic exposure.

The addition of bulky rubber balloons to rubber ETTs in the 1940s hindered or even made impossible their passage through the flange of the Magill blade. To get around this problem, Macintosh invented the curved blade in 1943. This blade was designed to control the tongue and sweep it to the left side of the mouth, creating sufficient room to pass the bulky tube/balloon combination. By the late 1940s, Macintosh tired of his design and reverted to the Magill blade, having invented the intubating stylet (gum elastic bougie or EI) to get around the problem. Macintosh inserted the EI down the flange of the paraglossally inserted Magill blade into the trachea, and then moved the blade to the center of the mouth, guiding the ETT into the trachea over the EI.

Techniques of Laryngoscopy

Preparation and Assistance

The decision to intubate implies that the airway manager has formulated a primary plan and backup plans should the primary plan fail. The primary plan is generally called "Plan A," whereas the backup plans are called "Plan B" and "Plan C." Plan A is almost always orotracheal intubation employing a laryngoscope.

Before embarking on the intubation attempt, the airway manager must ensure that the following are available:

- All of the equipment and medications needed for Plans A, B, and C
- Trained assistance
- Adequate suction

The assistant needs to be positioned on the right side of the patient and be trained and prepared to

- Pass equipment as needed to the airway manager.
- Hold the head in a position as stipulated.
- Apply Sellick's maneuver and laryngeal manipulation.
- Hold open the corner of the mouth during intubation.
- Remain in position until excused by the airway manager.

Fundamentals of Laryngoscopy

Laryngoscopy is two-handed procedure: the airway manager holds the laryngoscope in the left hand, and the right hand is placed under the patient's occiput to tilt the head back to open the mouth and lift and move the head during the laryngoscopy in an attempt to optimally visualize the glottis. Once the airway manager has the "best view" of the larynx, the assistant is asked to hold the head in that position with the left hand.

Positioning the Airway

Laryngoscopy will be more successful if the laryngoscopist assumes or creates a comfortable intubating position that allows inline visualization of the airway. This can be accomplished by adjusting either the height of the patient or the height of the intubator (stool, kneeling) to bring the airway into the laryngoscopist's central field of vision. Uncomfortable, contorted body positions lead to fatigue and unnecessarily complicate laryngoscopy.

Before placing the laryngoscope into the patient's mouth, the sniffing position is created by placing a pillow, folded towel, or sheet under the patient's head to facilitate slight forward flexion of the lower cervical spine on the chest and extension of the head on the neck ("sniffing the morning air" or "sipping English tea"; the "flex/extend" position) (Fig. 6-1). The "flex/flex" position provides better laryngeal exposure for some patients, whereas for others (e.g., the morbidly obese) the "extend/extend" position is better. Although there has been some controversy as to whether the sniffing position is best, it is generally accepted that this is the best *starting* position. The laryngoscopist's right-hand positioning of the head permits one to rapidly achieve the best position for intubation.

In the trauma victim, where inline stabilization of the cervical spine is recommended, or in patients with decreased cervical spine mobility, flexion of the lower cervical spine onto the chest and extension of the head on the neck may be impossible or inappropriate, thus making laryngoscopy more difficult. Patients with advanced cervical arthritis may have markedly reduced neck motion, which may also confound laryngoscopy.

Opening the Mouth

Once the optimal position for laryngoscopy has been achieved, the mouth is opened by tilting the head back with the right hand or by using the fingers of the right hand to "scissor" the mouth open. This latter maneuver is awkward because the scissoring fingers obstruct access to the right side of the mouth by the blade. In the event that mouth opening is limited, or the chest obstructs the handle preventing insertion, it may be necessary to remove the blade from the handle, insert the blade into the mouth, and then reattach the handle.

Handling the Laryngoscope

The laryngoscope handle should always be grasped in the left hand. Although laryngoscope manufacturers can supply devices for use with the right hand, they are difficult to acquire and both left- and right-handed care providers are advised to learn to hold the laryngoscope handle in their left hands.

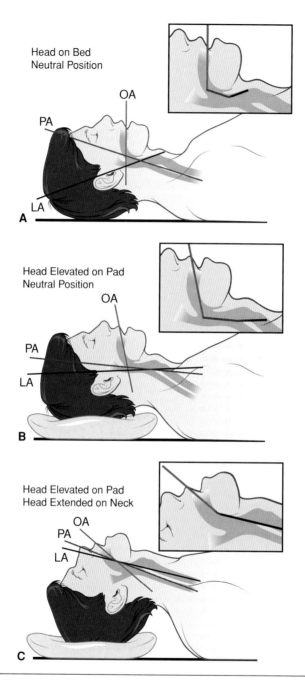

Figure 6-1 ● **A:** Anatomical neutral position. The oral axis (OA), pharyngeal axis (PA), and laryngeal axis (LA) are at greater angles to one another. **B:** Head, still in neutral position, has been lifted by a pillow flexing the lower cervical spine and aligning the PA and LA. **C:** The head has been extended on the cervical spine, aligning the OA with the PA and LA, creating the optimum sniffing position for intubation.

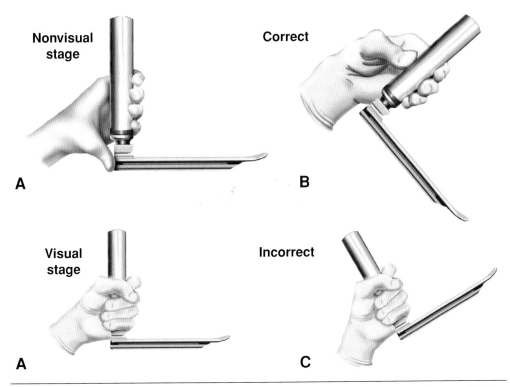

Figure 6-2 ● Laryngoscopy. **A:** Recommended grip of the laryngoscope. **B:** Technique of achieving greater glottic exposure. Note how the end of the laryngoscope handle is directed at approximately 45 degrees, and lift is applied longitudinally. **C:** Absence of the rocking motion will prevent dental injury and trauma.

To minimize trauma to airway structures, it is advisable during the blade insertion stage of laryngoscopy to hold the handle with the fingertips to maximize maneuverability and tactile fidelity, not clenched in the palm of the hand ("death grip") (Fig. 6-2). Once the tip of the laryngoscope blade is positioned where the operator wants it, the laryngoscope handle can be grasped using any familiar technique, including the death grip, as one applies elevation force to optimize laryngeal exposure. However, the expenditure of precious muscle strength during a phase of laryngoscopy where strength is not needed only serves to sap power from when it may be needed most as one tries to elevate the tongue and epiglottis to reveal the glottic opening.

If using a straight blade, the volar pad of the thumb may be positioned on the proximal end of the blade at the connection with the handle to facilitate advancement, particularly if the "insert blindly and withdraw technique" is being used.

Insertion of the Blade

There are two methods of inserting the laryngoscope blade into the mouth and over the tongue: the "look as you go" technique and the "insert blindly and withdraw technique." The former technique is the one usually employed with both straight and curved blades; the latter only with straight blades, and most often in infants.

Curved blades are intended to be advanced into the vallecula and depress the hyoepiglottic ligament to flip the epiglottis forward. This is crucial to the optimal visualization of the glottis with this blade, and failure to do so is a fundamental factor leading to

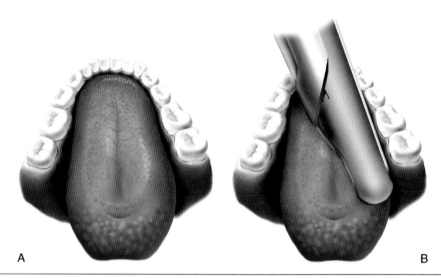

Figure 6-3 ● **A:** Oral Cavity. **B:** Initial anatomical relationship of the flange of the blade with the lingual surface of the molar teeth. Note there is no tongue between the flange of the blade and the teeth.

failure. The airway manager advances the curved blade over the tongue under direct vision until the tip of the epiglottis is visualized. At this point, the blade is gently "levered home" into the vallecula. Only after the tip of the blade is pressed firmly into vallecula does one "lift" the handle and blade to expose the glottis. Incomplete insertion may cause the posterior aspect of the tongue to "squeeze" out beneath the blade and force the epiglottis down over the glottis creating a grade 3B view (see Chapter 7).

Straight blades are intended to pick up the epiglottis whether inserted blindly or under direct vision ("look as you go" technique). Although the tip of the straight blade may be inserted into the vallecula, caution is advised if the blade has a sharp tip.

The blind insertion technique is generally faster than the look as you go technique. It also has the advantage of one knowing that the tip of the laryngoscope is beyond the glottis in the esophagus, eliminating the uncertainty that many infrequent intubators suffer when they intubate and cannot figure out "Am I too deep or too shallow?"

If one elects to use a blind insertion technique, there are two stages to the technique: a nonvisual insertion stage and a visual withdrawal stage. In the first stage (nonvisual) of this technique, the laryngoscope blade is fully inserted blindly, but gently, into the esophagus. Assuming the patient is totally paralyzed with maximum mandibular mobility, the laryngoscope blade is placed into the right side of the patient's mouth alongside the lingual surface of the right mandibular molar teeth (Fig. 6-3). This is an extremely important initial anatomical relationship in controlling the tongue. The laryngoscopist must be certain there is no tongue between the flanged surface of the blade and the lingual surface of the mandibular molar teeth before beginning laryngoscopy. If any tongue is seen, the laryngoscope should be removed and then replaced in the correct starting position. Failure to establish this starting position will compromise control of the tongue, potentially obstruct visualization of the glottic opening, and hinder passage of the ETT (Fig. 6-4). Blade insertion is generally much easier with the patient in the sniffing position rather than the neutral position. In the latter instance (most trauma patients), the laryngoscope blade must hug the anterior surface of the tongue as the blade compresses the tongue into the floor of the mouth and simultaneously opens the mandible and atraumatically advances through the oropharynx, posterior pharynx, and into the esophagus. This procedure is gentle, but requires some

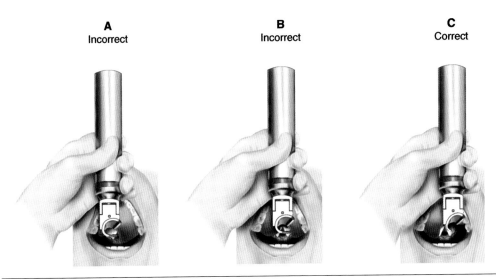

Figure 6-4 ● Tongue Control During Laryngoscopy. **A** and **B:** Poor visualization of the cords due to incorrect positioning of the blade. Note how the tongue folds over the blade and obscures the view. **C:** Correct positioning of the blade to control and move the tongue to the left, providing an optimal view for intubation.

muscle power. If more space is required to negotiate the posterior pharyngeal turn, it must be generated by further movement of the mandible as opposed to the neck.

Once the blade has been correctly positioned adjacent to the right mandibular molar teeth, its entire length is passed blindly and atraumatically into the patient's esophagus, traversing the base of the tongue, passing posterior to the epiglottis and cords, anterior to the posterior pharyngeal wall, and finally moving superiorly and anteriorly through the cervical esophagus into the proximal body of the esophagus. Active visualization of the posterior pharyngeal or laryngeal anatomy is neither possible nor required during this initial maneuver. As mentioned previously, the esophageal insertion is done completely by feel, with gentle pressure exerted by the volar pads of the fingers and thumb, allowing the laryngoscopist to feel the advancing tip of the laryngoscopic blade. Any perception of resistance during this maneuver requires immediate cessation of advancement, slight withdrawal and realignment superiorly, and then reinsertion. The tip of the advancing blade should move toward the midline during this insertion. The laryngoscopist can be assured that the application of cricoid pressure may need to be eased slightly to effect a complete atraumatic insertion.

As mentioned previously, with this initial position established, the cords will always be proximal to the tip of the laryngoscope blade, never distal (Fig. 6-5).

The second stage is totally visual. Under direct vision, the blade is slowly withdrawn from the esophagus to initially expose the glottis, the epiglottis (which can be picked up with the tip of either blade, providing maximum laryngeal exposure for successful intubation), and the base of the tongue (Fig. 6-6). It may require transient forearm muscle power to further elevate the tongue into the mandibular space just before intubation to achieve maximum glottic exposure.

Bimanual Laryngoscopy

Cormack and Lehane quantified the extent to which one is able to visualize the larynx, epiglottis, and upper airway during laryngoscopy (Fig. 6-7). Grades 1 and 2 are usually associated with low laryngoscopic failure rates, whereas grades 3 and 4 usually have higher

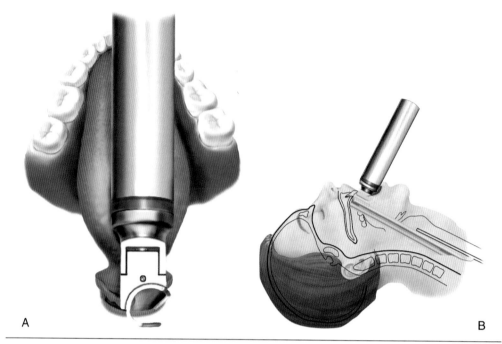

A

B

Figure 6-5 ● **A:** The initial starting position for the visual phase of laryngoscopy. **B:** Note that the blade is in the esophagus and the blade/handle junction is at the patient's teeth. Note the position of the cords proximal to the tip of the blade.

failure rates. Grade 3 has been further subdivided into grade 3A, where the epiglottis sits up, and grade 3B, where it remains flopped down over the glottis.

If the laryngoscopic view is less than adequate, reaching around to manipulate the larynx with the free right hand to apply firm backward, upward, and rightward pressure on the thyroid cartilage will most often improve the laryngeal view one full grade, producing maximum glottic exposure. This maneuver, which is distinct from cricoid pressure (Sellick's maneuver), is called the BURP maneuver (*Back*ward, *Up*ward, *Right*ward *Pressure*) or optimum external laryngeal manipulation (Fig. 6-8). Although this maneuver will often lead to improved visualization, the operator should always individualize the movement of the thyroid cartilage to optimize the laryngoscopic view.

Once the vocal cords are exposed and positioned optimally by the laryngoscopist, the assistant providing cricoid pressure with the right long finger and thumb can use the free right index finger to maintain this optimum view, and without releasing cricoid pressure, can perform a combined maneuver to give both Sellick's maneuver and BURP. This frees the laryngoscopist's right hand to insert the ETT.

Intubating the Trachea

Once the glottis has been identified, it is important that the laryngoscopist not lose sight of the target. The assistant, standing at the patient's right side applying Sellick's maneuver or Sellick-BURP with the right hand, should pull open the right side of the patient's mouth with the left index finger, providing generous access to the oropharynx and, most importantly, providing room for unimpeded passage of the ETT (Fig. 6-9). The ETT should be passed from the right side of the patient's mouth and must not be passed down the flange of the blade, if one is using a straight blade. If the ETT is mistakenly passed down the flange of the blade, it can become trapped, preventing advancement, or the cuff can be

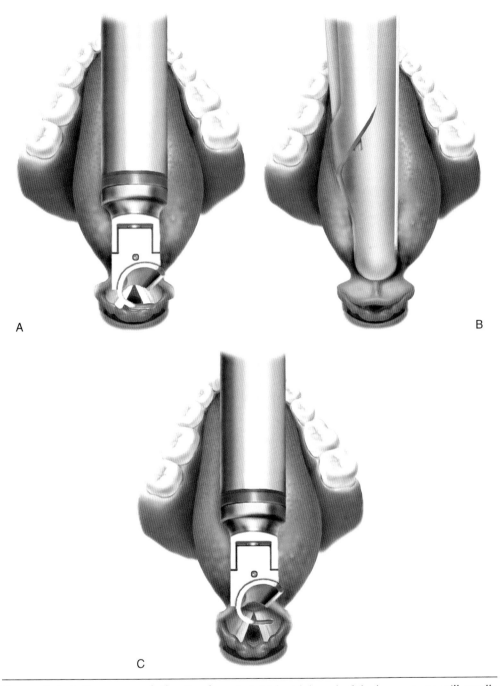

A

B

C

Figure 6-6 ● Exposure of The Cords. **A:** Initial withdrawal of the laryngoscope will usually expose the cords. If not, further withdrawal of the laryngoscope will disclose the epiglottis (**B**), which can be picked up and elevated (**C**), disclosing the glottic aperture.

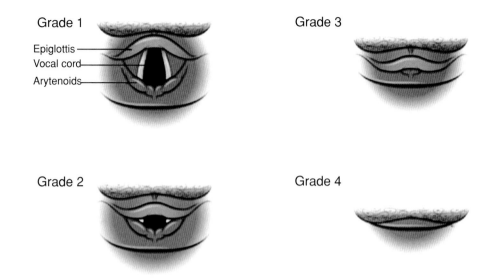

Grade 1

Epiglottis
Vocal cord
Arytenoids

Grade 3

Grade 2

Grade 4

Figure 6-7 ● Cormack-Lehane Laryngoscopic Grading System. Grade 1 is visualization of the entire glottic aperture. Grade 2 is visualization of just the arytenoid cartilages or the posterior portion of the glottic aperture. Grade 3 is visualization of only the epiglottis. Grade 4 is visualization of only the tongue or the tongue and soft palate.

lacerated. Entering from the right side of the patient's mouth prevents the loss of the target in the laryngoscopist's visual field.

As the ETT is initially passed into the right side of the patient's mouth, the bevel of the tube should lie in a horizontal position. The tube initially contacts the hard palate and then sweeps the soft palate as it is advanced toward the glottic opening occupying a position in the right peripheral field of vision. At the glottic opening, the bevel should be simultaneously rotated counterclockwise 90 degrees from a horizontal tube tip orientation to a vertical tube tip orientation so the narrowest dimension of the tube tip enters the glottis in alignment with the vocal cords (Fig. 6-10).

The angle that the stylet used in the ETT is bent is an individualized decision. It has, however, been shown to have an improved chance of passing beyond the glottis if the angle is less than 35 degrees. Following passage through the cords, the laryngoscope and the stylet are removed, and the balloon is inflated.

Endotracheal Tube Introducers

EIs are custom designed for Cormack Lehane grade 2 and 3 views. They are a fundamental piece of airway management equipment that must be part of every airway manager's skill set. As described previously, the EI employs a Seldinger-type technique. Crucial to success is the continuation of laryngoscopy during passage of the ETT over the EI.

EIs are ordinarily plastic, 60 to 70 cm in length, and incorporate a 30-degree deflection of the distal tip. The tip deflection enhances the anterior movement of the distal tip underneath the epiglottis, maximizing the chance it will pass into the glottis and hence the trachea, and permits the tactile appreciation of tracheal rings once placed in the trachea. Seventy-centimeter devices are easier to use than those 60 cm in length. A standard ETT is 30 cm in length, so 60 cm is exactly twice the length of an ETT; the added 10 cm of the 70-cm device facilitates grasping the proximal end of the EI as the ETT is advanced into the trachea. One manufacturer supplies a device with a hollow lumen to permit some degree

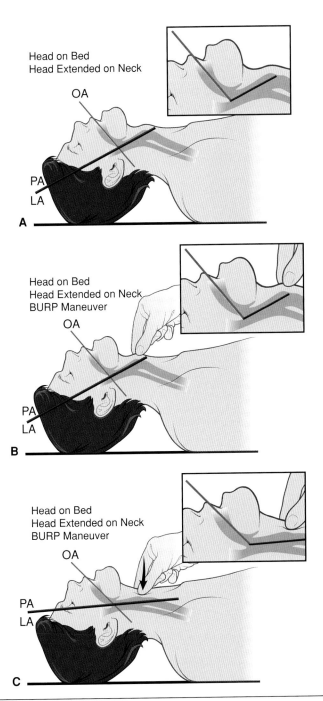

Figure 6-8 ● **A:** Relatively anteriorly placed larynx. **B:** BURP maneuver on the thyroid cartilage. **C:** BURP maneuver improves the laryngeal view for intubation.

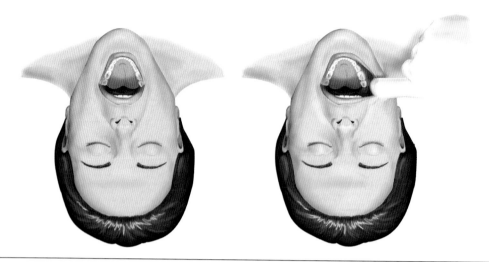

Figure 6-9 ● Retraction of the corner of the mouth by an assistant's index finger will provide ample room for unobstructed passage of the endotracheal tube.

of oxygenation in the event tube passage over the EI fails (Frova by Cook Critical Care, Bloomington, IN). Some EIs are reusable, whereas others are intended as single-use devices.

The EIs are labeled in centimeters, depicting the distance from the tip. The print on the EI is aligned on the same side of the EI as the tip deflection. Positioning the 25-cm mark of the EI at the patient's lip correlates with the tip of the EI at midtrachea. It is important to keep the writing and hence the deflected tip up (anterior) as the ETT is passed over the EI to minimize the chance of forcing the ETT posteriorly in the trachea, risking a posterior tracheal perforation.

Technique of Passing the EI

When using the EI, some laryngeal structure (epiglottis or better—grade 2 or 3) must be visible. *Under direct vision,* the EI is inserted behind the epiglottis, and an attempt is made to insert the tip through the glottis into the trachea. In a grade 2 view, the EI may be seen to enter the glottis. In a grade 3 view, the tip of the EI will not be seen to enter the glottis

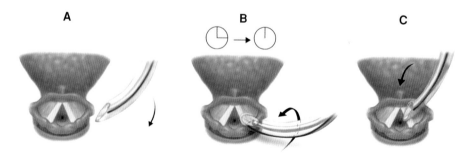

Figure 6-10 ● **The Endotracheal Tube is Rotated 90 Degrees Counterclockwise.** **(B)** as it is passed through the cords, changing the initial horizontal (widest) axis of the bevel **(A)** to the vertical (narrowest) axis **(C)**.

or trachea. Once in the trachea, the tip can often transmit a subtle click, click, click sensation generated by the tracheal rings as the EI is moved gently in and out of the airway. Feeling this sensation enhances your confidence that the EI is in the trachea; failing to sense it does not mean that the EI is not in the trachea. The tongue or other airway structures contacting the shaft of the EI may insulate against the transmission of the corrugated vibrations. In the case where tracheal rings cannot be felt, the EI should be gently advanced. If it is in the trachea, it will "hold up" at some point. Hold up will not occur if the EI is in the esophagus. In the event holdup occurs, withdraw the EI to 25 cm at the lips before advancing the ETT over the EI.

Failure of the ETT to pass easily over the EI into the trachea is most often due to the failure to maintain a "best laryngoscopic view" during the ETT insertion. Keeping the laryngoscope in place minimizes the angle the ETT/EI combination must negotiate and enhances the chance of successfully intubating the trachea.

As the ETT is passed over the EI, a gentle clockwise or counterclockwise twist as the bevel of the ETT reaches the glottis enhances passage. If the ETT gets hung up, rotate the tube 90 degrees, first to the right and then to the left. The tip of the ETT may be caught on the posterior commissure of the glottis, the anterior commissure of the cords, either cord, or the cricoid cartilage, although it is impossible to know the exact location. A similar experience may occur when the EI is passed. The possibilities and remedies are identical.

Once the ETT is in place, the intubating EI is removed, and tube position is confirmed.

CONFIRMING INTUBATION OF THE TRACHEA

Once the ETT has been placed, it is imperative to confirm that it is in the patient's trachea. Traditionally, one of the "gold standards" has been the direct visualization of the ETT passing through the vocal cords, but even this assertion has proven fallible. Probably the only "gold standard" is visualizing tracheal rings on fiberoptic bronchoscopy. The current standard is the detection of end-tidal carbon dioxide (CO_2), most commonly in emergency medicine, emergency medical services and hospital wards, and intensive care units using the colorimetric capnometer, which changes from purple to yellow in the presence of exhaled CO_2, or capnography in the operating room, where the presence of an appropriate waveform confirms tracheal placement.

When using a colorimetric end-tidal CO_2 detector, the color will quickly change from purple (poor) to yellow (yes). This color change should occur within one or two breaths, but in certain circumstances it may be delayed for up to six breaths. If the color change to yellow is not immediate, one has to be suspicious that the ETT is either in the esophagus or above the cords, rather than being properly positioned in the trachea. A color change to tan rather than to bright yellow may also indicate a supraglottic or esophageal location of the ETT tip. In this circumstance, several options are available to confirm the anatomical location of the tube: the laryngoscopy may be repeated to confirm that the tube is indeed properly positioned through the cords, a new colorimetric device may be tried, or the patient may be extubated and reintubated. If any doubt remains, the tube should be assumed to be in the esophagus.

In those clinical circumstances where CO_2 is not produced (e.g., prolonged cardiac arrest), the colorimetric detectors are of limited value and esophageal detecting devices (EDDs) may be used to confirm appropriate tube placement. There are two types of esophageal detecting devices: the piston syringe device and the self-inflating bulb device. Studies have shown that the sensitivity of the self-inflating bulb is greater than the piston syringe. The principle behind these devices relates to the anatomical differences between the trachea and the esophagus. The trachea is composed of anteriorly positioned cartilaginous rings that prevent the collapse of the airway into the ETT when the piston is aspirated or the compressed bulb is released and allowed to reinflate. Because the esophagus is a circumferentially muscular structure without any bony or cartilaginous support, placement of the ETT into the esophagus and aspiration of the syringe or release of the self-inflated bulb will invaginate the esophageal mucosa into the tube and prevent easy removal of the piston or rapid reinflation of the bulb. These devices are quite sensitive and specific, but again must be used in conjunction with other techniques to confirm proper placement of the ETT into the trachea.

Auscultation of the left supraclavicular area, left axilla, left chest, right chest, and epigastrium, respectively, are additive to end-tidal CO_2 and EDD confirmation techniques. The left side of the chest is preferentially auscultated first to confirm that a right mainstem intubation has not occurred. Fogging (condensation) of the ETT is a completely unreliable method of confirming tracheal intubation and should not be relied on. With the exception of bronchoscopic confirmation, none of these techniques taken alone guarantee proper placement of the ETT in the trachea. Thus, it is recommended that they all be done, especially in the arrested patient.

Chest x-rays are used primarily to assess for mainstem intubation and to evaluate tube position within the trachea, not to determine whether the ETT is in the trachea.

FAILED LARYNGOSCOPY AND INTUBATION

When tracheal intubation is unsuccessful, the patient should be ventilated with a bag and mask and high-flow oxygen if the saturations are below 90%. During this reoxygenation time, the laryngoscopist should systematically analyze the likely causes of the failure (Box 6-1). It makes no sense to attempt a second laryngoscopy without changing something in the procedure to improve chances for success. The following questions should be addressed:

- Is the patient in the optimum position for laryngoscopy and intubation? If the patient was placed in the sniffing position initially and the larynx still appeared quite anterior, reducing the degree of head extension could be helpful. In addition, it may even help to elevate and *flex* the patient's head with the laryngoscopist's free right hand (actually flex both the head and the neck) while performing laryngoscopy to create a better view of a true anterior airway.
- Would a different blade provide a better view? If the initial attempt at laryngoscopy was done with a curved blade, it may be advisable to change to a straight blade and vice versa. Alternatively, a different size blade of either type might be helpful.
- Is the patient adequately paralyzed? Laryngoscopy may have been attempted too soon after administering succinylcholine, or an inadequate dose of succinylcholine may have been administered. If the total time of paralysis has been such that the effect of succinylcholine is dissipating, then administration of a second full paralyzing dose of

---

BOX 6-1 Laryngoscopy: Common Errors Associated with Failed Attempts

- No tongue should be visible on the right side of the blade. If there is, remove the blade and reinsert it.
- Once the glottis is visualized using the left arm and hand, *keep it in view!* Do not relax the left hand/arm when you pick up the endotracheal tube with the right hand/arm.
- Keep your wing up. Although it is more comfortable to rest your elbow on the pillow or stretcher, once you have done that, all that you can do with the laryngoscope is lever it, pushing the target up and away from you.

succinylcholine is advisable. If this occurs, atropine must be available to treat poten-
tial bradycardia that occasionally accompanies repeat dosing of succinylcholine.
Appropriate paralysis can improve the view of laryngoscopy one full grade.
- Would external laryngeal manipulation (BURP) be helpful? Most often, BURP
improves the laryngeal view by one full grade.
- Is a more experienced laryngoscopist available? If so, a call for help may be in order.

EVIDENCE

1. **What is the best positioning of the airway for laryngoscopy?** Cormack and Lehane
(1) devised the most widely accepted system of categorizing the view of the larynx
achieved with an orally placed laryngoscope. More recently, Levitan et al. (2) devised
a scoring system to quantitate the percentage of glottic opening visible, which is
becoming used more frequently in the literature. The sniffing position (head extension, neck flexion) has been widely accepted as the optimum position for orotracheal
intubation, although Adnet et al. recently challenged this dogma, suggesting that
simple extension (head extension, neck extension) may be superior (3,4). For difficult intubations, there is even literature to support simple flexion (head flexion, neck
flexion) to optimize visualization (5,6). Although the question of optimal head positioning remains, it is likely that it will vary from patient to patient. This highlights
the importance of a two-handed technique for intubation, allowing for individualized adjustments during laryngoscopy.

2. **Is thyroid cartilage manipulation during laryngoscopy really necessary?** It has clearly
been shown that external laryngeal manipulation, one example of which is BURP,
improves laryngeal view grade by one full grade, on average (7–9). In addition, one
recent study demonstrated the importance of operator-directed laryngeal manipulation (as opposed to assistant-directed manipulation) in maximizing visualization of
the glottic structures (10). The importance of laryngoscopy being a bimanual technique is emphasized regardless of which direction the thyroid cartilage is displaced.

3. **Are EIs truly helpful?** The literature clearly supports the use of EIs to enhance success rates of intubation, particularly with grade 3 views (11–15). In one study, the
success rate improved from 66% to 96% after two attempts (14). Rotation of the tube,
usually 90 degrees counterclockwise, enhances ETT insertion success. In addition,
one study has shown a negative effect of Sellick's maneuver on the success of ETT
passage over the EI (16). Pathogenic bacteria may colonize both the Eschmann (Portex)
variety of EI and the plastic container it is housed in, emphasizing the importance of
sterilizing the device after each use (17). Although rare, bronchial perforation has been
reported with the device (18).

4. **Does it matter which laryngoscopic blade I use?** It is generally believed that one's
choice of a laryngoscope blade and the technique used to facilitate intubation is
best guided by personal choice and experience (3,19,20). The literature suggests
that straight blades improve laryngoscopic view (increased exposure of the vocal
cords), whereas curved blades provide better intubating conditions (more room to
maneuver) (20). The introduction of wider blades (e.g., Grandview) and use of
intubating stylets improves intubation success rates with the straight-blade technique (14). Regardless of the blade used, once visualization is obtained, the degree
of stylet induced ETT angulation can help or hinder passage through the larynx. One recent study demonstrated the optimal bend to be a 25- to 35-degree
angle (21).

   A modern Macintosh-type laryngoscope with a hinged tip that flexes when a
lever on the handle is depressed was introduced by McCoy and Mirakhur in 1993
(22). The mechanism of displacement of the tongue and elevation of the epiglottis is

similar to the Macintosh laryngoscope, in that the tip of the laryngoscope is inserted into the vallecula and the epiglottis is elevated indirectly by depressing the hyoepiglottic ligament. There have been many reports of conversion of grade 3 views to grade 1 or 2 (23). However, there have also been reports of failures (24).

5. **What are the various methods for confirming correct ETT placement?** Visualization of the ETT entering the larynx provides a reliable method of verifying correct position of the tube. Fiberoptic bronchoscopy remains the gold standard for verifying correct ETT placement in adults and pediatric patients by permitting the direct visualization of tracheal rings. This technique has also been used in the setting of emergency airway management (25–27). Auscultation of the chest for breath sounds and of the epigastrium for absence of air entry into the stomach and observation of chest motion during ventilation are common but notoriously inaccurate methods of ascertaining proper ETT placement. CO_2 detection and EDDs have become the standards of care to verify correct placement of the ETT in the trachea, although both techniques have shortcomings (28–43). As might be expected, CO_2 detection techniques tend to be less accurate in identifying correct placement of the ETT in patients with cardiac arrest, with reported false-negative rates (CO_2 not detected despite the tube being in the trachea) as high as 30% to 35% (32). In nonarrested patients, CO_2 detection is highly reliable, indicating correct placement 99% to 100% of the time (28,31,37). Soft drinks in the stomach containing CO_2 may mimic the exhaled CO_2 from the lungs for a few breaths, the so-called Cola complication; this confounding result ought not to persist beyond six breaths (42). The correct endotracheal placement of the tube can be evaluated by an EDD that consists of a self-inflating suction bulb or syringe and an attached adapter to fit it to a standard ETT connector. The collapsed bulb or syringe rapidly fills with air if the ETT is in the trachea; it does not inflate if the tube is in the collapsed esophagus with a specificity of about 99% (34,43). Lighted stylets have also been used to verify tracheal placement (44). In general, none of these techniques alone guarantee correct placement, and as many of them as possible should be used in every case.

REFERENCES

1. Cormack RS, Lehane J. Difficult tracheal intubation in obstetrics. *Anaesthesia* 1984;39:1105.
2. Levitan RM, Ochroch AE, Hollander J, et al. Assessment of airway visualization: validation of the percent of glottic opening (POGO) scale. *Acad Emerg Med* 1998;5:919–923.
3. Benumof JL. *The ASA difficult airway algorithm: new thoughts and considerations*. 51st Annual refresher course lectures and clinical update program, #235. American Society of Anesthesiologists; 2000.
4. Adnet F, Baillard C, Borron SW, et al. Randomized study comparing the "sniffing position" with simple head extension for laryngoscopic view in elective surgery patients. *Anesthesiology* 2001;95:836–841.
5. Hochman H, Zeitels SM, Heaton JT. Analysis of the forces and positions required for direct laryngoscopic exposure of the anterior cords. *Ann Otol Rhinol Laryngol* 1999;108:715–724.
6. Zeitels SM. Universal modular glottiscope system: the evolution of a century of design and technique for direct laryngoscopy. *Ann Otol Rhinol Laryngol* 1999;108(9 Pt 2, Suppl 179):2–24.
7. Knill RL. Difficult laryngoscopy made easy with a "BURP." *Can J Anaesth* 1993;40:279–282.
8. Benumof JL, Cooper SD. Quantitative improvement in laryngoscopic view by optimal external laryngeal manipulation. *J Clin Anesth* 1996;8:136–140.
9. Takahata O, Kubota M, Mamiya K, et al. The efficacy of the "BURP" maneuver during a difficult laryngoscopy. *Anesth Analg* 1997;84:419–421.

10. Levitan RM, Kinkle WC, Levin WJ, et al. Laryngeal view during laryngoscopy: a random-ized trial comparing cricoid pressure, backward-upward-rightward pressure, and bimanual laryngoscopy. *Ann Emerg Med* 2006;47:548–555.

11. Green DW. Gum elastic bougie and simulated difficult intubation. *Anaesthesia* 2003;58:391–392.

12. Henderson JJ. Development of the 'gum-elastic bougie.' *Anaesthesia* 2003;58:103–104.

13. Noguchi T, Kogak K, Shiga Y, et al. The gum elastic bougie eases tracheal intubation while applying cricoid pressure compared to a stylet. *Can J Anaesth* 2003;50:712–717.

14. Gataure PS, Vaughan RS, Latto IP. Simulated difficult intubation: comparison of the gum elastic bougie and the stylet. *Anaesthesia* 1996;51:935–938.

15. Combes X, LeRoux B, Suen P, et al. Unanticipated difficult airway in anesthetized patients: prospective validation of a management algorithm. *Anesthesiology* 2004;100:1146–1150.

16. McNelis U, Sandercombe A, Harper I, et al. The effect of cricoid pressure on intubation facilitated by the gum elastic bougie. *Anaesthesia* 2007;62(5):456–459.

17. Cupitt JM. Microbial contamination of gum elastic bougies. *Anaesthesia* 2000;55:466–468.

18. Viswanathan S, Campbell C, Wood DG, et al. The Eschmann tracheal tube introducer (gum elastic bougie). *Anesthesiol Rev* 1992;19:29.

19. Practice guidelines for management of the difficult airway. An updated report by the Amer-ican Society of Anesthesiologists Task Force on Management of the Difficult Airway. *Anes-thesiology* 2003;98:1269–1277.

20. Arino JJ, Velasco JM, Gasco C, et al. Straight blades improve visualization of the larynx while curved blades increase the ease of intubation: a comparison of the Macintosh, Miller, McCoy, Belscope and Lee-Fairview blades. *Can J Anaesth* 2003;50:501–506.

21. Levitan RM, Pisaturo JT, Kinkle WC, et al. Stylet bend angles and tracheal tube passage using a straight-to-cuff shape. *Acad Emerg Med* 2006;13:1255–1258.

22. McCoy EP, Mirakhur RK. The levering laryngoscope. *Anaesthesia* 1993;48:516–519.

23. Farling PA. The McCoy levering laryngoscope blade. *Anaesthesia* 1994;49:358.

24. Haridas RP. The McCoy levering laryngoscope blade. *Anaesthesia* 1996;51:91.

25. Nielsen LH, Kristensen J, Knudsen F, et al. Fibre-optic bronchoscopic evaluation of tracheal tube position. *Eur J Anaesthesiol* 1991;8:277–279.

26. Lee YS, Soong WJ, Jeng MJ, et al. Endotracheal tube position in pediatrics and neonates: comparison between flexible fiberoptic bronchoscopy and chest radiograph. *Zhonghua Yi Xue Za Zhi* (Taipei) 2002;65:341–344.

27. Hutton KC, Verdile VP, Yealy DM, et al. Prehospital and emergency department verifica-tion of endotracheal tube position using a portable, non-directable, fiberoptic bronchoscope. *Prehosp Disast Med* 1990;5:131–136.

28. Grmec S. Comparison of three different methods to confirm tracheal tube placement in emergency intubation. *Intensive Care Med* 2002;28:701–704.

29. Katz SH, Falk JL. Misplaced endotracheal tubes by paramedics in an urban emergency med-ical services system. *Ann Emerg Med* 2001;37:32–37.

30. Takeda T, Tanigawa K, Tanaka H, et al. The assessment of three methods to verify tracheal tube placement in the emergency setting. *Resuscitation* 2003;56:153–157.

31. Kelly JJ, Eynon CA, Kaplan JL, et al. Use of tube condensation as an indicator of endotra-cheal tube placement. *Ann Emerg Med* 1998;31:575–578.

32. MacLeod BA, Heller MB, Gerard J, et al. Verification of endotracheal tube placement with colorimetric end-tidal CO_2 detection. *Ann Emerg Med* 1991;20:267–270.

33. Hayden SR, Sciammarella J, Viccellio P, et al. Colorimetric end-tidal CO_2 detector for ver-ification of endotracheal tube placement in out-of-hospital cardiac arrest. *Acad Emerg Med* 1995;2:499–502.

34. Bozeman WP, Hexter D, Liang HK, et al. Esophageal detector device versus detection of end-tidal carbon dioxide level in emergency intubation. *Ann Emerg Med* 1996;27:595–599.

35. Cardoso MM, Banner MJ, Melker RJ, et al. Portable devices used to detect endotracheal intubation during emergency situations: a review. *Crit Care Med* 1998;26:957–964.

36. Tanigawa K, Takeda T, Goto E, et al. Accuracy and reliability of the self-inflating bulb to verify tracheal intubation in out-of-hospital cardiac arrest patients. *Anesthesiology* 2000;93: 1432–1436.

37. Li J. Capnography alone is imperfect for endotracheal tube placement confirmation during emergency intubation. *J Emerg Med* 2001;20:223–229.

38. Tanigawa K, Takeda T, Goto E, et al. The efficacy of esophageal detector devices in verifying tracheal tube placement: a randomized cross-over study of out-of-hospital cardiac arrest patients. *Anesth Analg* 2001;92:375–378.

39. Bhende MS, LaCovey DC. End-tidal carbon dioxide monitoring in the prehospital setting. *Prehosp Emerg Care* 2001;5:208–213.

40. Hendey GW, Shubert GS, Shalit M, et al. The esophageal detector bulb in the aeromedical setting. *J Emerg Med* 2002;23:51–55.

41. Tong YL, Sun M, Tang WH, et al. The tracheal detecting-bulb: a new device to distinguish tracheal from esophageal intubation. *Acta Anaesthesiol Sin* 2002;40:159–163.

42. Zbinden S, Schüpfer G. Detection of oesophageal intubation: the cola complication. *Anaesthesia* 1989;44:81.

43. Wee MY. The oesophageal detector device: assessment of a new method to distinguish oesophageal from tracheal intubation. *Anaesthesia* 1998;43:27–29.

44. Stewart RD, LaRosee A, Stoy WA, et al. Use of a lighted stylet to confirm correct endotracheal tube placement. *Chest* 1987;92:900–903.

7

Identification of the Difficult and Failed Airway

Michael F. Murphy and Ron M. Walls

DEFINITION OF THE DIFFICULT AND FAILED AIRWAY

Although both difficult and failed airways are discussed in this chapter, the two concepts are distinct. A difficult airway is one for which a preintubation examination has identified attributes that are likely to make laryngoscopy, intubation, bag-mask ventilation (BMV), the use of an extraglottic device (EGD; e.g., Combitube, laryngeal mask airway [LMA]), or surgical airway management more difficult than would be the case in an ordinary patient without those attributes. Identification of a difficult airway is a key component of the approach to airway management for any patient and is a key branch point on the main airway algorithm (see Chapter 2). The key reason for this is that, in general, one should not administer a neuromuscular blocking medication to a patient unless one has a measure of certainty that gas exchange can be maintained if laryngoscopy and intubation fail.

If a difficult airway is identified, the difficult airway algorithm is used, and the approach to management is different from that taken when the patient is not anticipated to have a difficult intubation (see Chapter 2).

A failed airway situation occurs when a provider has embarked on a certain course of airway management (e.g., rapid sequence intubation [RSI]) and has identified that intubation by that method is simply not going to succeed, requiring the immediate initiation of a rescue sequence (the failed airway algorithm, see Chapter 2). Certainly, in retrospect, a failed airway can be called a difficult airway because it has proven to be impossible to intubate, but the terms "failed airway" and "difficult airway" must be kept distinct because they represent different situations, require different approaches, and arise at different points in the airway management sequence. Furthermore, it is crucial that the airway manager recognize when a difficult airway has transitioned to a failed airway and use the correct management algorithm.

> *"The difficult airway is something one anticipates; the failed airway is something one experiences."*

Airways that are difficult to manage are fairly common in emergency practice, with some estimates being as high as 20% of all emergency intubations. However, the incidence of intubation failure is quite low, generally less than 1% for medical intubations and less than 3% for trauma intubations. The true incidence of the disastrous *"can't* intubate, *can't* oxygenate" (CICO) situation is unknown in emergency intubations, but is estimated to represent between 1 in 5,000 and 1 in 20,000 operating room intubations.

This chapter explores the concepts of the failed and the difficult airway in the setting of emergency intubation. Recognizing the difficult airway in advance and executing an appropriate and thoughtful plan, guided by the difficult airway algorithm (see Chapter 2) will minimize the likelihood that airway management will fail. Furthermore, recognizing the failed airway promptly will optimize the chances that the failing technique will be abandoned and the failed airway algorithm will guide an approach that is reasonably anticipated to succeed.

THE FAILED AIRWAY

A failed airway exists when either of the following conditions is met:

1. Failure to maintain acceptable oxygen saturations during or after one or more failed laryngoscopic attempts (CICO) *or*
2. Three failed attempts at orotracheal intubation by an experienced intubator, even when oxygen saturation can be maintained.

Clinically, the failed airway presents itself in two ways, depending on the urgency created by the situation:

1. There is not sufficient time to evaluate or attempt a series of rescue options, and the airway must be secured immediately because of an inability to maintain oxygen saturation by BMV. This is the CICO scenario (defined by the previous number 1).
2. There is time to evaluate and execute various options because the patient is in a *"can't* intubate, *can* oxygenate" situation (defined by the previous number 2).

The most important way to avoid airway management failure is to identify in advance those patients for whom difficulty can be anticipated with intubation, BMV, insertion of an EGD or cricothyrotomy.

The adage in anesthesia with respect to neuromuscular blockade and the orotracheal intubation of a patient who has some effective spontaneous ventilation has always been "Don't take anything away from the patient that you cannot replace," which can be truncated to "Don't burn any bridges." Although such advice is certainly sound in terms of elective anesthesia, this rigid principle is not always consistent with the realities of emergency airway management, where intubation is often required emergently regardless of the patient's underlying physiological condition or difficult airway attributes, and the approach must be chosen that is most likely to result in success. In fact, many patients with identified difficult airways are best managed using RSI, but the approach is customized and guided by the principles of the difficult airway algorithm (see Chapter 2).

THE DIFFICULT AIRWAY

The emergency airway algorithms were introduced in Chapter 2. When one is presented with a patient who requires intubation, the first decision is whether this is a crash airway. If it is not a crash airway, one must ask, "Is this a difficult airway?" Asking the question presumes that one has a framework with which to answer it.

In clinical practice, the difficult airway has five dimensions:

1. Difficult BMV
2. Difficult laryngoscopy
3. Difficult intubation
4. Difficult EGD
5. Difficult cricothyrotomy

These five dimensions can be reduced to four technical operations:

1. Difficult BMV
2. Difficult laryngoscopy and intubation
3. Difficult EGD
4. Difficult cricothyrotomy

One might think of these four operations as the four corners of a box, the difficult airway box (Fig. 7.1). According to the main emergency airway management algorithm, RSI is the method of choice for airway management in the event airway management difficulty is not anticipated. This requires a reliable and reproducible method for identifying the difficult airway. This evaluation must be expeditious, easy to remember, and complete. A distinct evaluation is required for difficult BMV, difficult laryngoscopy/intubation, difficult EGD, and difficult surgical airway management, and each evaluation must be applied to each patient before airway management is undertaken.

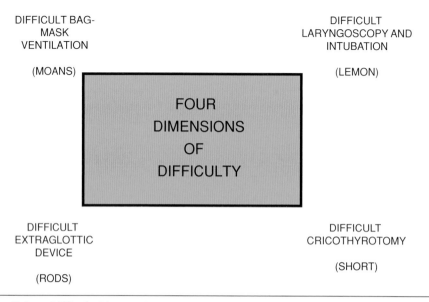

Figure 7-1 ● Difficult Airway Box. Note that the *four corners* represent the four dimensions of difficulty.

Difficult Bag-Mask Ventilation: MOANS

Chapter 5 highlights the importance of BMV in airway management, particularly as a rescue maneuver when orotracheal intubation has failed. If the airway manager is uncertain that neuromuscular blockade–facilitated orotracheal intubation (RSI) will be successful, he or she must be confident that BMV is possible, gas exchange through an EGD is possible, or, at the very least, a cricothyrotomy can rapidly be performed.

The validated indicators of difficult BMV can be easily recalled for rapid use in the emergency setting by using the mnemonic MOANS. Perhaps one can recall this mnemonic by picturing the obtunded, *moaning* patient as in need of BMV, or conversely, the involuntary *moans* that might escape the lips of the provider when he or she is confronted by a patient on whom BMV is not possible.

M *Mask seal:* Bushy beards, crusted blood on the face, or a disruption of lower facial continuity are the most common examples of conditions that may make an adequate mask seal difficult. Some experts recommend smearing a substance, such as KY jelly, on the beard as a remedy to this problem, although this action may simply make a bad situation worse in that the entire face may become too slippery to hold the mask in place.

O *Obesity/obstruction:* Patients who are obese (body mass index >26 kg/m²) are often difficult to ventilate adequately by bag and mask. Women in third-trimester gestation are also a prototype for this problem because of their increased body mass and the resistance to diaphragmatic excursion by the gravid uterus create elevated resistance to BMV. Pregnant or obese patients also desaturate more quickly, making the bag ventilation difficulty of even greater import (see Chapters 32 and 35). The difficulty bagging the obese patient is not caused solely by the weight of the chest and abdominal walls and the resistance by the abdominal contents to diaphragmatic excursion. Obese patients also have redundant tissues, creating resistance to airflow in the supraglottic airway. Similarly, patients with obstruction caused by angioedema, Ludwig's angina, upper airway abscesses (e.g., peritonsillar), epiglottitis, and others ought to be considered at this juncture. In general, edematous lesions (e.g., angioedema, croup, epiglottitis) are more amenable to bag and mask rescue if sudden obstruction occurs but not reliably so. Similarly, laryngospasm can usually be overcome with good bag and mask technique. In contrast, firm, immobile lesions such as hematomas, cancers, and foreign bodies are less amenable to rescue by BMV, which is unlikely to provide adequate ventilation or oxygenation if total obstruction arises in this context.

A   *Age:* Age older than 55 years is associated with a higher risk of difficult BMV, perhaps because of a loss of muscle and tissue tone in the upper airway. The age of 55 is not a precise cutoff, and some judgment can be applied with respect to whether the patient has relatively elastic (young) or inelastic (aged) tissue.

N   *No teeth:* An adequate mask seal may be difficult in the edentulous patient because the face tends to cave in. An option is to leave dentures (if available) in situ for BMV and remove them for intubation. Alternatively, gauze dressings may be inserted into the cheek areas via the mouth to puff them out in an attempt to improve the seal.

S   *Stiff:* This refers to patients whose lungs are themselves resistant to ventilation and require high ventilation pressures. These patients are primarily those with reactive airways disease with medium and small airways obstruction (asthma, chronic obstructive pulmonary disease) and those with pulmonary edema, acute respiratory distress syndrome, advanced pneumonia, or any other condition that reduces pulmonary compliance or increases airway resistance to BMV. A separate but unrelated S that connotes difficult BMV is a history of sleep apnea or snoring. This condition may not be detectable in the setting of an emergency intubation.

Difficult Laryngoscopy and Intubation: LEMON

The concept of difficult laryngoscopy and intubation is inextricably linked to poor glottic view. Cormack and Lehane introduced the most widely used system of categorizing the degree of visualization of the larynx during laryngoscopy, in which an ideal laryngoscopic view is designated grade 1 and the worst possible view grade 4 (Fig. 7.2). Cormack-Lehane (C-L) view grades 3 (epiglottis only visible) and 4 (no glottic structures at all visible) are highly correlated with difficult or failed intubation. C-L grades 1 (visualization of the entire

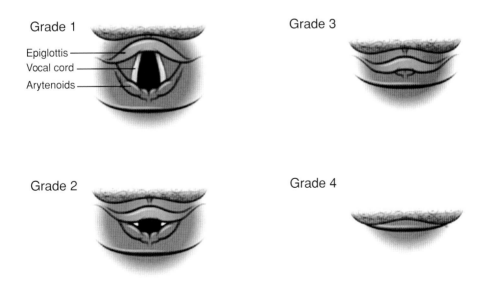

Figure 7-2 ● Cormack-Lehane laryngeal view grade system.

glottic aperture) and 2 (visualization of at least some portion of the cords or the arytenoids) are not typically associated with difficult intubation, although a patient with a grade 2 view in which only the arytenoids are visible is significantly more difficult to intubate than a patient with a grade 2 view in which any portion of the cords can be seen. Patients with a limited grade 2 view or a grade 3 view may greatly benefit by use of an endotracheal tube introducer such as the Eschmann introducer (EI), also known as the Eschmann stylet (or gum elastic bougie), or the Frova intubating stylet (see Chapter 6). The C-L grading system does not differentiate precisely the degree to which the laryngeal aperture is visible during laryngoscopy: a grade 2 view may reveal little of the vocal cords, or none at all if only the arytenoids are visible. This has led some authors to propose a 2a/2b system, wherein a 2a shows any portion of the cords and a 2b shows only the arytenoids. Grade 2b accounts for only about 20% of grade 2 views. However, when a grade 2b view occurs, two thirds of patients are difficult to intubate, whereas only about 4% of patients with grade 2a views are characterized as difficult intubations. A grade 1 view reveals the entire glottis and is associated with almost universal intubation success.

The question is often asked: how much of the cords must be visible during direct laryngoscopy to ensure intubation success? How much is *enough*? Although our discussion here focuses on direct laryngoscopy, many of the issues also apply, to some degree, to video laryngoscopy. The precise extent to which large-scale adoption of video laryngoscopy and other newer methods of intubation will transform our notions of difficult intubation is not known, but it is likely that a radical transformation will occur as direct laryngoscopy is gradually replaced by superior modern methods of intubation. In the context of emergency laryngoscopy, whether direct or by another method, one must first define *best attempt*. Updating concepts defined by Benumof, we might define the seven components of the best attempt as (a) performance by an adequately trained and experienced endoscopist, (b) adequate patient relaxation, (c) best possible positioning of the patient, (d) the use of external laryngeal manipulation (Backward, Upward, Rightward Pressure, or BURP), (e) length of the blade, (f) type of blade, and (g) type of laryngoscope. With this definition and no other confounding considerations, the optimal attempt at laryngoscopy may be achieved on the first attempt and should take no more than three attempts. Often, the circumstances of an emergency intubation preclude the first attempt being the best attempt. When an attempt at orotracheal intubation is unsuccessful and an additional attempt is contemplated, the operator should consider which of the seven attributes can be changed or improved on the subsequent attempt to enhance the chances of success.

Optimizing all seven components may not be possible in an emergency. For example, in the event the cervical spine is immobilized, it is not possible to place the patient in the sniffing position. Positioning the head and neck is an important step in optimizing conventional laryngoscopy as a prelude to orotracheal intubation. Although there is some debate about the relative role of simple head extension versus the sniffing position (head extension with neck flexion, see Chapter 6), in any case, optimal positioning of the patient for direct laryngoscopy improves laryngoscopic view. Patient positioning plays a much smaller role, if any, during video laryngoscopy.

Many researchers have attempted to determine with precision which patient attributes predict successful laryngoscopy and intubation and which predict failure. None have been able to do so. Lists of anatomical features, radiologic findings, and complex scoring systems have all been explored without success. In the absence of a proven and validated system that is capable of predicting intubation difficulty with 100% sensitivity and specificity, it is important to develop an approach that will enable a clinician to quickly and simply identify those patients who *might* be difficult to intubate so an appropriate plan can be made using the difficult airway algorithm. In other words, sensitivity (i.e., identifying all those who might be difficult) is more important than specificity (i.e., always being correct when identifying a patient as difficult) when we ask the question, "Does this patient's airway warrant using the difficult airway algorithm, or is it appropriate and safe to proceed directly to RSI?"

The mnemonic LEMON is a useful guide to identify as many of the risks as possible as quickly as possible to meet the demands of an emergency situation. The elements of the mnemonic are assembled from an analysis of the difficult airway prediction instruments in the elective anesthesia literature and are the subject of a validation study (NEAR III) by the investigators of the multicenter National Emergency Airway Registry project. The LEMON mnemonic is recalled by the popular idiom that a defective product is a "lemon"; thus, the difficult airway is a LEMON:

L *Look externally:* Although a gestalt of difficult intubation is not particularly sensitive (meaning that many difficult airways are not readily apparent externally), it is quite specific, meaning that if the airway looks difficult, it probably is. Most of the litany of physical features associated with difficult laryngoscopy and intubation (e.g., small mandible, large tongue, large teeth, short neck) are accounted for by the remaining elements of LEMON and so do not need to be specifically recalled or sought, which can be a difficult memory challenge in a critical situation. The external look specified here is for the "feeling" that the airway will be difficult. This feeling may be driven by a specific finding, such as external evidence of lower facial disruption and bleeding that might make intubation difficult, or it might be the ill-defined composite impression of the patient, such as the obese, agitated patient with a short neck and small mouth, whose airway appears formidable even before any formal evaluation (the rest of the LEMON attributes) is undertaken.

E *Evaluate the 3-3-2 rule:* This step is an amalgamation of the much-studied geometric considerations that relate mouth opening and the size of the mandible to the position of the larynx in the neck in terms of likelihood of successful visualization of the glottis by direct laryngoscopy. This relationship was first articulated by Patil in 1983, when he associated a thyromental distance of less than 6 cm with difficult intubation. The thyromental distance is the hypotenuse of a triangle, the axis being the antero-posterior length of the mandibular space, and the abscissa being the distance between the chin-neck junction (roughly the position of the hyoid bone indicating the posterior limit of the tongue) and the top of the larynx. The 3-3-2 rule accounts for the three geometric keys to successful visualization of the glottis by direct laryngoscopy:

- The mouth must open adequately to permit visualization past the tongue when both the laryngoscope blade and the endotracheal tube are within the oral cavity.
- The mandible must be of sufficient size (length) to allow the tongue to be displaced fully into the submandibular space.
- The glottis must be located a sufficient distance caudad to the base of the tongue that a direct line of sight can be created from outside the mouth to the vocal cords as the tongue is displaced inferiorly into the submandibular space.

The first "3," therefore, assesses mouth opening. A normal patient can open his or her mouth sufficiently to accommodate three of his or her own fingers between the upper and lower incisors. The second "3" evaluates the length of the mandibular space by ensuring the patient's ability to accommodate three of his or her own fingers between the tip of the mentum and chin-neck junction (hyoid bone) (Fig. 7.3A). The "2" assesses the position of the glottis in relation to the base of the tongue. The space between the chin-neck junction (hyoid bone) and the thyroid notch should accommodate two of the patient's fingers (Fig. 7.3B). Thus, in the 3-3-2 rule, the first 3 assesses the adequacy of oral access, and the second 3 addresses the dimensions of the mandibular space to accommodate the tongue on laryngoscopy. The ability to accommodate significantly more than or less than three fingers is associated with greater degrees of difficulty in visualizing the larynx at laryngoscopy: the former because the length of the oral axis is elongated; and the latter because the mandibular space may be too small to accommodate the tongue, requiring it to remain in the oral cavity or move posterior, obscuring the view of the glottis. Encroachment on the

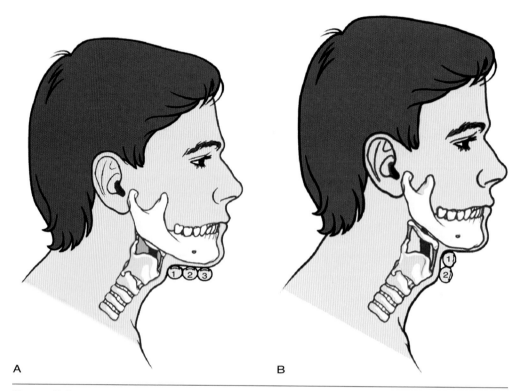

Figure 7-3 ● **A:** The second 3 of the 3-3-2 rule. **B:** The 2 of the 3-3-2 rule.

submandibular space by infiltrative conditions (e.g., Ludwig's angina) is identified during this evaluation. The final 2 identifies the location of the larynx in relation to the base of the tongue. If significantly more than two fingers are accommodated, meaning the larynx is distant from the base of the tongue, it may be difficult to visualize the glottis on laryngoscopy. Fewer than two fingers may mean that the larynx is tucked up under the base of the tongue and may be difficult to expose. This condition is often inaccurately called "anterior larynx."

M *Mallampati score:* Mallampati determined that the degree to which the posterior oropharyngeal structures are visible when the mouth is fully open and the tongue is extruded reflects the relationships among mouth opening, the size of the tongue, and the size of the oral pharynx, which defines access via the oral cavity for intubation, and that these relationships are loosely associated with intubation difficulty. Mallampati's classic assessment required that patients sit on the side of the bed, open their mouths as widely as possible, and protrude their tongue as far as possible without phonating. Figure 7.4 depicts how the scale is constructed. Although Class I and II patients are associated with low intubation failure rates, the importance with respect to the judgment of whether to use neuromuscular blockade rests with those in Classes III and IV, particularly Class IV where intubation failure rates may exceed 10%. By itself, the scale is neither sensitive nor specific; however, if it can be performed in an emergency, it may reveal important information about access to the oral cavity and the potential for difficult glottic visualization. Usually in the emergency situation, it is not possible to have the patient sit up and follow instructions. Therefore, a crude Mallampati measure is often all that can be assessed, by looking into the supine, obtunded patient's mouth with a tongue blade and light, or by using a lighted laryngoscope blade as a tongue depressor to gain an appreciation of how much mouth opening is present (at least in the

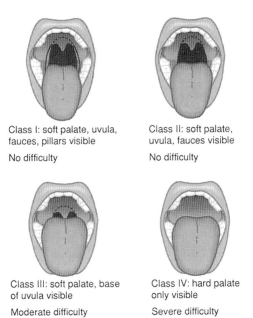

Class I: soft palate, uvula, fauces, pillars visible

No difficulty

Class II: soft palate, uvula, fauces visible

No difficulty

Class III: soft palate, base of uvula visible

Moderate difficulty

Class IV: hard palate only visible

Severe difficulty

Figure 7-4 ● The Mallampati Scale. In Class I, the oropharynx, tonsillar pillars and entire uvula are visible. In Class II, the pillars are not visible. In Class III, only a minimal portion of the oropharyngeal wall is visible and in Class IV the tongue is pressed against the hard palate.

preparalyzed state) and how likely the tongue and oral pharynx are to conspire to prevent successful laryngoscopy. Although not validated in the supine position using this approach, there is no reason to expect that the assessment would be any less reliable than the original method with the patient sitting and performing the maneuver actively.

O *Obstruction/obesity:* Upper airway obstruction should always be considered as a marker for a difficult airway. The four cardinal signs of upper airway obstruction are muffled voice (hot potato voice), difficulty swallowing secretions (because of either pain or obstruction), stridor, and a sensation of dyspnea. The first two signs do not ordinarily herald imminent total upper airway obstruction in adults, but critical obstruction is much more imminent when the sensation of dyspnea occurs. Stridor is a particularly ominous sign. The presence of stridor is generally considered to indicate that the circumference of the airway has been reduced to less than 50% of its normal calibre, or to a diameter of 4.5 mm or less. Upper airway obstruction should always be considered a difficult airway and managed with extreme care. The administration of even small doses of opioids and benzodiazepines, for sedation or to manage anxiety, may induce total obstruction as the stenting tone of the upper airway musculature relaxes, and upper airway instrumentation in the context of inflamed, irritated supraglottic tissues can induce laryngospasm. Either possibility argues for a "double setup" with cricothyrotomy backup during examination or planned awake intubation of a patient with upper airway obstruction. Chapter 30 deals with this topic in detail, particularly in relation to the management of the patient with upper airway obstruction, the selection of rescue interventions, and the timing of those interventions. Although it is controversial whether obesity per se is an independent marker for difficult laryngoscopy or whether obese patients simply have attributes that can be identified by detailed evaluation (e.g., Mallampati score, the 3-3-2 rule), obese patients frequently have poor glottic views by direct laryngoscopy, and obesity, in itself, should be considered to portend difficult laryngoscopy. Glottic view may be difficult whether a direct or video laryngoscope is used.

N   *Neck mobility:* The ability to position the head and neck is one of the seven factors necessary to the achievement of the optimal laryngoscopic view of the larynx. Cervical spine immobilization for trauma, by itself, may not create a degree of difficulty that ultimately leads one to avoid RSI after applying the thought processes of the difficult airway algorithm. However, cervical spine immobilization will make intubation more difficult and will compound the effects of other identified difficult airway markers. In addition, intrinsic cervical spine immobility, such as in cases of ankylosing spondylitis or rheumatoid arthritis, can make intubation by direct laryngoscopy extremely difficult or impossible and should be considered as a much more serious issue than the ubiquitous cervical collar (which mandates inline manual immobilization). Video laryngoscopy requires much less (or no) head extension, and may provide a superior glottic view when head extension or neck flexion is restricted. A recent study also showed reduced cervical spine movement during intubation using the Shikani optical stylet versus direct laryngoscopy.

Difficult Extraglottic Device: RODS

Extraglottic airway devices have emerged as invaluable rescue airway management devices, in addition to their role in routine airway management in the operating room. Devices such as the intubating LMA (Fastrach) and the esophageal tracheal Combitube (Combitube) have a substantial volume of literature attesting to their utility as rescue devices in emergency medical services, emergency medicine, the critical care unit, and anesthesia.

Studies have identified factors that predict difficulty in placing an EGD and providing adequate gas exchange. These can be assessed using the mnemonic RODS.

R   *Restricted mouth opening:* Depending on the EGD to be employed, more or less oral access may be needed.
O   *Obstruction:* Upper airway obstruction at the level of the larynx or below. An EGD will not bypass this obstruction.
D   *Disrupted or distorted airway:* At least in as much as the "seat and seal" of the EGD may be compromised. Seal may be exceedingly difficult or impossible to achieve in the face of a fixed flexion deformity of the neck, or with the upper airway distortion of angioedema, for example.
S   *Stiff lungs or cervical spine:* Ventilation with an EGD may be difficult or impossible in the face of substantial increases in airway resistance (e.g., deadly asthma) or decreases in pulmonary compliance (e.g., pulmonary edema). There are reports of difficult LMA insertion in patients with limited neck movement.

Difficult Cricothyrotomy: SHORT

There are no absolute contraindications to performing an emergency cricothyrotomy (see Chapter 16). However, some conditions may make it difficult or impossible to perform the procedure, making it imperative to identify those conditions in advance and allowing consideration of alternatives rather than simply relying on a rapidly performed cricothyrotomy as a rescue technique. The mnemonic SHORT is used to quickly assess the patient for features that may indicate that a cricothyrotomy might be difficult. The mnemonic can be recalled by remembering that a patient with a *short* neck is difficult to perform a surgical airway on, or that time is *short* when cricothyrotomy is indicated. The SHORT mnemonic is applied as follows:

S   *Surgery (or other airway disruption):* The anatomy may be subtly or obviously distorted, making the airway difficult to find or impeding access to the anterior portion of it (e.g., halo device after spine surgery).
H   *Hematoma (includes infection/abscess):* A hematoma (postoperative or traumatic) or an infective process in the pathway of the cricothyrotomy may make the procedure technically difficult, but should never be considered a contraindication in a life-threatening situation.

O   *Obesity (includes any access problem):* Obesity should be considered a surrogate for any problem that makes percutaneous or open surgical access to the anterior neck problematic, such as a very short neck; large, descending pannus; and subcutaneous emphysema. Careful palpation of the relevant landmarks (see Chapter 16) will identify these issues.

R   *Radiation distortion (and other deformity):* Past radiation therapy may distort and scar tissues making the procedure difficult, or fixed flexion deformity of the spine may limit the working access to the anterior landmarks.

T   *Tumor:* Tumor, either in or around the airway, may present difficulty, both from access and bleeding perspectives.

SUMMARY

- When intubation is indicated, the most important question is "Is this airway difficult?" Considerations of pharmacologic agents for RSI, for example, do not come into play until the patient has been thoroughly assessed for difficulty (MOANS, LEMON, RODS, and SHORT) and the appropriate issues addressed using the algorithms.

- MOANS is always crucially important. The ability to oxygenate a patient with a bag and mask turns a potential CICO situation requiring urgent cricothyrotomy into a "*can't* intubate, *can* oxygenate" situation, in which many rescue options can be considered. The ability to prospectively identify and avoid situations in which bag ventilation will be difficult or impossible is critical to avoiding unnecessary emergency cricothyrotomy.

- When cricothyrotomy is necessary, the possibility will have virtually always been identified in advance, and application of SHORT will permit the operator to be mentally and physically prepared for the surgical airway.

- No single indicator, combination of indicators, or even weighted scoring system of indicators can be relied on to guarantee success or predict inevitable failure for oral intubation. Application of a systematic method to identify the difficult airway and then analysis of the situation to identify the best approach, given the anticipated degree of difficulty and the skill, experience, and judgment of the individual performing the intubation, will lead to the best decisions regarding how to manage the particular clinical situation. In general, it is better to err by identifying an airway as potentially difficult, only to subsequently find this not to be the case, than the other way around.

EVIDENCE

1. **What is the incidence of difficult and failed airway?** In anesthesia practice, the incidence of the failed airway has been identified as 1:2,230 (0.05%) in surgical patients (1) and in approximately 1:280 (0.36%) of parturients for cesarian section under general anesthesia (2). The largest single-center series in the emergency medicine literature has demonstrated a failure rate for RSI of approximately 1% (3). Emerging numbers from the multicenter NEAR project show cricothyrotomy rates of approximately 0.5% in medical cases and 2.3% in trauma (4).

2. **How reliable are the factors we evaluate in predicting difficult intubation?** Many studies have attempted not only to define the features that may predict difficulty, but also to precisely define those airways where failure will occur. The goal has been to attempt to precisely divide the population into those who can be safely anesthetized

and paralyzed and those who ought to be intubated while awake. The landmark publication in 1956 by Cass et al. (5) identified those anatomical features that may predict difficult intubation. This work coincided with the introduction of paralytic agents into anesthetic practice in the late 1940s and early 1950s. Many subsequent investigators attempted to deliver tools that could accurately predict failure (6–13). Although all failed to craft a formula or identify a specific predictor for failure, Mallampati had a measure of success in that he identified oral access as a crucial feature of the assessment for difficulty (13). Langeron, in particular, contributed greatly to the scientific validation of those features, predicting difficult BMV with his study published in 2000 (14,15).

3. **Is there any evidence that positioning the airway prior to intubation improves the view of the glottis?** Cormack and Lehane (16) devised the most widely accepted system of categorizing the view of the larynx achieved with an orally placed laryngoscope. The sniffing position has been widely accepted as the optimum position for orotracheal intubation (17), although Adnet et al. (18) more recently challenged this dogma, suggesting that simple extension may be sufficient or possibly even superior. In attempting to provide a framework or an approach to answering the question of optimum positioning of the head and neck, Levitan et al. (19) devised a scoring system to quantify the percentage of glottic opening visible during a best laryngoscopy, although this scale has yet to gain widespread acceptance.

4. **What is the evidence that stridor indicates a critically narrowed airway?** Stridor is of particular significance in the setting of an *acute airway problem,* where progression of the pathophysiological process may precipitate total airway obstruction that cannot be rescued. Stridor is a characteristic sign in disorders such as croup. Its significance in this condition is attenuated by the fact that we know children with croup seldom progress in an unpredictable manner to total airway obstruction. Stridor is also seen in many chronic ear, nose, and throat disorders, but again is much less significant in this setting due to the nonprogressive or slowly progressive nature of the disorder. The presence of stridor in the setting of an acute upper airway disorder is generally considered to indicate that the circumference of the airway has been reduced to less than 50% of its normal calibre (20), or to a diameter of 4.5 mm or less (21).

5. **Is there any evidence to support the use of RODS to predict difficulty in placing an extraglottic device?** The first three letters are as much a matter of common sense as evidence. However, there is good evidence that ventilation with an EGD may be difficult or impossible in the face of substantial increases in airway resistance (e.g., deadly asthma) or decreases in pulmonary compliance (e.g., pulmonary edema) (22). Furthermore, there are reports of difficult LMA insertion in patients with limited neck movement (23,24).

REFERENCES

1. Samsoon GLT, Young JRB. Difficult tracheal intubation: a retrospective study. *Anaesthesia* 1987;14:17–27.

2. Rocke DA, Murray WB, Rout CC, et al. Relative risk analysis of factors associated with difficult intubation in obstetric anesthesia. *Anaesthesiology* 1992;77:67.

3. Sakles JC, Laurin EG, Rantapaa AA, et al. Airway management in the emergency department: a one-year study of 610 tracheal intubations. *Ann Emerg Med* 1998;31:325–332.

4. Bair AE, Filbin MR, Kulkarni RG, et al. The failed intubation attempt in the emergency department: analysis of prevalence, rescue techniques, and personnel. *J Emerg Med* 2002;23: 131–140.

5. Cass NM, James NR, Lines V. Difficult direct laryngoscopy complicating intubation in anaesthesia. *BMJ* 1956;1:488–490.

6. Bellhouse CP, Dore C. Criteria for estimating likelihood of difficulty of endotracheal intubation with the MacIntosh laryngoscope. *Anaesth Intensive Care* 1988;16:329.

7. Savva D. Prediction of difficult tracheal intubation. *Br J Anaesth* 1994;73:149.

8. Tse JC, Rimm EB, Hussain A. Predicting difficult endotracheal intubation in surgical patients scheduled for general anesthesia: a prospective blind study. *Anesth Analg* 1995;81:254.

9. El-Ganzouri AR, McCarthy RJ, Tuman KJ, et al. Preoperative airway assessment: predictive value of a multivariate risk index. *Anesth Analg* 1996;82:1197–204.

10. Oates JD, MacLeod AD, Oates PD, et al. Comparison of two methods for predicting difficult intubation. *Br J Anaesth* 1991;66:305.

11. Rose DK, Cohen MM. The airway: problems and predictions in 18,500 patients. *Can J Anesth* 1994;41:372–383.

12. Mallampati SR. Clinical sign to predict difficult tracheal intubation (hypothesis). *Can Anesth Soc J* 1983;30:316.

13. Mallampati SR, Gatt SP, Gugino LD, et al. A clinical sign to predict difficult intubation: a prospective study. *Can Anesth Soc J* 1985;32:429.

14. Langeron O, Masso E, Hurax C, et al. Prediction of difficult mask ventilation. *Anaesthesiology* 2000;92:1229.

15. Wilson ME, Spiegelhalter D, Robertson JA, et al. Predicting difficult intubation. *Br J Anaesth* 1988;61:211.

16. Cormack RS, Lehane J. Difficult tracheal intubation in obstetrics. *Anaesthesia* 1984;39:1105.

17. Benumof JL. *The ASA difficult airway algorithm: new thoughts and considerations*. In: Hagberg CA. Handbook of difficult airway management. Philadelphia: Churchill Livingstone; 2000;31–48.

18. Adnet F, Baillard C, Borron SW, et al. Randomized study comparing the "sniffing position" with simple head extension for laryngoscopic view in elective surgery patients. *Anesthesiology* 2001;95:836–841.

19. Levitan RM, Ochroch AE, Hollander J, et al. Assessment of airway visualization: validation of the percent of glottic opening (POGO) scale. *Acad Emerg Med* 1998;5:919–923.

20. Mason RA, Fielder CP. The obstructed airway in head and neck surgery. *Anaesthesia* 1999;54:625–628.

21. Donlon J Jr. *Anesthetic and airway management of laryngoscopy and bronchoscopy*. St. Louis, MO: Mosby; 1996.

22. Buckham M, Brooker M, Brimacombe J, et al. A comparison of the reinforced and standard laryngeal mask airway: ease of insertion and the influence of head and neck position on oropharyngeal leak pressure and intracuff pressure. *Anaesth Intensive Care* 1999;27:628–631.

23. Ishimura H, Minami K, Sata T, et al. Impossible insertion of the laryngeal mask airway and oropharyngeal axes. *Anesthesiology* 1995;83:867–869.

24. Olmez G, Nazaroglu H, Arslan SG, et al. Difficulties and failure of laryngeal mask insertion in a patient with ankylosing spondylitis. *Turk J Med Sci* 2004;34:369–352.

8

Sedation and Anesthesia for Awake Intubation

Michael F. Murphy

DESCRIPTION

Humans protect their airway at virtually any cost. In fact, it is generally impossible to get even a glimpse of the glottis with a laryngoscope in a fully awake and aware patient. This is why the *"awake"* methods of laryngoscopy referred to in the difficult airway algorithm always enclose the term *awake* in quotation marks, meaning that although the patient may be nominally aware, his or her sensibilities are attenuated by local anesthesia, sedation, or both.

Ordinarily, local anesthesia and sedation are used concurrently for diagnostic or therapeutic upper airway interventions in patients. If the patient is uncooperative or when time is of the essence, systemic sedation dominates and less local anesthesia is used. Cooperative patients requiring nonemergent diagnostic maneuvers tend to receive more local anesthesia and less systemic sedation because there is sufficient time to dry the airway of secretions and perform the various local anesthesia techniques.

Awake laryngoscopy has two main roles, both of which apply to patients with anticipated difficult intubation: (a) to determine whether intubation will be feasible, thus facilitating a decision regarding the use of neuromuscular blocking agents, and (b) to intubate, particularly in circumstances in which the patient's airway may be deteriorating, as in angioedema or upper airway burns or trauma ("the dynamic airway"). An awake look intended to determine the feasibility of intubating the trachea nasally or orally can be accomplished in two ways. First, a flexible fiberoptic bronchoscope or nasopharyngoscope inserted through the nostril may be used to determine if nasal intubation is feasible or to locate the glottis in patients suffering from blunt or penetrating neck trauma to determine if orotracheal intubation will be possible. Topical nasal anesthesia and minimal, if any, sedation are usually all that is required. Second, a standard or video laryngoscope blade is inserted into the mouth as for a direct laryngoscopy, with the intention of confirming that glottic visualization (and, thus, orotracheal intubation) is possible.

Substantial local anesthesia of the mouth, oropharynx, and hypopharynx, or very deep sedation, is usually required to obtain an adequate view of the glottis using this technique. If the glottis is adequately visualized, then the airway manager may elect to proceed immediately to an awake intubation or withdraw the laryngoscope and perform rapid sequence intubation (RSI). The approach will be dictated by the clinical circumstance. In general,

- If the difficult airway is dynamic (i.e., evolving) and is the reason for the intubation, then it is usually advisable to intubate the patient during the awake direct laryngoscopy, if possible, because the airway may deteriorate significantly over time or as a result of the direct laryngoscopy. A good rule of thumb is, if the airway might change, intubate it when you have the chance.
- If the difficult airway is chronic (e.g., cervical rheumatoid arthritis) and is not the reason for the airway crisis but simply a confounder to the intubation, then it is reasonable to withdraw the laryngoscope and perform a proper RSI, in the knowledge that the airway is not going to deteriorate further while the RSI is being done.

An awake intubation is more invasive and requires greater degrees of local anesthesia, sedation, or, usually, both.

INDICATIONS AND CONTRAINDICATIONS

Awake intubation is indicated when the individual responsible for airway management is not confident that gas exchange will be assured by any or all of these techniques if the patient is rendered apneic: bag-mask ventilation (BMV), extraglottic device (EGD), or intubation. This is particularly important if an awake laryngoscopy has confirmed that intubation will be challenging. Sedation, upper airway local anesthesia, or both may be indicated for the insertion of nasal and oral airways or an extraglottic rescue device, such as a laryngeal mask airway or Combitube.

Similarly, sedation or local anesthesia of the upper airway may be indicated to facilitate upper airway evaluation (e.g., endoscopy) to identify the location of foreign bodies and remove them, identify a cause of hoarseness, evaluate airway integrity in blunt and penetrating neck trauma, diagnose epiglottitis in a patient with throat pain out of keeping with the oropharyngeal examination, and others.

There are really no contraindications to the use of local anesthetic agents and systemic sedation to enable upper airway evaluation, particularly in an emergency. However, there are some precautions with respect to the choice of sedative agents and how they are used.

SEDATION TECHNIQUES

An awake look in an emergency airway situation relies almost *entirely* on the intravenous (IV) titration of systemically active sedation. There is usually not enough time to produce adequate local anesthesia of the oropharynx and the hypopharynx for a patient to tolerate an awake look procedure without at least a moderate level of sedation. The level of sedation sought is similar to that used for painful procedures in the emergency department, such as reduction of a dislocated shoulder or drainage of a deep cutaneous abscess.

A variety of sedating-type medications may be used, including midazolam, propofol, etomidate, ketamine, and others. In the emergent situation, when judicious chemical restraint is required to permit airway examination of combative and intoxicated patients, haloperidol, a butyrophenone, can be immensely helpful. IV doses of 2 to 10 mg in the adult can be carefully titrated to effect at 3 to 5 minute intervals.

Two medications have been employed in anesthetic practice that may show promise for use in the emergency department awake look situation: remifentanil and dexmedetomidine. Remifentanil is an ultrashort-acting medication that, given by bolus injection or by infusion, has a rapid onset and offset, both measured in tens of seconds rather than minutes. The drug is supplied in 1-mg ampules and is ordinarily diluted in 100 mL of saline to make a concentration of 10 mcg/mL. The median dose of remifentanil that is required to produce loss of consciousness when administered over 2 minutes is 12 mcg/kg; at doses ≤5 mcg/kg, no subjects lost consciousness. It has been recommended that dosing should be calculated on lean body mass and reduced by as much as 50% to 70% in the elderly. Remifentanil, therefore, appears to be very easily titrated. Muscle rigidity has not been observed with infusions up to 0.5 mcg/kg/minute or bolus doses of 25 to 200 mcg. Anecdotally, remifentanil infusion appears to attenuate both the gag reflex and laryngeal reflexes, and can facilitate airway anesthesia. It may be particularly useful in patients with hyperactive gag reflexes, and in the presence of excess secretions, remifentanil may be an invaluable adjunct in awake intubation. Remifentanil may prove to be an exception to the general rule that sedatives cannot or should not be used to compensate for poor regional anesthesia of the airway.

Dexmedetomidine is an alpha-2 agonist that is indicated for the induction of general anesthesia and performance of sedation. It has virtually no respiratory depressant functions, although it may produce profound bradycardia. Infusion by itself and in combination with ketamine has been used for awake fiberoptic intubation. Dexmedetomidine may be a desirable drug for use with fiberoptic intubation, but experience is limited.

Agent selection depends on the clinical situation, medication availability, and familiarity of the sedating professional with the medication. In general, it is best to achieve sedation for airway examination by the same methods used for other procedures so the airway manager is using those agents with which he or she is most familiar and in similar doses.

All agents classified as sedative hypnotics (e.g., benzodiazepines, barbiturates, propofol, and, to some extent, etomidate) cause respiratory depression in a dose-dependent fashion, as do the opioids such as fentanyl and morphine, particularly when use in conjunction with sedative hypnotic agents. Patients with borderline ventilatory drive or barely compensated respiratory failure may be rendered apnoeic by relatively small doses of these agents. Sedative and opioid analgesic agents also produce some degree of muscle relaxation. Patients with upper airway obstruction may become totally obstructed if these agents cause any loss of upper airway muscle tone, and the operator should always be prepared to proceed directly to a surgical airway when sedation and local anesthesia are undertaken on a patient with partial or impending airway obstruction (see Chapter 7).

Levels of sedation lighter than deep general anesthesia are associated with increased intubation difficulty and failure rates. In addition, deep general anesthesia defeats the fundamental purposes of an awake approach (i.e., the maintenance of spontaneous ventilation and active airway protection while one explores alternatives to induction and paralysis).

Ketamine is a dissociative agent and, in doses exceeding 1 mg/kg IV, has respiratory and cardiovascular depressant properties. It may also sensitize the larynx to laryngospasm in the face of laryngeal inflammatory disorders. However, in low to moderate doses, it stimulates respiration, causes mild elevation in heart rate and blood pressure, and maintains muscle tone. Thus, on balance, in the setting of an airway emergency, it may be the best agent to choose to enable the patient to tolerate the evaluation and to continue breathing. The method is to titrate the ketamine in 10- to 20-mg aliquots IV until the patient will tolerate an awake look. The patient may be dissociated but ordinarily will continue to breathe spontaneously and maintain patency of the airway. Some authors advocate a combination of ketamine and propofol drawn up in the same syringe to make a concentration of 5 mg/mL of each (5 mL of 10 mg/mL ketamine plus 5 mL of 10 mg/mL of propofol in a 10-mL syringe) titrated 1 to 2 mL at a time. Although this method administers two agents in a fixed combination, it appears to be effective and safe, and the two drugs are compatible in the same syringe. Alternatives include balanced use of a benzodiazepine (e.g., midazolam) and an opioid (e.g., fentanyl), intravenously titrated etomidate, or other agents used for painful, stimulating procedures. All agents require continuous vigilance with respect to airway patency and adequacy of ventilation.

LOCAL ANESTHESIA TECHNIQUES

Local anesthesia of the airway may be produced topically, by injection, or by combining these two techniques. The selection of a local anesthetic agent will depend on the properties of the agent and how it is supplied (concentration and preparation—aqueous, gel, or ointment). Although the provision of profound local anesthesia in a highly cooperative patient may enable the airway to be visualized and the trachea to be intubated even without sedation, significant systemic sedation will almost always be necessary in the emergency setting.

Determination of the maximum safe dose of local anesthetic agents applied topically to the mucous membrane of the airway is difficult and must take into account the method of topical administration. Traditional dosage guidelines may be excessively conservative when some or all of the drug is administered by aerosol or atomizer inhalation based on the available evidence, with respect to serum levels and toxicity occurrences. However, caution must be exercised, and a precalculated dose should not be exceeded. As always, clinical judgment is required, and meticulous attention to detail should be employed when lidocaine is applied to the airway such that effective anesthesia is achieved without producing toxicity.

The Nose

Topical anesthesia with vasoconstriction is the technique of choice for the nose.

- Using bayonet nasal forceps, place an *agent-soaked* cotton ball along the floor of the nose toward the back of the inferior turbinate (see Fig. 4-1). Place a second ball just

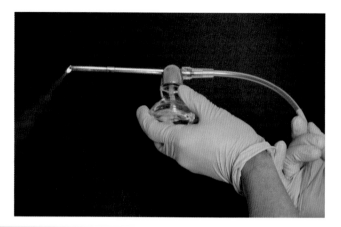

Figure 8-1 ● De Vilbiss Atomizer.

anterior to that, another up against the front of the middle turbinate, and a final one in the vestibule of the nose. It is advisable to place a suture through the cotton balls before placing them. The suture facilitates easy retrieval. Alternatively, surgical patties (strings already attached) or nasal tampons can be used. Some prefer to place a dry nasal Xomed or Merocel wick along the floor of the nose and then inject the agent through a plastic IV cannula along the length of the wick, leaving the soaked wick in place for 10 minutes.

- Adequate topical anesthesia of the *dried* upper airway can often be achieved by nebulizing a mixture of 4 cc of 4% lidocaine with 1 cc of 1% phenylephrine. This procedure typically takes 10 to 15 minutes, though, and may still require some augmentation by topical spray during the procedure. Note that this approach will administer 160 mg of lidocaine topically, so it must be dose adjusted for small adults and children (toxic dose of lidocaine is 4 mg/kg).
- Alternatively, one may elect to use a DeVilbiss atomizer (Fig. 8-1) or a MAD (Fig. 8-2) to atomize the agent into the nostril while asking the patient to sniff. Atomization produces larger droplets than nebulization. The result is that more of the medication rains out in the upper airway with atomizers than nebulizers, producing a denser block.

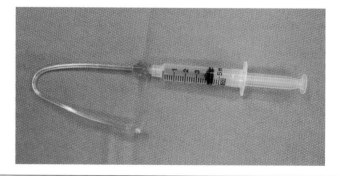

Figure 8-2 ● Mucosal Atomization Device (MAD). The syringe forces the local anesthetic solution through the atomizing tip, resulting in a very fine mist, which can be synchronized with the patient's inspiration.

- Vasoconstriction is probably important. Not only does it enlarge nasal passageways, but it may also reduce the risk of mucosal damage and bleeding and enhance the effectiveness of the topical block. Phenylephrine (Neosynephrine) 0.25% solution, or oxymetazoline (Afrin) sprayed and sniffed into the nostrils 2 to 3 minutes before the local anesthetic agent is applied is effective. Alternatively, one can prepare tetracaine 0.45% with epinephrine 1:25,000 (40 mcg/mL) or use 4% cocaine (40 mg/mL) applied by either of the previous methods. The maximum safe dose of tetracaine is 50 to 80 mg; for cocaine, 1 to 3 mg/kg, although toxic reactions have been reported with as little as 20 to 30 mg.
- Virtually all local anesthetic agents are effective when used topically in the nose. However, cocaine 4% and tetracaine 0.45% are particularly effective because of their ability to deeply penetrate tissues and eliminate the deep pressure-type pain commonly associated with inserting devices through the nose. Lidocaine is effective, particularly the 4% aqueous solution (discussed previously), although it tends to cause an intense burning dysesthesia when applied and produces less deep anesthesia, and at 40 mg/mL, toxicity can occur as the volume increases. Most consider 3 to 4 mg/kg applied to a mucosal surface to be a safe maximum dose for lidocaine.

The Mouth

Topical anesthesia of the oral cavity reduces the discomfort generated by grasping the tongue with gauze and pulling it forward to control it and draw the epiglottis forward during a procedure such as bronchoscopic intubation. Secretion of saliva can be eliminated by using an antimuscarinic agent such as glycopyrrolate (Robinul) (0.01 mg/kg intramuscularly or IV; usual adult dose 0.4–0.8 mg). This approach will enhance the block of the oral cavity, tongue, oropharynx, and hypopharynx by permitting superior penetration of the local anesthetic agent. If there is sufficient time (20 minutes is required for this medication to effectively dry the oropharyngeal secretions), it is always advisable to administer glycopyrrolate as part of the local anesthesia of the upper airway.

- The mouth is best anesthetized topically by having the patient gargle and swish with a 4% aqueous solution of lidocaine. The gargling augments the anesthesia of the oro- and hypopharynx.
- An atomizer can also be used to spray the structures of the oral cavity.

The Oropharynx and Hypopharynx

Begin by having the patient gargle, swish, and then spit out 30 mL of 4% lidocaine. For the most part, the sensory supply of the oro- and hypopharyngeal areas is via the glossopharyngeal nerve (see Chapter 4). The best way to achieve local anesthesia of these areas that is sufficiently dense to permit laryngoscopy or awake intubation is to use a technique that blocks this nerve at the base of the palatopharyngeal arch (posterior tonsillar pillar; see Fig. 4-4). Two techniques are commonly used:

- A 23-gauge angled tonsillar needle with 1 cm of exposed needle tip is inserted 0.5 cm behind the midpoint of the posterior tonsillar pillar and directed laterally and slightly posteriorly (Fig. 8-3). Two cc of 2% lidocaine is then deposited following a negative aspiration test. Although this block can be effective, it is not widely used because of the proximity of the carotid artery. A risk of carotid injection up to 5% has been noted.
- A safer way is to use a topical technique. The oral cavity and the pharynx must be thoroughly dry for any topical technique to work. Put 5 mL of 5% lidocaine ointment on the end of a tongue depressor. Have the patient sitting erect and pull the tongue out using gauze. Apply the lidocaine ointment as far back on the base of the

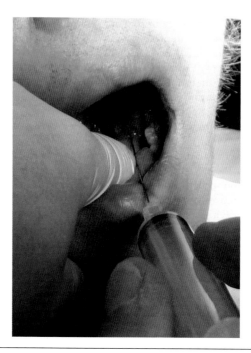

Figure 8-3 ● Glossopharyngeal Nerve Block: insertion point for a 23-gauge angled tonsillar needle.

tongue as possible using the tongue depressor, as one would apply butter or jam to a piece of toast. Put the tongue back in the mouth and wait 15 minutes. The ointment will liquefy as it warms and will run into the area at the base of the palatopharyngeal arch, penetrating the mucosa to reach the glossopharyngeal nerve. It will also run into the valleculae and pyriform recesses to block the superior branch of the internal laryngeal nerve, producing laryngeal anesthesia.

The Larynx

The drying imperative does not apply to the larynx. Topical local anesthesia of this structure can be provided using a manual spray device, an atomizer, or a nebulizer to spray 4 to 6 mL of 4% lidocaine aqueous. Alternatively, one can block the superior laryngeal branch of the vagus nerve (see Fig. 4-6):

- The internal branch of the superior laryngeal nerve can be blocked as it runs just deep to the mucosa in the pyriform recess using Jackson forceps to hold a cotton pledget soaked in 4% lidocaine against the mucosa for about 1 minute (Fig. 8-4).
- This block can also be performed using an external approach to the nerve as it perforates the thyrohyoid membrane just below the greater cornu of the hyoid bone. A 21- to 25-gauge needle is passed medially through skin to contact the hyoid bone as posteriorly as possible. The needle is then walked caudad off the hyoid. Resistance may be appreciated as the thyrohyoid membrane is perforated. Following aspiration to rule out entry into the pharyngeal lumen or a vessel, 3 cc 2% lidocaine can be injected. If the hyoid cannot be palpated or if palpation produces undue patient discomfort, then the thyroid cartilage can be used as a landmark. The needle is then walked cephalad from a point on the thyroid cartilage about one-third of the distance from the midline to the greater cornu. Complications again include intra-arterial injection, hematoma, and airway distortion.

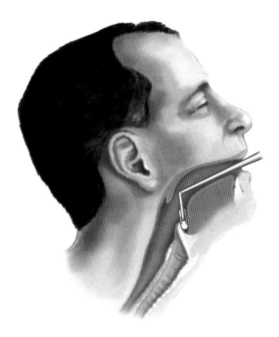

Figure 8-4 ● Use of Jackson Cross-over Forceps to Perform a Transmucosal Superior Laryngeal Nerve Block. A cotton pledget, soaked in 4% lidocaine, is held against the mucosa for about 1 minute.

The Trachea

The trachea is best anesthetized topically. Again, drying beforehand is unnecessary. Local anesthetic agent can be sprayed into the trachea using a handheld spraying device, an atomizer, a fiberoptic scope with a working channel, or a nebulizer.

- Tracheal and laryngeal anesthesia can be produced by puncturing the cricothyroid membrane and injecting local anesthetic agent directly into the trachea. A 5-mL syringe containing 3 mL of 4% lidocaine aqueous is attached to a 20-gauge IV catheter over a needle device. It may be helpful to cut the plastic cannula to about 1.5 cm in length to minimize tracheal stimulation and coughing. A small area of skin is anesthetized over the cricothyroid membrane using a 25- to 27-gauge needle TB or insulin syringe to create a wheal. The needle/IV cannula/syringe combination is then inserted into the trachea through the wheal, aspirating for air during insertion. Once the air column is entered, the cut plastic cannula is threaded in over the needle, and the needle is discarded. The lidocaine is injected at end exhalation with the subsequent inspiration and cough facilitating downward and upward spread of the anesthetic, reaching the cords in 95% of cases.

SUMMARY

- Topical anesthesia of the mouth, oropharynx, and hypopharynx will not be fully successful unless the mucous membranes are first dried by the administration of glycopyrrolate.
- An awake look in the context of a difficult airway is primarily accomplished by using IV agents, supplemented by local anesthetic agents. Titrate ketamine or other appropriate sedation agents as for sedation/analgesia for a painful procedure.

- Use benzodiazepines, propofol, and opioids with extreme caution in patients with impending airway obstruction.

EVIDENCE

1. **Is there any evidence for the use of ketamine and propofol together?** The combination of ketamine and propofol for procedural sedation is a relatively new idea. The anesthesia literature (1–3) describes how this combination is used.
2. **What are the pharmacodynamics of local anesthetic agents?** The physicochemical characteristics of the local anesthetic agents define their clinical behavior, such as their onset time, potency, and duration of action. Detailed descriptions of these agents and their properties are found in the literature (4–7).
3. **Does cocaine cause coronary vasoconstriction?** It is well known that recreational cocaine use is associated with coronary spasm leading to myocardial ischemia and infarction as well as sudden death (8). It is important to realize that medically administered cocaine to produce nasal vasoconstriction has produced similar complications (9–11).
4. **What is the greatest risk when I am doing an injection glossopharyngeal block?** Mongan and Culling (12) described the inadvertent intracarotid injection of a local anesthetic agent during an attempted glossopharyngeal block followed by an immediate seizure.
5. **Can local anesthesia of the upper airway cause airway obstruction?** Extensive clinical experience with lidocaine has shown it to be an effective topical agent for airway anesthesia and to have a wide margin of safety. However, in the presence of pre-existing airway compromise, topical anesthesia and instrumentation of the airway can be associated with complete airway obstruction, probably due in part to laryngospasm in response to the stimulation of the irritated airway. Whenever one applies topical anesthesia or performs instrumentation of an inflamed, compromised airway, one must be prepared to perform a surgical airway. In certain cases, an awake cricothyrotomy or tracheostomy under local anesthesia may be preferable (13–15).

REFERENCES

1. Mortero RF, Clark LD, Tolan MM, et al. The effects of small dose ketamine on propofol sedation: respiration, postoperative mood, perception, cognition and pain. *Anesth Analg* 2001;92:1465–1469.
2. Badrinath S, Avrramov MN, Shadrick M, et al. The use of a ketamine-propofol combination during monitored anesthesia care. *Anesth Analg* 2000;90:858–862.
3. Frey K, Sukhani R, Pawlowski J, et al. Propofol versus propofol-ketamine sedation for retrobulbar nerve block: comparison of sedation quality, intraocular pressure changes, and recovery profiles. *Anesth Analg* 1999;89:317–321.
4. Cathrall W, Mackie K. Local anesthetics. In: Hardman JC, Linbird LE, Molinoff PS, et al., eds. *Goodman and Gilman's the pharmacological basis of therapeutics*, 9th ed. New York: McGraw-Hill; 1996:331–347.
5. Ritchie JM, Greene NM. Local anesthetics. In: Gilman AG, Goodman LS, Oilman A, eds. *Goodman and Gilman's the pharmacological basis of theraputics*, 6th ed. New York: Macmillan; 1980:300–320.
6. Lewin NA, Goldfrank LR, Weisman RS. Cocaine. In: Goldfrank LR, Weisman RS, Flomenbaum NE, et al., eds. *Goldfrank's toxicologic emergencies*, 3rd ed. Norwalk, CT: Appleton-Century-Crofts; 1986:477–485.

7. Morris IR. Pharmacologic aids to intubation and the rapid sequence induction. *Emerg Med Clin North Am* 1988;6:753–768.

8. Minor RL Jr, Scott BD, Brown DD, et al. Cocaine induced myocardial infarction in patients with normal coronary arteries. *Ann Intern Med* 1992;115:797–806.

9. Lange RA, Cigarroa RG, Yancy CW Jr, et al. Cocaine induced coronary artery vasoconstriction. *N Engl J Med* 1989;321:1557–1562.

10. Ross GS, Bell J. Myocardial infarction associated with inappropriate use of topical cocaine as treatment for epistaxis. *Am J Emerg Med* 1992;10:219–222.

11. Laffey JG, Neligan P, Ormonde G. Prolonged perioperative myocardial ischemia in a young male: due to topical intranasal cocaine? *J Clin Anesth* 1999;11:419–424.

12. Mongan PD, Culling RD. Rapid oral anesthesia for awake intubation. *J Clin Anesth* 1992;4:101–105.

13. Ho AMH, Chung DC, To EWH, et al. Total airway obstruction during local anesthesia in a non-sedated patient with a compromised airway. *Can J Anesth* 2004;51(8):838–841.

14. Wong DT, McGuire GP. Management choices for the difficult airway [author reply]. *Can J Anesth* 2003;50(6):624.

15. Mason RA, Fielder CP. The obstructed airway in head and neck surgery [editorial]. *Anaesthesia* 1999;54:625–628.

9

Blind Intubation Techniques

Steven A. Godwin

DESCRIPTION

Blind intubation techniques are those methods of airway management that do not provide direct visualization of the larynx during the intubation process. Both blind nasotracheal intubation (NTI) and digital tracheal intubation (DTI) use indirect indicators of airway identification in lieu of direct vision laryngoscopy. NTI relies on listening to and feeling air movement, whereas DTI depends on the provider's ability to use tactile senses to distinguish airway anatomy as the tube is inserted. Other methods of airway management that do not require direct visualization of the glottis, but that do require specialized equipment, such as lighted stylets and gum elastic bougies, are discussed in other chapters.

I.   **Blind Nasal Intubation**

Although NTI was widely used in emergency departments (EDs) in the past, it is rapidly being supplanted by superior techniques of oral intubation with neuromuscular blockade, even in the prehospital setting. In general, NTI has a number of serious drawbacks, and few advantages when compared to the other techniques that are now commonly used for emergency airway management. NTI has largely fallen out of favor in the ED because it takes longer, has a higher failure rate, has a higher complication rate, and requires smaller tube sizes than oral rapid sequence intubation (RSI). However, despite these inherent problems, NTI is still considered an important skill because it may be useful in certain difficult airway situations, particularly in departments without fiberoptic capability.

A. *Indications and contraindications*

As clinicians become more facile and comfortable with neuromuscular blockade and a variety of other approaches, the one remaining indication for NTI may be the spontaneously breathing patient with an identified difficult airway, for whom RSI is judged to be inadvisable (see Chapters 2 and 7). NTI is achieved by listening to the patient's spontaneous respirations through the tube and, therefore, should not be attempted in the apneic patient. It is relatively contraindicated in combative patients; in those with anatomically disrupted or distorted airways (e.g., neck hematoma, upper airway tumor); in cases of increased intracranial pressure; in the context of severe facial trauma with suspected basal skull fracture; in upper airway infection, obstruction, or abscess; and in the presence of coagulopathy. NTI should be performed with great reservation on any patient who needs rapid intubation because, despite optimistic claims to the contrary, intubation usually requires several minutes to complete using this technique, and significant oxygen desaturation can occur. Therefore, it is a poor choice for patients with respiratory failure, such as the asthmatic patient in extremis, who cannot be oxygenated during the protracted intubation attempt. In addition, one of the primary indications for NTI in the past, the multiply injured patient with potential cervical spine injury, has been discarded, and oral RSI with inline stabilization is now the recommended route (see Chapter 27).

B. **Technique**

1. Preoxygenate the patient with 100% oxygen as for RSI (see Chapter 3), if possible. Try to avoid bagging with positive pressure if spontaneous ventilation is adequate.

2. Choose the nostril to be used. Inspect the interior of the naris, with particular reference to the septum and turbinates. It may help to occlude each nostril in turn and listen to the flow of air through the orifices. If there appears to be no clear favorite, the right naris should be selected because it better facilitates passage of the tube with the leading edge of the bevel laterally placed.

3. Instill two or three drops of Neo-Synephrine or oxymetazoline nasal solution into each nostril. This will vasoconstrict the nasal mucosa and makes tube passage easier. The incidence of epistaxis may also be reduced. It may also be helpful to soak

two or three cotton-tipped applicators in the vasoconstrictor solution and place them gently and fully into the naris until the tip touches the nasopharynx. This provides vasoconstriction at the area that is often most difficult to negotiate blindly with the endotracheal tube (ETT). Nasal topical anesthesia may then be placed as time permits. Insertion of a 4% cocaine pack or instillation of 2% lidocaine jelly will provide anesthesia for the nose. The oral cavity can be sprayed with 4% lidocaine or a similar spray, and, if desired, the pharynx may be anesthetized similarly. An alternative is to nebulize a solution of 4 mL of 4% lidocaine with 1 mL of 0.5% Neo-Synephrine in a gas-powered nebulizer, as one would do with albuterol. This takes approximately 5 to 10 minutes but provides excellent anesthesia and is well tolerated. Still another suggested method involves insertion of an absorbent nasal tampon (as is used for epistaxis) and application of several milliliters of 2% lidocaine with 1:100,000 epinephrine. Cricothyroid puncture with instillation of 5 to 10 mL of 1% to 2% lidocaine is often advocated. This technique is reasonably simple and effective but usually produces coughing, perhaps an undesirable result. Importantly, complete anesthesia of the glottis may not be desirable in all cases. Advancing the tube during the inspiratory phase of a cough sometimes allows immediate intubation of an otherwise elusive trachea. If the patient is awake, explain the procedure. This is a crucial step that is often neglected. If the patient becomes combative during intubation, the attempt must cease because epistaxis, turbinate damage, or even pharyngeal perforation may ensue. A brief, reassuring explanation of the procedure, its necessity, and anticipated discomfort may avert this undesirable situation.

4. Lubricate the tube and the nostril. The use of 2% lidocaine jelly has been advocated, but it is not in contact with the nasal mucosa long enough to result in anesthesia. However, the jelly is an adequate lubricant and is not harmful, so it is a reasonable choice.

5. Select the appropriate size of ETT. In general, the tube should be the largest one that will fit through the nostril without inducing significant trauma. In most patients, a tube with an ID of 6.0 to 7.5 cm will suffice. A smaller tube will fit through a difficult or tight space better than a larger tube. Test the ETT cuff for leaks.

6. Because the patient is often seated, it is probably easiest for a right-handed person to intubate from the patient's left side. This allows the right hand to be used for the intubation, while the left hand manipulates the location of the larynx and provides feedback to the right hand. By leaning slightly forward between the two hands, the operator can listen to the breath sounds and guide the tube into place. If the patient is supine, the operator will position him- or herself immediately above the patient's head. Positioning the head as for oral intubation is worthwhile, however. The so-called sniffing position, with the neck flexed on the body and the head extended on the neck, optimizes the alignment of the mouth and pharynx with the vocal cords and trachea. Care must be taken to avoid overextending the neck, which causes the tube to pass anteriorly to the epiglottis. A small towel may be placed behind the patient's occiput to help maintain this relationship.

7. Some advise gently inserting a gloved and lubricated little finger into the chosen nostril as deeply as possible to check for patency and to dilate the nostril to accept the tube as atraumatically as possible. The intubation sequence begins by gently inserting the ETT into the nostril with the leading edge carefully avoiding the rich vascular area of the anterior septum. For consistency, the remainder if this discussion assumes a right naris intubation by a right-handed operator. The tube should be turned so that the leading edge of the bevel is "out" (i.e., away from the septum). This will minimize the chances of septum injury and epistaxis. This also orients the natural curve of the ETT tube with the natural curve of the airway. The major nasal airway is located below the inferior turbinate and place-

ment of the ETT should follow the floor of the nose backward. The tip of the tube should be directed caudad at an approximately 10-degree angle to follow the gently downsloping floor of the nose (see Chapter 4). This entire process should be done slowly and with meticulous care. Once the nasal portion of the airway is navigated, inciting epistaxis is unlikely. When the tip of the tube approaches the posterior pharynx, resistance will often be felt, particularly if the leading edge of the ETT enters the depression in the nasopharynx where the eustachian tube enters. At this point, it is possible to penetrate the nasopharyngeal mucosa with the ETT and dissect submucosally if care is not taken (see Chapter 4). If this occurs, the ETT should be removed and the alternate nostril attempted. In the event that this anatomical structure cannot be navigated, the insertion of a stylet into the ETT with a gentle C-shaped curve and reinserting the curve will keep the ETT off the post nasopharynx and is usually successful. Often, rotating the proximal end of the ETT 90 degrees toward the left nostril once this resistance is felt will facilitate "turning the corner" by orienting the leading edge of the ETT away from the depression. Once the oropharynx is successfully entered, restore the tube to the original orientation and proceed.

8. The tube should now be advanced until the breath sounds are best heard through it (usually approximately 3–5 cm). At this point, the distal tip of the tube is positioned immediately above the vocal cords. This process may be facilitated by occluding the opposite naris and closing the mouth.

9. Simultaneous with an inspiratory effort by the patient, advance the tube gently but firmly 3 to 4 cm while applying laryngeal pressure with the left hand. The vocal cords abduct during inspiration and are most widely separated at this time.

10. When the tube is advanced, one of three things will occur. If the trachea is entered, a series of long, wheezy coughs will usually emanate from the patient. Inflation of the cuff and a few ventilations with an end-tidal carbon dioxide (CO_2) detector will confirm intratracheal placement. If the trachea is not entered, the tube either will slide easily down the esophagus or will come to an abrupt halt as it tries to pass anterior to the vocal cords or abuts against the anterior wall of the larynx. In the former case, the patient will not cough, and ventilation through the tube will be better heard over the stomach than over the lungs. End-tidal CO_2 will not be detected. If the tube has passed down the esophagus, it is necessary to bring the distal tip of the tube further anteriorly. Withdraw the tube until the breath sounds are well heard again. Then extend the patient's head slightly and try again. If the intubation is being performed on a patient with possible cervical spine trauma, movement is impossible, and the intubation should be reattempted without any change in patient position. In the event the ETT repeatedly passes anterior to the larynx, flex the head on the neck.

11. Inflate the cuff and confirm position with an end-tidal CO_2 detection device. *Do not administer neuromuscular blocking agents to a patient who has undergone NTI unless tracheal tube placement has been confirmed by end-tidal CO_2 detection.* Breath sounds are never reliable as an indicator of tracheal placement, but this is particularly true in the spontaneously breathing patient who has undergone nasoesophageal intubation, whose own breath sounds will continue to be heard over the lungs, even when the ETT is being bag ventilated. A chest radiograph should also be obtained. If the presence of the tube or inflation of the cuff leads to prolonged coughing by the patient, administer 2 mL of 2% lidocaine solution through the ETT during an inspiration. This will often dramatically improve tube tolerance in seconds.

12. Only 60% to 70% of intubations will succeed on the first attempt. The "blind" nature of the procedure requires adjustment and attention to feedback. If the intubation is proving extremely difficult, consider the various options in Box 9-1.

BOX 9-1 Nasotracheal Intubation: Techniques

- The "Endotrol" tube, which has a ringlike apparatus connected to the distal end to allow anterior deflection of the tip of the tube, may be extremely helpful in such cases.
- If the tube has met with a "dead end," it is anterior to the cords or abutted against the anterior wall of the trachea. It may be possible to ascertain by palpation with the left hand whether the tube is off to the left, off to the right, or anterior in the midline. If the tube is truly anterior, slight withdrawal of the tube until breath sounds are well heard followed by slight flexion of the head should facilitate passage. This is a common pitfall. When a first attempt fails, the operator often continues to further extend the neck in an attempt to succeed, each extension making the situation anatomically more impossible. If it is believed that the tube is off to the left or right in addition to being anterior, withdraw the tube, flex the head slightly (if possible), and turn the head slightly in the direction to which the distal tip of the tube was off the midline. For example, if the distal end of the tube was off to the right, turning the head to the right will cause the distal end of the tube to swing to the left (i.e., toward the midline), which is the desired corrective direction. Alternatively, if it is desirable to keep the patient's head in the midline, the proximal end of the endotracheal tube (ETT) may be rotated to the side where the distal end was detected to achieve this effect.
- Inflation of the cuff as the tube lies in the oropharynx may aid in alignment of the ETT with the glottic opening. The tube is then advanced until it meets resistance at the cords, and then the cuff is deflated prior to being pushed through the cords during inspiration. Inflation of the cuff is felt to lift the end of the tube away from the esophagus and into alignment with the vocal cords.
- Use of a guide such as a nasogastric tube or ETT changer in combination with the previously described inflated cuff technique may improve success rates. With this method, after the ETT has been advanced with the cuff inflated to meet resistance at the laryngeal opening, the nasogastric tube is inserted through the ETT. The inflated cuff allows for alignment of the outlet of the ETT with the vocal cords, and the nasogastric tube will slide through the outlet, through the glottis, and into the trachea. As the nasogastric tube slides through the glottis, coughing may occur, suggesting proper placement. The cuff can then be deflated and guided into the trachea over the nasogastric tube, which is then withdrawn from the ETT.
- Pass a fiberoptic laryngoscope or bronchoscope through the tube into the trachea (see Chapter 12).
- Pass a lighted stylet through the tube to assist in locating the glottis (see Chapter 11).
- Change to a new tube, perhaps one that is 0.5 to 1.0 mm ID smaller. The tube often becomes warm and soft during the intubation attempt and is no longer capable of being appropriately manipulated.
- Use a laryngoscope and Magill forceps. This may require conditions that are not present (i.e., the ability to insert a laryngoscope into the mouth and visualize the vocal cords).
- Grasp the tongue with a piece of gauze and pull it forward, or sit the patient up (if possible). This may improve the angle at the back of the tongue.
- Abandon the attempt. Prolonged attempts are associated with hypoxemia and glottic edema caused by local trauma. Either situation can worsen the situation substantially. Repeated attempts are not significantly more successful than the first. In 10% to 20% of cases, nasotracheal intubation will simply not be possible.
- In an unconscious patient, the nasal passage may be dilated with a nasopharyngeal airway or a gloved small finger if problems are encountered trying to get the tube through the naris. Again, a smaller tube may be advisable.

II. Digital Tracheal Intubation

DTI is a tactile intubation technique in which the intubator uses his or her fingers to direct an ETT into the larynx. The technique has gained limited utility in clinical practice. It is not easy to perform, especially if the intubator has small hands or short fingers, nor is it aesthetically pleasing. However, in certain failed airway circumstances in an austere environment, DTI may be an option.

A. *Indications and contraindications*

DTI may be indicated:

1. In situations with poor lighting, difficult patient position, disrupted airway anatomy, or potential C-spine instability. Many of these situations are more likely in the prehospital setting (e.g., a patient trapped in a automobile).

2. If laryngoscopy equipment is unavailable or not working.

3. When visualization of the larynx is impossible (e.g., blood secretions) and no alternative devices or techniques are possible.

4. In failed intubation in an austere environment without rescue airway devices.

The patient must be sufficiently obtunded to prevent a biting injury to the intubator. Generally, this technique should only be considered in a patient who is frankly comatose and unresponsive or who has arrested.

B. *The technique of tactile digital intubation is as follows:*

1. Have an assistant use a gauze sponge to gently but firmly retract the tongue.

2. Insert a stylet in the ETT and bend the ETT/stylet at a 90-degree angle just proximal to the cuff, as for a lighted stylet intubation (see Chapter 11), and place the ETT/stylet into the mouth.

3. Slide the index and long fingers of the nondominant hand palm down along the tongue positioning the ETT/stylet on the palmar surface of the hand.

4. Identify the tip of the epiglottis with the tip of the long finger and direct it anteriorly.

5. Use the index finger to gently direct the ETT/stylet into the glottic opening.

C. *Success rates and complications*

Perhaps the most substantial limitation in performing this technique successfully is the length of the intubator's fingers relative to the patient's oropharyngeal dimensions. Biting injuries or unintentional dental injuries to the hand with the risk of infectious disease transmission may occur. The technique has only infrequently been used in the ED and most authors agree that some degree of experience is needed to perform this skill in an efficient and effective manner.

The two major tips for performing this technique are to have an assistant retract the tongue, thereby allowing the intubator the best access to the epiglottis and to ensure that the patient is sufficiently obtunded to tolerate airway manipulation.

EVIDENCE

1. **Although historically recommended as the primary method for difficult airway management, NTI is an infrequently performed procedure for patients requiring emergent airway management and is now less commonly selected as a rescue method:** Because RSI has become the method of choice for intubation of emergency patients, fewer physicians routinely perform NTI. In a recent review, of 610 intubations performed in a large ED with a Level I trauma center, Sakles et al. (1) reported only 8 (1.3%) NTIs. Of these patients, two attempts were unsuccessful. A review of ED intubations from 30 hospitals as part of the National Emergency Airway Registry (NEAR) databank project, identified 207/7,712 (2.7%) patients that required the use of rescue techniques and/or additional personnel. Rescue RSI was performed after failure of an alternative technique in 102/207 (49%) patients, whereas NTI was used

as a rescue in 36/207 (17%) of patients. Although there were a greater number of rescue intubations with NTI than fiberoptic devices, 10/207 (4.8%), Bair et al. (2) emphasized the rapid growth in the use of fiberoptics over other methods for both primary and rescue airway management. Although still an important backup skill to maintain, NTI has a diminished role in emergency airway management.

2. **When no other alternatives are available, NTI may be performed safely in facial trauma, but clinicians should be aware of rare, yet devastating, possible complications:** Historically, facial trauma was believed to be an absolute contraindication for NTI due to the perceived associated risk of intracranial placement in the presence of cribriform plate disruption. There have been two reported cases of intracranial placement of a nasotracheal tube after facial trauma (3,4). These case reports have been criticized for demonstrating the outcome of poor technique rather than the presence of facial trauma as the cause of these injuries (5). At least one study has been published evaluating the risk of NTI in the presence of facial trauma. This retrospective review of 311 patients with intubation in the presence of facial fractures found that 82 patients underwent NTI (6). The authors found no episodes of intracranial placement, significant epistaxis requiring nasal packing, esophageal intubation, or osteomyelitis. Although there is no evidence that facial trauma is not a contraindication for NTI, in the modern era of RSI and the availability of multiple alternative airway devices, the indications for NTI in the ED setting are limited.

3. **Cuff inflation, neutral head position, and use of ETTs with directional tip control provide added benefit to increase success rates for NTI in both normal and difficult airways:** A number of improvements to the technique for passage of the nasotracheal tube through oropharynx and into the glottis have been suggested over the years. The most studied and successful aid to NTI appears to be the addition of cuff inflation during passage of the tube through the oropharynx until the outlet abuts the glottic opening. A prospective randomized trial evaluating successful NTI with the cuff inflated versus deflated technique demonstrated the inflated cuff technique to be superior. The results showed that 19/20 (95%) patients were intubated with the cuff inflated. In contrast, only 9/20 (45%) patients were intubated with the cuff deflated (7). A separate study compared success rates for NTI and fiberoptic bronchoscope in patients with an immobilized cervical spine with ASA I and II status airways while undergoing elective surgery. The authors reported that there was no significant difference in success rates between the groups. The study concluded that ETT cuff inflation could be used as an alternative to fiberoptic bronchoscopy in patients with an immobilized cervical spine (8), but this conclusion is not warranted by this small study, and both techniques are highly operator dependant. Other studies have demonstrated increased success with NTI using a neutral head position (9) and ETTs with directional tip control (10). However, in the immobilized trauma patient without other identified difficult airway attributes (see Chapter 7), RSI will still be considered the primary method of airway management. In the context of specific difficult airway attributes that argue against administering a paralytic agent, either fiberoptic intubation or NTI, performed with the patient spontaneously breathing, may be appropriate (see Chapters 2 and 7).

REFERENCES

1. Sakles JC, Lauren EG, Rantapaa AA, et al. Airway management in the emergency department: a one year study of 610 tracheal intubations. *Ann Emerg Med* 1998;31(3):325–332.

2. Bair AE, Filbin MR, Kulkarni RG, et al. The failed intubation attempt in the emergency department: analysis of prevalence, rescue techniques, and personnel. *J Emerg Med* 2002;23(2):131–140.

3. Horellou MF, Mathe D, Feiss P. A hazard of naso-tracheal intubation. *Anaesthesia* 1978;33:78.

4. Marlow FJ, Goltra DQ Jr, Schabel SI. Intracranial placement of a nasotracheal tube after facial fracture: a rare complication. *J Emerg Med* 1997;15:187–191.

5. Walls RM. Blind nasotracheal intubation in the presence of facial trauma—is it safe? *J Emerg Med* 1997;15:243–244.

6. Rosen CL, Wolfe RE, Chew SE, et al. Blind nasotracheal intubation in the presence of facial trauma. *J Emerg Med* 1997;15:141–145.

7. Van Elstraete AC, Pennant JH, Gajraj NM, et al. Tracheal tube inflation as anaid to blind nasotracheal intubation. *Br J Anaesth* 1993;70:691–693.

8. Van Elstraete AC, Mamie JC, Mehdaoui H. Nasotracheal intubation in patients with immobilized cervical spine: a comparison of tracheal tube cuff inflation and fiberoptic bronchoscopy. *Anesth Analg* 1998;87(2):400–402.

9. Chung Y, Sun M, Wu H. Blind nasotracheal intubation is facilitated by neutral head position and endotracheal tube cuff inflation in spontaneously breathing patients. *Can J Anesth* 2003;50(5):511–513.

10. O'Conner RE, Megargel RE, Schnyder ME, et al. Paramedic success rate for blind nasotracheal intubation is improved with the use of an endotracheal tube with directional tip control. *Ann Emerg Med* 2000;36:328–332.

10

Extraglottic Devices

Michael F. Murphy

INTRODUCTION

The first laryngeal mask airway (LMA) was introduced in 1981 as an alternative to mask anesthesia. It quickly became apparent that this device was not only easier to use than a mask, but it was also more effective than the existing alternative, a face mask, and less invasive than an endotracheal tube (ETT). The esophageal tracheal Combitube (ETC or Combitube) has been in use since 1987. In concept, it is similar to the LMA. It provides a direct conduit for gas exchange that is easier to use and more effective than a bag and a mask, and less invasive than an ETT. The success these devices have enjoyed has spawned the evolution of similar devices attempting to mimic or improve on their safety; ease of use; and ability to facilitate spontaneous, assisted, or mechanical ventilation.

The terminology referring to these devices has been confusing. Some authors have referred to them as *supraglottic* devices (SGDs), although only certain designs are truly supraglottic (e.g., LMAs, CobraPLA [perilaryngeal airway], Pharyngeal Airway Express or PAXpress). The term *retroglottic device* (RGD) or *infraglottic device* (IGD) has been used to refer to those devices that pass behind and beyond the larynx to enter the upper esophagus (e.g., ETC, King LT airway, Rusch EasyTube). The following taxonomy emerges as reasonably descriptive of the class: the general term for this family of devices is *extraglottic device* (EGD). There are two subclasses: a SGD, which sits above and surrounds the glottis (e.g., LMA), and a RGD, or an IGD, which enters the upper esophagus (e.g., Combitube). These devices are supplied in reuseable and single-use variants.

EGDs differ from face mask gas delivery apparatus in that they are inserted through the mouth to a positon where they provide a direct conduit for air to flow into the lungs. They vary in size and shape, and most have balloons or cuffs that when inflated provide a reasonably tight seal in the upper airway to permit positive-pressure ventilation with variable limits of peak airway pressure.

Although bag-mask ventilation (BMV) is relatively simple in concept, it is difficult or impossible to perform in selected patients (see Chapter 7), even in the hands of experts. Use of an EGD is a more easily acquired skill than BMV for the nonexpert airway practitioner.

Tracheal intubation is the "gold standard" for effective ventilation and protection from aspiration, but the skill is not easily mastered or maintained. The EGDs are a viable alternative to tracheal intubation in many emergency settings, particularly in prehospital care.

Finally, airway management difficulty and failure are associated with significant morbidity and mortality. Certain EGDs have a potential role in both the difficult (LMA) and failed (most EGDs) airway.

Thus, the indications for these devices have expanded over the past two decades to include using the devices:

- As an airway rescue when BMV is difficult and ETT has failed
- As a "single attempt" rescue device performed simultaneously with preparation for cricothyrotomy in the "*can't* inbutate, *can't* oxygenate" (CICO) failed airway (see Chapter 2)
- As an easier and more effective alternative to BMV in the hands of basic life support providers
- As an alternative to endotracheal intubation by advanced life support providers
- As an alternative to endotracheal intubation for elective airway management in the OR for appropriately selected patients
- As a conduit to facilitate endotracheal intubation (e.g., LMA Fastrach, Cookgas intubating laryngeal airway [ILA]).

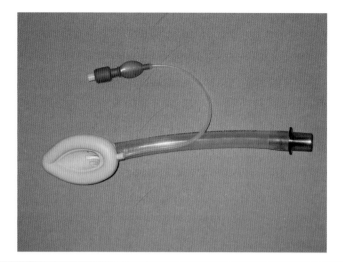

Figure 10-1 • **LMA Classic.** Note the aperture bars at the end of the plastic tube intended to limit the ability of the epiglottis to herniate into this opening.

THE SUPRAGLOTTIC CLASS

The LMA Classic (Fig. 10-1) serves as the prototype for much of the supraglottic class, although other designs also exist. Variants of this original design, also made by the Laryngeal Mask Company Limited, include both reuseable and nonreuseable (disposable) devices:

- Fastrach or intubating LMA (ILMA; reuseable and disposable) (Fig. 10-2)
- LMA Supreme (disposable) (Fig. 10-3)
- LMA ProSeal (reuseable)

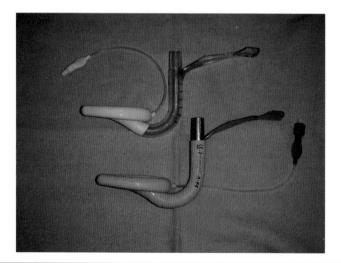

Figure 10-2 • **LMA Fastrach or Intubating LMA (ILMA).** Both the reuseable and disposable variants are pictured. The most unique feature of this device that confers a particular advantage is the handle to permit positioning in the hypopharynx to improve airway seal and the capacity for adequate gas exchange. This factor may be crucial in rescuing a failed airway.

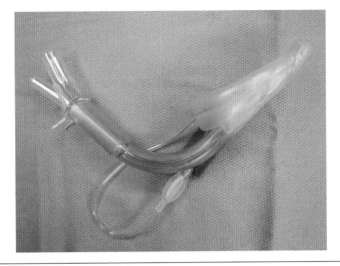

Figure 10-3 ● LMA Supreme.   The rigid construction of the tube and the curvature of the device enhance insertion characteristics and the immediacy of the seal obtained once inflated.

- LMA Unique (disposable variant of the LMA Classic)
- LMA Flexible (reinforced tube variant of the LMA Classic)
- LMA CTrach, a videocapable variant of the LMA Fastrach (Fig. 10-4)

Other SGDs (both original designs and LMA derived) include:

- A variety of disposable LMA Classic–type designs (e.g., Portex, Solus)
- Ambu LMA (ALMA; disposable and reuseable) (Fig. 10-5)
- CobraPLA (disposable) (Fig. 10-6)
- Pharyngeal Airway Express (PAXpress) (Fig. 10-7)
- Cookgas ILA (reuseable) and Air Q (disposable) (Fig. 10-8A and B)

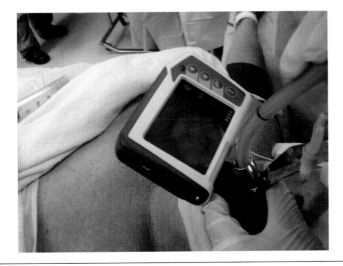

Figure 10-4 ● LMA CTrach.

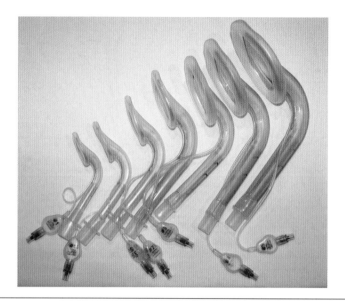

Figure 10-5 ● **Ambu LMA (ALMA).** This is the family of ALMAs.

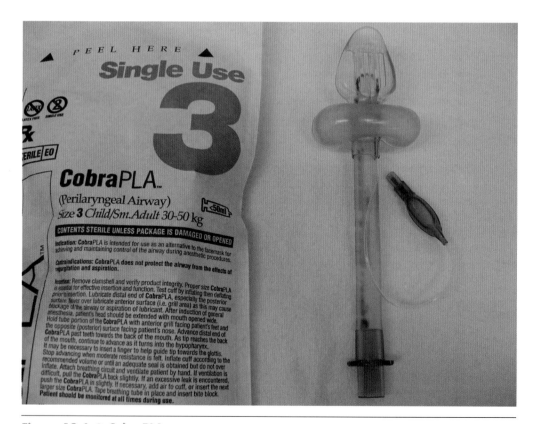

Figure 10-6 ● CobraPLA.

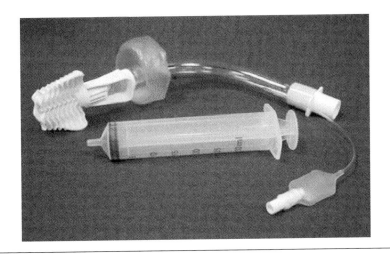

Figure 10-7 ● PAXpress.

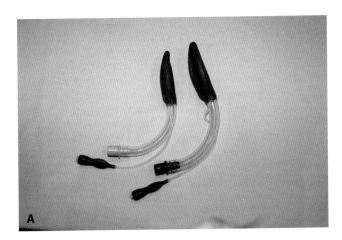

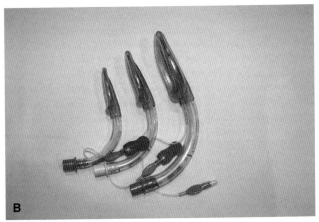

Figure 10-8 ● **A:** The reuseable Cookgas ILA. **B:** The disposable Air Q variant.

LARYNGEAL MASK COMPANY LIMITED DEVICES

The original LMA was introduced into clinical practice in 1981 and looks like an ETT equipped with an inflatable, elliptical, silicone rubber collar (laryngeal mask) at the distal end (Fig. 10-1). The laryngeal mask component is designed to surround and cover the supraglottic area, providing upper airway continuity. Two rubber bars cross the tube opening at the mask end to prevent herniation of the epiglottis into the tube portion of the LMA. The LMA Classic is a multiuse (reuseable) device.

The disposable and much less expensive variety of this device is called the LMA Unique. The LMA Flexible incorporates a nonkinkable design ("wire reinforced") in the tube portion of the device to prevent kinking as the device warms. We do not recommend it for management of the emergency airway.

The LMA ProSeal incorporates an additional lumen through which one can pass a suction catheter into the esophagus or stomach. It also has a higher sealing pressure capacity than the LMA Classic (28 cm H_2O vs. 24 cm H_2O), theoretically conferring an advantage for ventilating patients requiring higher airway pressures, although the difference may not be clinically significant. Because of its expense, relative difficulty in insertion, and marginal benefit in the emergency situation, the LMA ProSeal does not currently have a place in emergency airway management.

A recently introduced disposable device called the LMA Supreme has compelling design characteristics that may make it suitable for emergency airway rescue, although evidence to support this contention is limited. It is the easiest of the Laryngeal Mask Company Limited devices to insert (comparable to the ALMA), seals readily, and, like the LMA ProSeal, has a channel through which a gastric tube can be passed. This device can be considered as a replacement for BMV and endotracheal intubation in the hands of nonexpert airway managers.

The LMA Fastrach, also called the ILMA, is the most important version of the LMA for rescue emergency airway management because it combines the high insertion and ventilation success rate of the other LMAs with specially designed features to facilitate blind intubation. The LMA Fastrach has an epiglottic elevating bar and a rigid guide channel that directs an ETT anteriorly into the larynx, enhancing the success rate of blind intubation. The LMA Fastrach device is a substantial advance in airway management, particularly as a rapidly attempted rescue device in the CICO situation while preparations for cricothyrotomy are underway. The LMA Fastrach is supplied in both reuseable and disposable forms.

The LMA devices are easy to use, produce little in the way of adverse cardiovascular responses on insertion, and, as mentioned previously, have the potential to play a significant role in both routine and rescue emergency airway management. Ventilation success rates near 100% have been reported in operating room (OR) series, but patients with difficult airways were excluded, so the emergency airway ventilation success rate is probably somewhat lower. Intubation success rates through the ILMA are consistently in the 95% range, significantly better than through the standard LMA (about 80%). However, an LMA does not constitute *definitive airway management*, defined as a protected airway (i.e., a cuffed ETT in the trachea) unless one is successful at passing an ETT through the device into the trachea. Although they do not reliably prevent the regurgitation and aspiration of gastric contents, LMAs confer some protection of the airway from aspiration of blood and saliva from the mouth and pharynx.

The patient must have effective topical airway anesthesia (see Chapter 8) or be significantly obtunded (e.g., by RSI medications) to tolerate insertion of these devices. The LMA Classic and the LMA Fastrach are fairly expensive but can be autoclaved and reused. The disposable models, LMA Unique, LMA Supreme, and the LMA Fastrach, are much less expensive.

The LMA CTrach is an LMA Fastrach with a video capability that transmits the image at the distal end of the device to a screen mounted on the airway component. It has the same indications and insertion technique as an LMA Fastrach. The expense and learning curve of the device are unlikely to be acceptable to most emergency and emergency medical services (EMS) providers.

Indications and Contraindications

The standard LMA is now widely used in anesthetic practice instead of mask anesthesia, and the LMA Fastrach is becoming incorporated into difficult airway management.

The LMA and LMA Fastrach have two principal roles in rescue emergency airway management: (a) as a rescue device in a *"can't* intubate, *can* oxygenate" situation, or (b) as a single attempt to effect gas exchange in the CICO failed airway as one concurrently prepares to perform a cricothyrotomy (see Chapter 2). Any attempt to rescue the patient's airway with an LMA, however, must not delay the initiation of the cricothyrotomy.

The handle of the LMA Fastrach permits easier insertion of the device and allows for its manipulation to achieve optimum seal once the cuff is inflated. Thus, if one operator (or an assistant) is opening the cricothyrotomy tray, the principal airway manager can be placing the LMA Fastrach without risk of delay and increased duration of hypoxia. The LMA Fastrach can be used as a rescue device for a CICO airway when laryngeal pathology is not the reason BMV and endotracheal intubation have been unsuccessful. These devices have been used successfully in pediatrics, by novice intubators, during cardiopulmonary resuscitation, and in EMS.

Technique: LMA Fastrach

The LMA Fastrach comes in three sizes: no. 3, no. 4, and no. 5. The no. 3 will fit a normal-size 10- to 12-year-old child and small adults, and is recommended for persons weighing approximately 30 to 50 kg. Most average-size women will require a no. 3. Larger women and smaller men will take a no. 4, recommended for patients weighing 50 to 70 kg, and larger men will generally require a no. 5, recommended for those weighing more than 70 kg. For patients on the borderline between one mask size and another, it is generally advisable to select the larger mask because it provides a better seal.

The intention is to rescue a patent airway initially and recover the oxygen saturations by ventilating through the LMA Fastrach device. Once the saturations are adequate, endotracheal intubation through the device using the silicone-tipped ETT (although conventional ETTs can be used as well) that comes with the device can be accomplished. This can be done blindly or by using a fiberoptic scope or a lighted stylet (e.g., Trachlight). When using the Trachlight (see Chapter 11), it is helpful to remove the rigid metal stylet and and then mount the silicone-tipped LMA Fastrach ETT on the light-tipped wand. The result is instantaneous verification of successful tracheal intubation using the transillumination attribute of the Trachlight.

Select the appropriate-size LMA Fastrach. Deflate the cuff of the mask, and apply a water-soluble lubricant to the anterior and posterior surfaces and the greater curvature of the bend in the metal "stem." Inflating the mask, and then deflating it while pressing the ventral surface of the inflatable collar firmly against a flat surface, produces a smoother and "flipped-back" leading edge (this is a feature of all Laryngeal Mask Company Limited device collars [Fig. 10-9]) and thus enhances the insertion performance. Hold the device in the dominant hand by the metal handle and open the airway. Insert the collar in the mouth, ensuring that the curved silicone-coated metal tube portion of the device is in contact with the chin and the mask tip is flat against the palate before rotation (Fig. 10-9).

1. Rotate the mask into place with a circular motion, maintaining firm pressure against the palate and posterior pharynx (Fig. 10-10A–C). Insert the device until resistance is felt and only the metal end of the silicone-coated tube protrudes from the airway.
2. Inflate the cuff of the LMA Fastrach and hold the metal handle firmly in the dominant hand, using a "frying pan" grip. Ventilate the patient with a ventilation bag, attached to the LMA Fastrach using the other hand. While ventilating, manipulate the mask with the dominant hand by lifting slightly as if to pull the mask toward

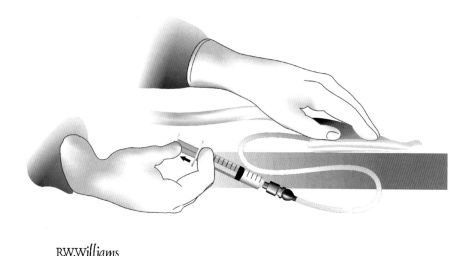

R.W.Williams

Figure 10-9 ● Correct method of deflating the LMA cuff.

the ceiling over the patient's feet (Fig. 10-11). This will provide a good mask seal and will ensure that the mask is correctly positioned for intubation. Best mask positioning will be identified by essentially noiseless ventilation, almost as if the patient is being ventilated through a cuffed ETT.

3. Visually inspect and inflate the silicone-tipped ETT that is supplied with the LMA Fastrach to verify cuff integrity and symmetry. *Fully deflate* cuff (important), lubricate the ETT liberally, and pass it through the LMA Fastrach. With the black vertical line on the ETT facing the operator (indicates that the bevel will be oriented with the narrowest part advancing in an anatomically advantageous orientation through the cords), insert the ETT to the 15-cm-depth marker, which corresponds to the transverse black line on the silicone-tipped ETT. This indicates that the silicone tip of the tube is about to emerge from the LMA Fastrach, pushing the epiglottic elevating bar up to lift the epiglottis. Use the handle to gently lift the LMA Fastrach as the ETT is advanced (Fig. 10-11). Carefully advance the ETT until intubation is complete. Do not use force of the ETT. Inflate the ETT cuff and confirm intubation. Then deflate the cuff on the LMA Fastrach.

4. Most of the time in the emergency situation, the LMA Fastrach and ETT are both left in situ. However, the LMA Fastrach can be removed fairly easily, leaving just the ETT in place. The key to successful removal of the mask is to remember that one is attempting to keep the ETT precisely in place and to remove the mask over it. First remove the 15-mm connector from the ETT. Then immobilize the ETT with one hand and gently ease the deflated LMA Fastrach out over the ETT with a rotating motion until the proximal end of the mask channel reaches the proximal end of the ETT. Use the stabilizer rod provided with the device to hold the ETT in position as the LMA Fastrach is withdrawn over the tube (Fig. 10-12). Remove the stabilizer rod from the LMA Fastrach and grasp the ETT at the level of the incisors (Fig. 10-13). *The stabilizer bar must be removed to allow the pilot balloon of the ETT to pass through the LMA Fastrach* (Fig. 10-14). Failure to do so may result in the pilot balloon being avulsed from the ETT, rendering the balloon incompetent and necessitating reintubation, preferably over an ETT changer.

Technique: LMA Classic, LMA Unique, and LMA Supreme

Although the LMA Classic, LMA Unique, and LMA Supreme can be rapidly inserted as primary airway management devices, or to rescue a failed airway with ventilation success rates comparable to that of the LMA Fastrach, they are not as effective as the LMA Fastrach for facilitating intubation. In fact, the LMA Fastrach is often easier to insert because

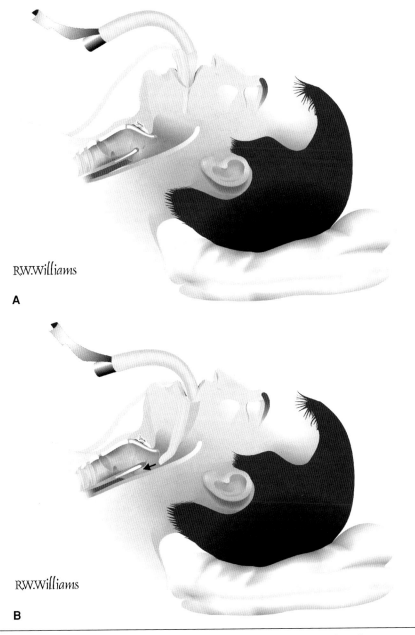

R.W.Williams

A

R.W.Williams

B

Figure 10-10 ● A–C: Insertion of the LMA Fastrach. Note that only a short segment of the tubular portion of the device extends beyond the lips. (*continued*)

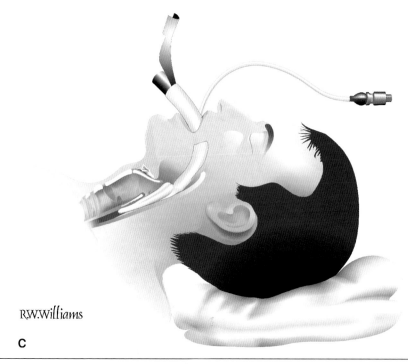

R.W.Williams

C

Figure 10-10 ● **(Continued)** This metal tube accepts a bag-mask device fitting to enable bag-mask ventilation.

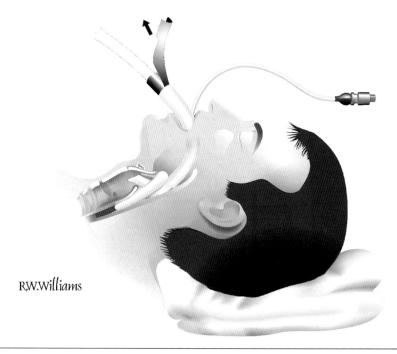

R.W.Williams

Figure 10-11 ● Lift the handle of the LMA Fastrach as the endotracheal tube is about to pass into the larynx to improve the success rate of intubation. This is called the Vergese maneuver after Dr. Archie Brain's associate Dr. Chandy Vergese.

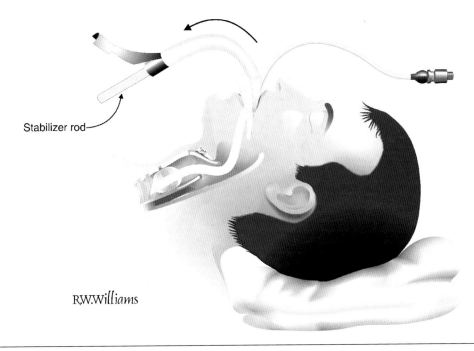

Figure 10-12 ● Use of the stabilizer rod to ensure the endotracheal tube is not inadvertently dragged out of the trachea as the LMA Fastrach is removed.

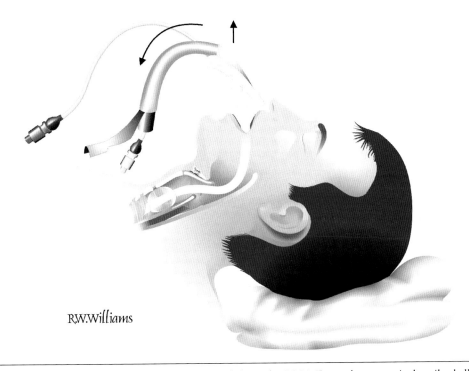

Figure 10-13 ● The stabilizer rod is removed from the LMA Fastrach to permit the pilot balloon of the endotracheal tube (ETT) to go through the LMA Fastrach and prevent it from being avulsed from the ETT.

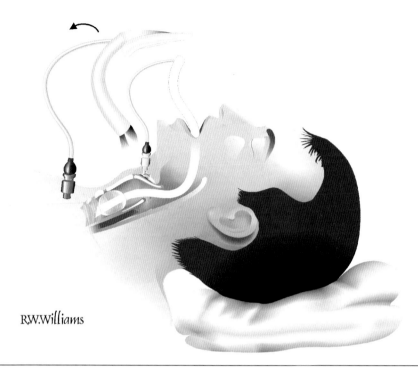

R.W.Williams

Figure 10-14 ● The pilot balloon of the endotracheal tube emerges from the end of the LMA Fastrach intact.

of the handle and metal tube design. Select the appropriate size of LMA as described previously for the LMA Fastrach. Unlike the LMA Fastrach, the LMA Classic and the LMA Unique have smaller sizes (1, 1.5, 2, and 2.5) available for use in infants and children. The LMA Supreme is available in sizes 3 to 5.

1. Place the device so that the collar is on a flat surface and inflate; then deflate the mask by aspirating the pilot balloon (Fig. 10-9). Completely deflate the cuff and ensure that it is not folded. The collar is designed to flip backward so the epiglottis is not trapped between the collar and the glottic opening. Lubricate both sides of the LMA with water-soluble lubricant to facilitate insertion.
2. Open the airway by using a head tilt as one would in basic airway management, if possible. Some, including the device inventor, recommend that a jaw lift be performed to aid insertion.
3. Insert the LMA into the mouth with the laryngeal surface directed caudally and the tip of your index or long finger resting against the cuff-tube junction (Fig. 10-15). Press the device onto the hard palate (Fig. 10-16) and advance it over the back of the tongue as far as the length of your index or long finger will allow (Fig. 10-17). Then use your other hand to push the device to its final seated position (Fig. 10-18), allowing the natural curve of the device to follow the natural curve of the oro- and hypopharynx to facilitate its falling into position over the larynx. The dimensions and design of the device allow it to wedge into the esophagus with gentle caudad pressure and to stop in the appropriate position over the larynx.
4. Inflate the collar with air—20 mL, no. 3; 30 mL, no. 4; 40 mL, no. 5—or until there is no leak with bag ventilation (Fig. 10-19). If a leak persists, ensure that the tube of the LMA emerges from the mouth in the midline, ensure that the head and neck

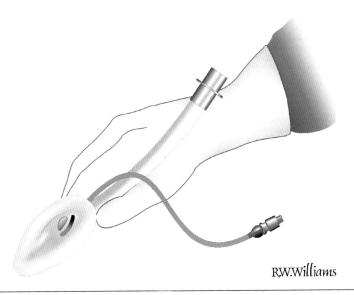

R.W.Williams

Figure 10-15 ● Correct position of the fingers for LMA insertion.

are in anatomical alignment (i.e., neither flexed nor extended), reinsert the device, or go to the next larger size.

Complications and Limitations

Unfortunately, the distal collar tip of the Laryngeal Mask Company Limited devices tends to "roll up" on insertion, creating a partial "insertion block" hindering optimal placement.

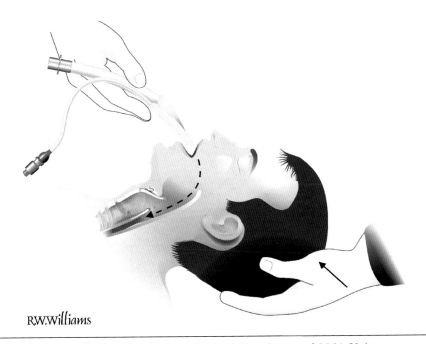

R.W.Williams

Figure 10-16 ● Starting insertion position for the LMA Classic and LMA Unique.

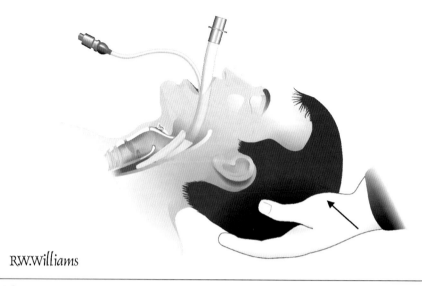

R.W.Williams

Figure 10-17 ● Insert the LMA to the limit of your finger length.

This feature also likely contributes to pharyngeal abrasion and bleeding that is often seen with these devices. Some authorities recommend partial inflation of the cuff to minimize tip roll, although there is little evidence that this helps. Insertion of the LMA Classic and LMA Unique "upside down" and rotating into place once in the hypopharynx has also been described and is preferred by some. This author prefers the deflated cuff, jaw lift, hard palate press technique.

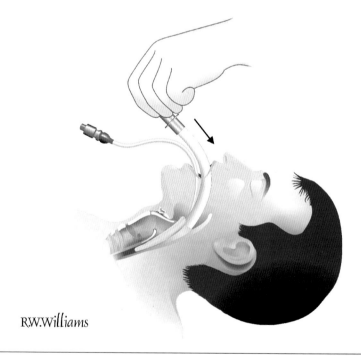

R.W.Williams

Figure 10-18 ● Complete the insertion by pushing the LMA in the remainder of the way with your other hand.

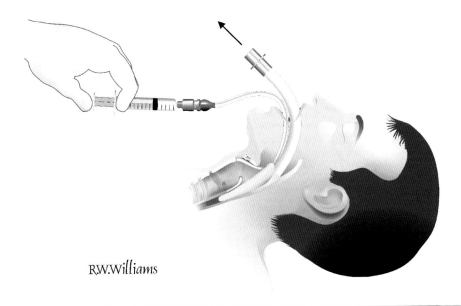

R.W.Williams

Figure 10-19 ● Inflate the collar of the LMA.

Achieving a seal sufficient to enable positive-pressure ventilation with an LMA may be difficult. Keeping the tube portion of the device in the midline and altering the position of the head in neck from flexion (more usual) to neutral or extension may be of help. Overall, ventilation success rates are very high with all LMA-type devices. Optimal positioning improves ventilatory effectiveness and, in the case of the LMA Fastrach, facilitates intubation.

The LMA does not prevent the aspiration of gastric contents, serving to emphasize its role as a temporizing measure only. This limits its usefulness in prehospital and emergency airway care beyond that of a temporizing measure, except when the LMA Fastrach is used to achieve intubation. Cricoid pressure has variously been reported to hinder and help in achieving proper seat and seal of the LMA.

OTHER SUPRAGLOTTIC DEVICES

Disposable LMA-type Designs

Several manufacturers produce disposable devices that appear almost identical to the LMA Classic. Although they do not incorporate the epiglottic obturator bars seen in the LMA Classic and LMA Unique, the effect of their absence is not clear. These devices have the same indications, contraindications, insertion techniques, and complictions as similar Laryngeal Mask Company Limited devices.

The ALMA device (Fig. 10-5) has several unique design features that confer particular insertion and seal advantages:

- The device is semi-inflated in the package. This feature provides an "immediate seal" once inserted, eliminating the inflation step and speeding the time to ventilation.
- The leading tip of the inflatable collar is reinforced and "spatulated" to minimize tip roll and improve insertion characteristics.
- The tube incorporates a curve that is flexible at the curved portion and more rigid proximally to improve insertion characteristics.

Recently, the manufacturer softened the plastic in the curved portion of the tube in response to concerns that this portion of the tube might compress the hypopharyngeal mucous membrane and lead to ischemia. In this author's experience, this device and the LMA Supreme are the most easily inserted and rapid to seal of the disposable LMA-type devices.

Cookgas ILA and Air Q

Like the LMA Fastrach, the Cookgas ILA device (Fig. 10-8A) is a supraglottic ventilatory device that also permits endotracheal intubation. Conventional ETTs are used for intubation as opposed to a unique ETT as is supplied with the LMA Fastrach. The Air Q (Fig. 10-8B) is a disposable version of the Cookgas ILA.

CobraPLA

The CobraPLA (Fig. 10-6) consists of a breathing tube with a circumferential inflatable cuff proximal to the ventilation outlet portion, a 15-mm standard adapter, and a distal widened "cobra head," which holds soft tissues apart and allows ventilation of the trachea. Once in place, the cobra head should lie in front of the laryngeal inlet. Inside the cobra head is a ramp that directs breathing gases into the trachea. Over the distal, anteriorly placed breathing hole of the cobra head, there is a soft grill. This feature helps direct the epiglottis off the cobra head anteriorly. The bars of the grill are flexible enough to allow the passage of an ETT. The cuff is shaped to reside in the hypopharynx at the base of the tongue, and when inflated, raises the base of the tongue exposing the laryngeal inlet, as well as effecting an airway seal. The CobraPLA is available in eight sizes according to the weight of the patient. The no. 3 is used for most female patients, the no. 4 for most men, and the no. 5 for larger men. When one is unsure of size, or when learning placement technique, it is advisable to pick the *smaller size*. The manufacturer supplies suggested age ranges for each size and cuff inflation volumes.

The lack of evidenciary support has hindered the application of this device in emergency airway management, routine or rescue.

Pharyngeal Airway Express

The PAXpress (Fig. 10-7) is a recently introduced SGD. It has not found its way into mainstream use, particularly in emergency airway management, due to a variety of factors, including a relatively high incidence of mucosal trauma. In addition, mucosal pressures may exceed pharyngeal perfusion pressure, and the PAXpress produces more marked changes in hemodynamic variables as compared with those produced by the LMA. Further studies are required to evaluate the safety and indications of this new extraglottic airway.

THE INFRA(RETRO)GLOTTIC CLASS

This class includes the following devices:

- ETC, or Combitube (Fig. 10-20)
- King LT airway (or laryngeal tube airway) (Fig. 10-21)
- Rusch EasyTube (Fig. 10-22)
- LaryVent (LV)
- Airway management device (AMD)

These devices are intended to be placed blindly into the esophagus. The Combitube, the King LT airway (called the laryngeal tube airway in some jurisdictions, e.g., Europe), and the EasyTube share a dual balloon design feature. One balloon seals the esophagus and the

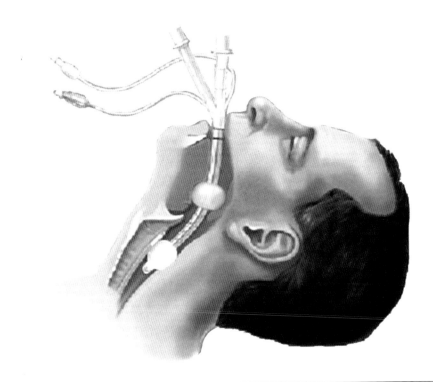

Figure 10-20 ● The Combitube Inserted and Seated. Note how the laryngeal aperture is trapped between the two balloons.

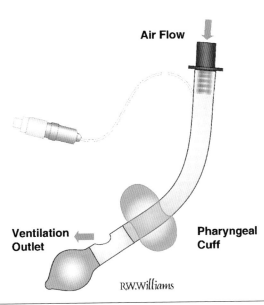

Figure 10-21 ● The King LT airway. Note that there is only one pilot balloon to inflate both balloons.

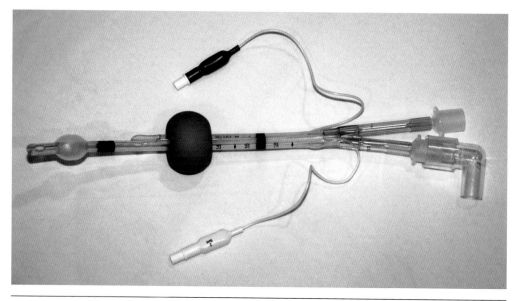

Figure 10-22 ● Rusch EasyTube.

other the oropharynx, trapping the larynx between the two. The Combitube and the Easy-Tube employ two separate pilot balloons to enable independent balloon inflation; the King LT has a single pilot balloon. The LaryVent and the AMD have not achieved a body of evidence at the time of writing to recommend their use in emergency airway management and are thus not further discussed.

These devices share three indications in emergency airway management practice:

1. As a substitute for BMV in the hands of basic life support providers
2. As a substitute for endotracheal intubation when endotracheal intubation is not possible (e.g., patient entrapment) or providers are not sufficiently skilled to perform it
3. As a rescue device in the failed airway, simultaneous with preparation to perform a cricothyrotomy

These devices also share the following contraindications:

- Responsive patients with intact airway-protective reflexes
- Patients with known esophageal disease
- Caustic ingestions
- Upper airway obstruction due to laryngeal foreign bodies or pathology

These modern retroglottic devices represent a dramatic improvement over the esophageal obturator airway and the esophageal gastric tube airway of the 1970s and 1980s, which have no place in modern emergency airway management. A substantial advantage of the modern devices is that they do not require facility with BMV as did the obsolete devices.

Combitube

The Combitube (Fig. 10-20) has been in clinical use for a much longer period of time than any of the other RGDs and has therefore accumulated the largest body of evidence describing its indications, contraindications, benefits, and risks. This is an important factor that distinguishes the Combitube from the other devices, particularly as costs are compared.

The Combitube is a dual-lumen, dual-cuff, disposable airway intended to be inserted into the esophagus, although it can be accommodated by the trachea if it is inadvertently placed there, and will function adequately in the short term as an ETT. The Combitube is supplied in two sizes: 37F SA (small adult), to be used in patients 4 to 5.5 feet tall, and 41F, which is for use in patients more than 5.5 feet tall. There is no Combitube suitable for use in children less than 4 feet tall. In addition to the indications listed previously, use of the Combitube has been described in upper gastrointestinal or upper airway hemorrhage that threatens airway and tracheal patency and in a case of severe facial burns.

Insertion Technique

Insertion of the Combitube is a blind technique, although a laryngoscope may be used, permitting insertion under direct vision.

1. With the patient supine (insertion is possible in any position) and the head and neck in a neutral position, lift the tongue and jaw upward ("jaw lift") with the nondominant hand.
2. Insert the device in the midline, allowing the curve of the device to follow the natural curve of the airway, and advance the device until the alveolar ridge is between the imprinted black bands on the device. Moderate force is required to enable the device to pass through the pharyngeal constrictor muscles into the esophagus. Substantial resistance should prompt the operator to withdraw and readvance. Inflate the proximal large oropharyngeal balloon with approximately 100 mL of air (Combitube 37F: 85 mL) via the blue pilot balloon labeled #1.
3. Inflate the white distal balloon with 5 to 15 mL of air (Combitube 37F: 5–12 mL) via the white pilot balloon labeled #2.
4. Begin ventilation using the longer blue connecting tube. The presence of air entry into the lung, the detection of end-tidal carbon dioxide, and the absence of gastric insufflation by auscultation indicate that the Combitube is in the esophagus, which occurs with virtually every insertion. The incidence of inadvertent tracheal intubation is less than 5%. Aspiration of gastric contents and gastric decompression is possible by passing the provided suction tube through the clear connecting tube into the stomach.
5. The absence of breath sounds in the chest, end-tidal carbon dioxide, and the presence of gastric insufflation by auscultation indicates that the Combitube is in the trachea (a distinctly rare event), and ventilation should be performed through the shorter clear connection tube.
6. The absence of any sounds on auscultation may indicate that the device has been inserted too far and should be repositioned after the proximal balloon is deflated.

Complications

The Combitube has been shown to be an effective airway management device that is easy to position properly. The Combitube appears in one study to be superior to the LMA Classic in the prehospital setting, and it has been shown to be a useful airway rescue device in the event of a failed intubation. However, like the LMA, it does not provide optimum protection against aspiration (although aspiration has never been reported), and its merit relative to the LMA Fastrach is unknown. Complications are rare and mostly related to upper airway hematomas, pyriform perforation, and perforation of the esophagus.

Increased cuff volumes are required at times to achieve a seal sufficient to permit adequate ventilation. As cuff volume is increased, the pressure transmitted to the mucosa is increased to the point where mucosal perfusion may be compromised, particularly where the cuff is adjacent to rigid anatomical structures such as the cervical spine (pharyngeal balloon) and the larynx (esophageal balloon). Over time, this may lead to ischemic mucosal injury. A high rate of success with few complications has been reported in prehospital use for cardiac arrest victims.

Finally, it should be noted that the pharyngeal balloon on the Combitube (as opposed to the Rusch EasyTube or the King LT airway) is made of latex.

OTHER RETROGLOTTIC DEVICES

The King LT airway

The King LT airway (King Systems Corp, Noblesville, IN; also known as the laryngeal tube airway, predominantly in Europe) (Fig. 10-21) is a newly developed multiuse (King LT) and disposable (King LT-D), latexfree, single-lumen silicon tube with oropharyngeal and esophageal low-pressure cuffs with a ventilation outlet between the two cuffs. It is supplied in blind distal tip and open distal tip variants to permit gastric decompression. A single pilot balloon is employed to inflate both balloons simultaneously, which is technically easier to use than the Combitube inflation system. However, it is also this feature that may lead to the fact that this device's airway seal capability is sometimes lost following insertion necessitating a deflation of the balloons and repositioning, a feature that is not common with the Combitube.

The device is available in pediatric and adult sizes in Europe; however, at the writing of this chapter, the pediatric-size devices were not available in the United States.

The King LT is inserted similarly to the Combitube, although there is usually less resistance on insertion. When seated, it works in a fashion that is very similar to that of the Combitube. Ventilation and oxygenation capabilities seem to be similar to the LMA and Combitube.

Rusch EasyTube

The Rusch EasyTube (Fig. 10-22) is a dual-lumen tube designed for difficult or emergency airway intubation and ventilation. It was approved for use in the European Union in 2003 and for use in the United States by the U.S. Food and Drug Administration in 2005. Like the Combitube, the EasyTube creates a viable airway, regardless of whether it is placed in the trachea or in the esophagus. When placed in the esophagus, the EasyTube allows the passage of a fiberoptic scope, a suction catheter, or a tracheal tube introducer through the more proximally terminating lumen. It is suggested by the manufacturer that the risk of tracheal trauma relative to the Combitube is reduced due to the single-lumen diameter of the device at the distal tip.

The EasyTube is supplied in only two sizes (28F and 41F) as opposed to the Combitube, which is supplied in 37F and 41F sizes. Again, the manufacturer claims that this allows the 28F EasyTube to be employed in older children. Finally, the EasyTube is latex free.

At present, there is little published evidence with respect to the indications, contraindications, success rates, and complications associated with this device. However, it has compelling design features that may make it useful as an airway rescue device similar to the Combitube and the King LT airway.

EVIDENCE

Supraglottic Class

1. **Is the LMA effective in difficult and failed airway management?** There is ample evidence that LMAs are useful in emergency airway management, both for the management of the difficult airway and rescue of the failed airway (1–13), provided one is concurrently preparing to undertake a surgical airway.

2. **What success rates have been achieved intubating through the LMA Fastrach?** Success rates for blind intubation through the LMA Fastrach range from 70% to 95% (14–16), and coupling the device with a Trachlight produces success rates of 100% (17–19). Some studies have described the technique of coupling the LMA Fastrach or LMA Classic with a fiberscope to ensure intubation success in both infants and adults (20,21).

3. **Is the LMA effective in the pediatric population?** There is ample evidence that the LMA is appropriate and widely accepted as a rescue device in children (22–25). Some authors have described guidelines for selecting the appropriate size in children (23), and the manufacturer provides a pocket card to guide clinicians.

4. **How easy is it for nonexperts to successfully use these LMA devices?** A variety of authors have described successful insertion and use of the device by basic rescuer nonmedical personnel (26,27), paramedics, nurses, and respiratory therapists (28–30), and naive airway managers (28). Some of the EMS literature has questioned the ease of use of the device as a primary method of airway management in EMS (31), although analysis has shown that training is key to its successful use (31–36).

5. **Are these devices acceptable airway management devices for patients undergoing cardiopulmonary resuscitation (CPR)?** Numerous studies have demonstrated that the LMA (and Combitube) is at least as effective as other methods of airway management for patients requiring CPR (30,37).

6. **Can the LMA fail to provide adequate ventilation, and what complications with short-term use might I expect?** The LMA may fail to provide a seal sufficient to permit adequate ventilation, often attributed to the sensitivity of the seal to head and neck position (38–40). The head and neck should be neutral to slightly flexed, the tube of the LMA in the midline, and the natural anterior curve of the device maintained during ventilation (41). Insufflation of the stomach may occur (42). Although the LMA may not offer total protection from the aspiration of regurgitated gastric contents (43–48), it does offer protection from the aspiration of material produced above the device (49). This material that accumulates above the cuff of an ETT is suspected to be a major cause of ventilator-associated pneumonia in ventilated intensive care unit patients. Cricoid pressure may or may not interfere with proper functioning of an LMA (50,51), although in practice each case is evaluated individually. Negative-pressure pulmonary edema (mentioned previously) is caused by a patient sucking hard to inspire against an obstruction. Fluid is sucked into the alveolar spaces. This complication has been reported with patients biting down on the LMA (52) and can be prevented by placing folded gauze flats between the molar teeth on either side. This also serves to keep the device in the midline, enhancing the seal.

7. **Are there any comprehensive reviews that I might find useful?** Comprehensive reviews of the use of the LMA in emergency medicine and rescue airway management are available (53,54).

Retroglottic Class

1. **What is the status of the Combitube with respect to its use as a rescue airway device?** The Combitube has been identified as a rescue airway device for the failed airway by authoritative bodies in the United States and Canada (1,2). Its use is well described in the anesthesia, resuscitation, emergency medicine, and EMS literature both as a first-line device and as a device to be used in the face of a difficult or failed airway (55–61). Several authors have identified the Combitube as a valuable adjunct in CPR (62–64), performing as well as or better than the LMA and BMV.

2. **What kind of airway management success rates have been reported with the Combitube?** Success rates of 98% to 100% are regularly reported in these studies. The ease of insertion (65–69) and adequacy of ventilation by physicians and nonphysician providers is well established (70–72).

3. **Has the Combitube been successful in the management of the difficult or failed airway?** The device is useful in the management of the difficult airway (73) and in rescuing a failed airway (74–76) while one prepares to undertake a cricothyrotomy.

4. **Has the Combitube been used in any unusual situations?** It has been demonstrated to protect the airway, control bleeding, and permit ventilation in a case of craniofacial trauma associated with severe bleeding (77) and to secure an airway in a case of severe facial burns preventing intubation (78).

5. **What precautions should I be aware of with this device?** It is unclear whether the Combitube provides protection against the aspiration of gastric contents (79). The downside of the Combitube includes reports of potentially serious complications related to its use, particularly pyriform sinus perforation (80–84) and esophageal perforation (85–89). A word of caution: Mucosal pressures exerted by the inflated balloons may exceed mucosal perfusion pressure, leading to mucosal ischemia (90).

6. **Has the King LT airway been demonstrated to be similarly effective in nonemergency airway management as the LMA and Combitube?** Simple handling, possible aspiration protection, and availability in newborn to adult sizes are considered to be advantages of this airway device (91–94).

7. **Does the King LT have a place in EMS as an airway management device?** There is some evidence that this device is easily learned by EMS personnel and provides more effective ventilation than bag-mask devices (95–97).

8. **Is the King LT airway useful as an emergency airway adjunct?** The evidence that the King LT is useful as a rescue airway or in patients where intubation has failed is limited and for the most part is based on case reports (98–100). However, a recent publication provides compelling evidence that this device may well be of use in the difficult and failed airway (101).

9. **Are there potential problems that I ought to be aware of with this device?** As with the Combitube, mucosal compression by the inflated balloons may lead to mucosal ischemic injury (90,102).

REFERENCES

1. Crosby ET, Cooper RM, Douglas MJ, et al. The unanticipated difficult airway with recommendations for management. *Can J Anaesth* 1998;45:757–776.

2. American Society of Anesthesiologists Task Force on Management of the Difficult Airway. Practice guidelines for management of the difficult airway: an updated report by the American Society of Anesthesiologists Task Force on Management of the Difficult Airway. *Anesthesiology* 2003;98(5):1269–1277.

3. Foley LJ, Ochroch EA. Bridges to establish an emergency airway and alternate intubating techniques. *Crit Care Clin* 2000;16:429–444.

4. Cooper JR Jr. Use of a LMA and a sequential technique for unanticipated difficult intubations. *Anesthesiology* 2002;97:1326.

5. Parmet JL, Colonna-Romano P, Horrow JC, et al. The laryngeal mask airway reliably provides rescue ventilation in cases of unanticipated difficult tracheal intubation along with difficult mask ventilation. *Anesth Analg* 1998;87:661–665.

6. Fukutome T, Amaha K, Nakazawa K, et al. Tracheal intubation through the intubating laryngeal mask airway (LMA-Fastrach) in patients with difficult airways. *Anaesth Intensive Care* 1998;26:387–391.

7. Brimacombe J, Berry A, Van Duren P. Use of a size 2 LMA to relieve life-threatening hypoxia in an adult with quinsy. *Anaesth Intensive Care* 1993;21:475–476.

8. King CJ, Davey AJ, Chandradeva K. Emergency use of the laryngeal mask airway in severe upper airway obstruction caused by supraglottic oedema. *Br J Anaesth* 1995;75:785–786.

9. Defalque RJ, Hyder ML. Laryngeal mask airway in severe cervical ankylosis. *Can J Anaesth* 1997;44:305–307.

10. Jones JR. Laryngeal mask airway: an alternative for the difficult airway. *AANA J* 1995;63:444–449.

11. Brain AI. Use of the LMA in the unstable cervical spine. *Singapore Med J* 2001;Suppl 1:46–48.

12. DeMello WF, Kocan M. The laryngeal mask in failed intubation. *Anaesthesia* 1990;45:689.

13. Brimacombe J, Berry A. LMA for failed intubation. *Can J Anaesth* 1993;40:802–803.

14. Rosenblatt WH, Murphy M. The intubating laryngeal mask: use of a new ventilating-intubating device in the emergency department. *Ann Emerg Med* 1999;33:234–238.

15. McQuibban GA. LMA-Fastrach. *Can J Anaesth* 1998;45:95–96.

16. Fukutome T, Amaha K, Nakazawa K, et al. Tracheal intubation through the intubating laryngeal mask airway (LMA-Fastrach) in patients with difficult airways. *Anaesth Intensive Care* 1998;26:387–391.

17. Agro F, Hung OR, Cataldo R, et al. Lightwand intubation using the Trachlight: a brief review of current knowledge. *Can J Anaesth* 2001;48:592–599.

18. Agro F, Brimacombe J, Carassiti M, et al. Lighted stylet as an aid to blind tracheal intubation via the LMA. *J Clin Anesth* 1998;1:263–264.

19. Agro F, Brimacombe J, Carassiti M, et al. Use of a lighted stylet for intubation via the laryngeal mask airway. *Can J Anaesth* 1998;45:556–560.

20. Kannan S, Chestnutt N, McBride G. Intubating LMA guided awake fibreoptic intubation in severe maxillo-facial injury. *Can J Anaesth* 2000;47:989–991.

21. Bandla HP, Smith DE, Kiernan MP. Laryngeal mask airway facilitated fibreoptic bronchoscopy in infants. *Can J Anaesth* 1997;44:1242–1247.

22. Loke GP, Tan SM, Ng AS. Appropriate size of laryngeal mask airway for children. *Anaesth Intensive Care* 2002;30:771–774.

23. Park C, Bahk JH, Ahn WS, et al. The laryngeal mask airway in infants and children. *Can J Anaesth* 2001;48:413–417.

24. Tobias JD. The laryngeal mask airway: a review for the emergency physician. *Pediatr Emerg Care* 1996;12:370–373.

25. Paterson SJ, Byrne PJ, Molesky MG, et al. Neonatal resuscitation using the laryngeal mask airway. *Anesthesiology* 1994;80:1248–1253.

26. Levitan RM, Ochroch EA, Stuart S, et al. Use of the intubating laryngeal mask airway by medical and nonmedical personnel. *Am J Emerg Med* 2000;18:12–16.

27. Burgoyne L, Cyna A. Laryngeal mask vs. intubating laryngeal mask: insertion and ventilation by inexperienced resuscitators. *Anaesth Intensive Care* 2001;29:604–608.

28. Choyce A, Avidan MS, Patel C, et al. Comparison of laryngeal mask and intubating laryngeal mask insertion by the naive intubator. *Br J Anaesth* 2000;84:103–105.

29. Davies PR, Tighe SQ, Greenslade GL, et al. Laryngeal mask airway and tracheal tube insertion by unskilled personnel. *Lancet* 1990;336:977–979.

30. Grayling M, Wilson IH, Thomas B. The use of the laryngeal mask airway and Combitube in cardiopulmonary resuscitation: a national survey. *Resuscitation* 2002;52:183–186.

31. Rumball CJ, MacDonald D. The PTL, Combitube, laryngeal mask, and oral airway: a randomized prehospital comparative study of ventilatory device effectiveness and cost-effectiveness in 470 cases of cardiorespiratory arrest. *Prehosp Emerg Care* 1997;1:1–10.

32. Miller GT. LMA Fastrach. EMS discovers the intubating laryngeal mask airway. *J Emerg Med Serv* 2002;27:68–74.

33. Dries D, Frascone R, Molinari P, et al. Does the ILMA make sense in HEMS? *Air Med J* 2000;20:35–37.

34. Martin SE, Ochsner MG, Jarman RH, et al. Use of the laryngeal mask airway in air transport when intubation fails. *J Trauma* 1999;47:352–357.

35. Sasada MP, Gabbott DA. The role of the laryngeal mask airway in pre-hospital care. *Resuscitation* 1994;28:97–102.

36. Pennant JH, Walker MB. Comparison of the endotracheal tube and laryngeal mask in airway management by paramedical personnel. *Anesth Analg* 1992;74:531–534.

37. Samarkandi AH, Seraj MA, el Dawlatly A, et al. The role of laryngeal mask airway in cardiopulmonary resuscitation. *Resuscitation* 1994;28:103–106.

38. Zavattaro M, LMA failure. *Anaesth Intensive Care* 1996;24:119.

39. Okuda K, Inagawa G, Miwa T, et al. Influence of head and neck position on cuff position and oropharyngeal sealing pressure with the laryngeal mask airway in children. *Br J Anaesth* 2001;86:122–124.

40. Keller C, Brimacombe J. The influence of head and neck position on oropharyngeal leak pressure and cuff position with the flexible and the standard laryngeal mask airway. *Anesth Analg* 1999;88:913–916.

41. Brimacombe J, Berry A. Leak reduction with the LMA. *Can J Anaesth* 1996;43:537.

42. Latorre F, Eberle B, Weiler N, et al. Laryngeal mask airway position and the risk of gastric insufflation. *Anesth Analg* 1998;86:867–871.

43. Cassinello F, Rodrigo FJ, Munoz-Alameda L, et al. Postoperative pulmonary aspiration of gastric contents in an infant after general anesthesia with laryngeal mask airway (LMA). *Anesth Analg* 2000;90:1457.

44. Brimacombe JR, Berry A. The incidence of aspiration associated with the laryngeal mask airway: a meta-analysis of published literature. *J Clin Anesth* 1995;7:297–305.

45. Ismail-Zade IA, Vanner RG. Regurgitation and aspiration of gastric contents in a child during general anaesthesia using the laryngeal mask airway. *Paediatr Anaesth* 1996;6:325–328.

46. Brimacombe J, Berry A. LMA-related aspiration in children. *Anaesth Intensive Care* 1994;22:313–314.

47. Asai T. Aspiration and the LMA. *Can J Anaesth* 1992;39:746.

48. Barker P, Langton JA, Murphy PJ, et al. Regurgitation of gastric contents during general anaesthesia using the laryngeal mask airway. *Br J Anaesth* 1992;69:314–315.

49. Rosenblatt W. Personal communication.

50. Aoyama K, Takenaka I, Sata T, et al. Cricoid pressure impedes positioning and ventilation through the laryngeal mask airway. *Can J Anaesth* 1996;43:1035–1040.

51. Brimacombe J, White A, Berry A. Effect of cricoid pressure on ease of insertion of the laryngeal mask airway. *Br J Anaesth* 1993;71:800–802.

52. Bhavani-Shankar K, Hart NS, Mushlin PS. Negative pressure induced airway and pulmonary injury. *Can J Anaesth* 1997;44:78–81.

53. Pollack CV Jr. The laryngeal mask airway: a comprehensive review for the emergency physician. *J Emerg Med* 2001;20:53–63.

54. Berry AM, Brimacombe JR, Verghese C. The laryngeal mask airway in emergency medicine, neonatal resuscitation, and intensive care medicine. *Int Anesthesiol Clin* 1998;36:91–109.

55. Mercer M. The role of the Combitube in airway management. *Anaesthesia* 2000;55:394–395.

56. Gaitini LA, Vaida SJ, Agro F. The esophageal-tracheal Combitube. *Anesthesiol Clin North Am* 2002;20:893–906.

57. Idris AH, Gabrielli A. Advances in airway management. *Emerg Med Clin North Am* 2002;20:843–857.

58. Agro F, Frass M, Benumof JL, et al. Current status of the Combitube: a review of the literature. *J Clin Anesth* 2002;14:307–314.

59. Keller C, Brimacombe J, Boehler M, et al. The influence of cuff volume and anatomic location on pharyngeal, esophageal, and tracheal mucosal pressures with the esophageal tracheal Combitube. *Anesthesiology* 2002;96:1074–1077.

60. Shuster M, Nolan J, Barnes TA. Airway and ventilation management. *Cardiol Clin* 2002;20:23–35.

61. Agro F, Frass M, Benumof J, et al. The esophageal tracheal Combitube as a non-invasive alternative to endotracheal intubation: a review. *Minerva Anestesiol* 2001;67:863–874.

62. Grayling M, Wilson IH, Thomas B. The use of the laryngeal mask airway and Combitube in cardiopulmonary resuscitation: a national survey. *Resuscitation* 2002;52:183–186.

63. Gabrielli A, Layon AJ, Wenzel V, et al. Alternative ventilation strategies in cardiopulmonary resuscitation. *Curr Opin Crit Care* 2002;8:199–211.

64. Frass M, Staudinger T, Losert H, et al. Airway management during cardiopulmonary resuscitation—a comparative study of bag-valve-mask, laryngeal mask airway and Combitube in a bench model. *Resuscitation* 1999;43:80–81.

65. Levitan RM, Kush S, Hollander JE. Devices for difficult airway management in academic emergency departments: results of a national survey. *Ann Emerg Med* 1999;33:694–698.

66. Lefrancois DP, Dufour DG. Use of the esophageal tracheal Combitube by basic emergency medical technicians. *Resuscitation* 2002;52:77–83.

67. Ochs M, Vilke GM, Chan TC, et al. Successful prehospital airway management by EMT-Ds using the Combitube. *Prehosp Emerg Care* 2000;4:333–337.

68. Tanigawa K, Shigematsu A. Choice of airway devices for 12,020 cases of nontraumatic cardiac arrest in Japan. *Prehosp Emerg Care* 1998;2:96–100.

69. Rumball CJ, MacDonald D. The PTL, Combitube, laryngeal mask, and oral airway: a randomized prehospital comparative study of ventilatory device effectiveness and cost-effectiveness in 470 cases of cardiorespiratory arrest. *Prehosp Emerg Care* 1997;1:1–10.

70. Calkins MD, Robinson TD. Combat trauma airway management: endotracheal intubation versus laryngeal mask airway versus Combitube use by Navy SEAL and Reconnaissance Combat Corpsmen. *J Trauma* 1999;46:927–932.

71. Yardy N, Hancox D, Strang T. A comparison of two airway aids for emergency use by unskilled personnel: the Combitube and laryngeal mask. *Anaesthesia* 1999;54:181–183.

72. Dorges V, Ocker H, Wenzel V, et al. Emergency airway management by non-anaesthesia house officers—a comparison of three strategies. *Emerg Med J* 2001;18:90–94.

73. Staudinger T, Tesinsky P, Klappacher G, et al. Emergency intubation with the Combitube in two cases of difficult airway management. *Eur J Anaesthesiol* 1995;12:189–193.

74. Blostein PA, Koestner AJ, Hoak S. Failed rapid sequence intubation in trauma patients: esophageal tracheal Combitube is a useful adjunct. *J Trauma* 1998;44:534–537.

75. Enlund M, Miregard M, Wennmalm K. The Combitube for failed intubation—instructions for use. *Acta Anaesthesiol Scand* 2001;45:127–128.

76. Della Puppa A, Pittoni G, Frass M. Tracheal esophageal Combitube: a useful airway for morbidly obese patients who cannot intubate or ventilate. *Acta Anaesthesiol Scand* 2002;46:911–913.

77. Morimoto F, Yoshioka T, Ikeuchi H, et al. Use of esophageal tracheal Combitube to control severe oronasal bleeding associated with craniofacial injury: case report. *J Trauma* 2001;51:168–169.

78. Wagner A, Roeggla M, Roeggla G, et al. Emergency intubation with the Combitube in a case of severe facial burn. *Am J Emerg Med* 1995;13:681–683.

79. Mercer MH. An assessment of protection of the airway from aspiration of oropharyngeal contents using the Combitube airway. *Resuscitation* 2001;51:135–138.

80. Urtubia RM, Gazmuri RR. Is the Combitube traumatic? *Anesthesiology* 2003;98:1021–1022.

81. Urtubia RM, Carcamo CR, Montes JM. Complications following the use of the Combitube, tracheal tube and laryngeal mask airway. *Anaesthesia* 2000;55:597–599.

82. Oczenski W, Krenn H, Dahaba AA, et al. Complications following the use of the Combitube, tracheal tube and laryngeal mask airway. *Anaesthesia* 1999;54:1161–1165.

83. Moser MS. Piriform sinus perforation during esophageal-tracheal Combitube placement. *J Emerg Med* 1999;17:129.

84. Richards CF. Piriform sinus perforation during esophageal-tracheal Combitube placement. *J Emerg Med* 1998;16:37–39.

85. Krafft P, Nikolic A, Frass M. Esophageal rupture associated with the use of the Combitube. *Anesth Analg* 1998;87:1457.

86. Krafft P, Frass M, Reed AP. Complications with the Combitube. *Can J Anaesth* 1998;45: 823–824.

87. Walz R, Bund M, Meier PN, et al. Esophageal rupture associated with the use of the Combitube. *Anesth Analg* 1998;87:228.

88. Vezina D, Lessard MR, Bussieres J, et al. Complications associated with the use of the esophageal-tracheal Combitube. *Can J Anaesth* 1998;45:76–80.

89. Klein H, Williamson M, Sue-Ling HM, et al. Esophageal rupture associated with the use of the Combitube. *Anesth Analg* 1997;85:937–939.

90. Ulrich-Pur H, Hrska F, Krafft P, et al. Comparison of mucosal pressures induced by cuffs of different airway devices. *Anesthesiology* 2006;104:933–938.

91. Dorges V, Ocker H, Wenzel V, et al. The Laryngeal Tube S: a modified simple airway device. *Anesth Analg* 2003;96:618–621.

92. Genzwuerker HV, Hilker T, Hohner E, et al. The laryngeal tube: a new adjunct for airway management. *Prehosp Emerg Care* 2000;4:168–172.

93. Dorges V, Ocker H, Wenzel V, et al. The laryngeal tube: a new simple airway device. *Anesth Analg* 2000;90:1220–1222.

94. Agro F, Cataldo R, Alfano A, et al. A new prototype for airway management in an emergency: the laryngeal tube. *Resuscitation* 1999;41:284–286.

95. Kette F, Reffo I, Giordani G, et al. The use of laryngeal tube by nurses in out-of-hospital emergencies: preliminary experience. *Resuscitation* 2005;66:21–25.

96. Kurola J, Harve H, Kettunen T, et al. Airway management in cardiac arrest—comparison of the laryngeal tube, tracheal intubation and bag-mask-ventilation in emergency medical training. *Resuscitation* 2004;61:149–153.

97. Asai T, Hidaka I, Kawachi S. Efficacy of the laryngeal tube by inexperienced personnel. *Resuscitation* 2002;55:171–175.

98. Asai T. Use of the laryngeal tube for difficult fiberoptic tracheal intubation. *Anaesthesia* 2005;60:826.

99. Matioc A, Olson J. Use of the laryngeal tube in two unexpected difficult airway situations: lingual tonsillar hyperplasia and morbid obesity. *Can J Anesth* 2004;51:1018–1021.

100. Genzwuerker H, Dhonau S, Ellinger K. Use of the laryngeal tube for out-of-hospital resuscitation. *Resuscitation* 2002;52:221–224.

101. Winterhalter M, Kirchhoff K, Groschel W, et al. The laryngeal tube for difficult airway management: a prospective investigation in patients with pharyngeal and laryngeal tumours. *Eur J Anaesthesiol* 2005;22:678–682.

102. Keller C, Brimacombe J, Kleinsasser A, et al. Pharyngeal mucosal pressures with the laryngeal tube airway versus ProSeal laryngeal mask airway. *Anasthesiol Intensivmed Notfallmed Schmerzther* 2003;38:393–396.

11

Lighted Stylet Intubation

Michael F. Murphy and Orlando R. Hung

DESCRIPTION

Although direct vision laryngoscopy and intubation has been proven over the years to be reliable and relatively easy, the accurate and prompt placement of an endotracheal tube (ETT) remains a major challenge in some patients, even in the hands of experienced laryngoscopists. It has been estimated that between 1% and 3% of patients present with difficult airways, leading to difficult endotracheal intubation under direct vision using a laryngoscope (see Chapter 7). In fact, it is impossible to intubate some patients using this technique, emphasizing the key role of cricothyrotomy in emergency airway management.

ETTs can be placed into the trachea nonsurgically in the following ways:

- Under direct vision (via a laryngoscope) or indirect vision (via GlideScope or a Bullard laryngoscope)
- With an indirect indicator, such as listening to and feeling air movement in "blind" nasal intubation, transillumination of light in the neck with lighted stylets and bronchoscopes, and tactile digital intubation
- With a guide, such as an intubating laryngeal mask airway or an intubating guide (e.g., Eschmann introducer)
- Blindly, without an indicator

Lighted stylet intubation is of use in those situations where conventional laryngoscopy has failed to provide visualization of the larynx sufficient to allow direct vision intubation. In general, there must be adequate ventilation and oxygenation to allow time for the use of the lighted stylet (i.e., "*can't* intubate, *can* oxygenate" situation).

The light-guided intubation technique relies on the transillumination of the soft tissues of the neck to indicate intratracheal tube placement. It was first used in Japan in 1959 by Yamamura and colleagues for nasal intubation. This technique takes advantage of the anterior location of the trachea, relative to the esophagus. With the light bulb of a lighted stylet placed at the tip of the ETT, a well-defined, circumscribed glow can readily be seen in the anterior neck area when the tip of the ETT enters the trachea through the glottic opening. However, if the tip of the ETT is in the esophagus, the light glow is diffuse and not easily seen.

Although the light-guided intubation technique had shown some promise, it was not widely used until the 1970s, following the introduction of the Flexilum (Concept Corporation, Clearwater, FL). The Tubestat (Concept Corporation, Clearwater, FL) was developed in the early 1980s, following minor refinements of the original Flexilum design. Despite these improvements, difficulties persisted with the use of these devices, mostly related to the degree of transillumination that could be achieved. A lighted stylet device from Vital Signs (Vital Light) has the advantage of low cost, but is lacking some desirable features. Any fiberoptic device (rigid or flexible) with distal light emission can be used to intubate using this principle. The Shikani optical stylet is another example and is discussed in Chapter 13.

The Trachlight (Laerdal Medical Corp., Wappinger Falls, NY) lighted stylet has incorporated many modifications to improve the transillumination features of the light, and has the flexibility to allow oral and nasal intubation (Fig. 11-1). Although there are several acceptable and approved lighted stylets available, the Trachlight seems to be superior, based on its features and adaptability. The remainder of this discussion refers to the Trachlight.

INDICATIONS AND CONTRAINDICATIONS

The "*can't* intubate, *can't* oxygenate" situation is a relative contraindication to Trachlight intubation because of the time required, unless the operator has considerable skill and experience with the device and the intubation attempt can be made in parallel with preparations for cricothyrotomy. As with conventional intubation techniques, this technique requires

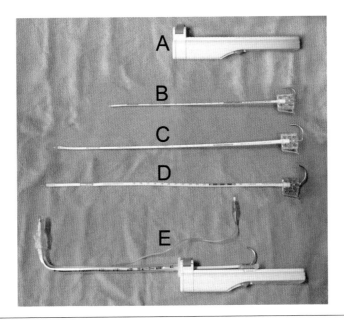

Figure 11-1 ● Laerdal Trachlight Handle (A) and three sizes of wands: infant (B), pediatric (C), and adult (D). The wand and rigid internal stylet combination has been attached to the handle and an endotracheal tube (ETT) loaded onto the wand (E). Note the point of connection of the ETT to the handle.

moderate to substantial sedation and/or local anesthesia of the airway; it has been successfully used both for primary intubations during rapid sequence intubation (RSI) and as a rescue device.

As with all procedures, practice in a controlled setting is important to develop facility with the device to allow predictable success rates. It has been demonstrated that this technique is easier to teach and the skill is easier to maintain than is conventional laryngoscopy. The Trachlight also appears to produce less airway trauma and physiological disturbance than conventional laryngoscopy. For the foreseeable future, the majority of emergency physicians will undoubtedly continue to prefer the laryngoscope to the Trachlight. However, this device may serve as a valuable rescue device in the *"can't* intubate, *can* oxygenate" situation. The Trachlight ought to be considered a primary device when orotracheal intubation by other techniques is judged to be difficult or impossible (e.g., limited mouth opening, cervical spine mobility) or because of inability to visualize the glottis, particularly if a fiberoptic device is not available. The device can be used to facilitate both nasotracheal and orotracheal intubation. If the Trachlight is used to attempt nasotracheal intubation, transillumination replaces the use of audible breath sounds to guide the tip of the ETT into the glottic opening, making the technique possible in apneic patients.

This technique is contraindicated when there is reasonable suspicion that the anatomy of the airway is abnormal or shifted from the midline. Laryngeal pathology generally mandates intubation by direct visualization and so it is also a contraindication to this technique.

TECHNIQUE

The Trachlight device consists of two parts: a reusable handle and a disposable, malleable lighted stylet, recommended by the manufacturer to be limited to ten uses (Fig. 11-2). The

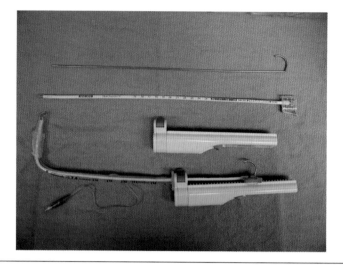

Figure 11-2 ● Trachlight handle, flexible lighted wand, and rigid internal stylet disassembled with an endotracheal tube.

power control circuitry and batteries are within the handle. The Trachlight requires three AAA standard alkaline batteries, which are easily changed by opening the cover on the handle. A female connector with a locking lever located on the front of the handle accepts and secures the standard 15-mm male connector of ETTs. The stylet consists of a durable, flexible plastic tube with a bright light bulb at one end. The light bulb is sufficiently bright to permit transillumination and intubation under ambient light in most cases and offers a wide degree of illumination at its tip. The light begins to blink after 30 seconds to prevent the bulb from overheating. Within the plastic sheath is a removable, malleable, metal stylet, and affixed to the end of the stylet opposite the light is a rigid plastic connector with a release arm, which attaches the stylet assembly to the handle (Fig. 11-2). This connector can be adjusted and slides along the handle to accommodate ETTs of varying lengths. During intubation, the ETT and the wand become pliable when the rigid stylet is retracted. This feature facilitates the advancement of the tube into the trachea.

1. **Preparation.** To ensure easy retraction during intubation, the internal rigid stylet of the wand should be well lubricated, preferably with a silicone fluid (Endoscopic Instrument Lubricant, ACMI) that will not dry over time. Similarly, the external wall of the wand should be lubricated with a water-soluble lubricant. Cut the ETT to 26 cm for orotracheal intubation by removing, and then reattaching, the ETT connector. This step makes the device easier to maneuver into the airway. Insert the wand into the ETT with the light just protruding from the end of the ETT so that it can be felt as you palpate the opening at the distal end of the ETT. Some recommend aligning the centimeter numbers of the wand with those in the ETT, but the transillumination is better with the light just emerging from the distal end of the tube. For most patients, the ETT-Trachlight (ETT-TL) combination should be bent just proximal to the ETT cuff where the words "bend here" are located on the wand. In very large or very small patients, the bend may have to be more proximal or more distal, respectively. The correct length for this distal limb of the ETT-TL combination is the distance from the base of the tongue to the cricothyroid membrane. This length corresponds externally to the distance from the angle of the mandible to the cricothyroid membrane, and the bend in the ETT-TL combination can easily be compared externally with these landmarks. The bend should be a sharp right angle, mimicking the shape of a field hockey

stick. For a nasotracheal intubation, the length of the distal limb ought to correspond to the distance from the back of the nasopharynx to the cricothyroid membrane, externally represented by the distance from the tragus of the ear to the cricothyroid membrane. The bend is a gentler sweep and slightly greater than 90 degrees to bring the tip sufficiently anterior to enter the glottis when the ETT is introduced nasally. For nasal intubation, some authors advocate leaving the rigid stylet in place; others recommend removing it entirely. Removing the stylet reduces the control one has over the distal end of the tube, and if this practice is followed, the use of an Endotrol control tip nasotracheal tube is recommended. Whether oral or nasal intubation is planned, the tip of the ETT should also be lubricated with a water-soluble lubricant.

2. ***Positioning.*** With the intubator standing at the head of the patient, the neck is bared to allow maximal visualization of the patient's anterior neck during intubation. The technique can also be performed from the side of the patient. Usually, the patient's head and neck are placed in a *neutral* position, although it may be necessary to extend the head slightly to optimize visualization (Fig. 11-3). In obese patients or patients with an extremely short neck, placing a pillow under the shoulder and neck may be helpful, if possible, but the problems presented by these anatomical variations can also often be overcome by changing the angle of the tube bend or the length of the distal (bent portion) ETT.

3. ***Ambient lighting.*** In general, patients can be intubated easily under ambient lighting conditions. Dimming the light or shading the neck to optimize visualization of the transilluminated glow may be necessary in those with generous subcutaneous tissue or darkly pigmented skin.

Technique of Intubation

With the patient lying supine, the lower alveolar ridge and mentum are grasped and lifted upward using the intubator's nondominant hand. This lifts the tongue and epiglottis upward to facilitate the intubation. Alternatively, the thumb of the nondominant hand can be placed in the mouth along the patient's tongue to lift the tongue upward and forward as the interphalangeal joint of the thumb is flexed. The nondominant hand must be kept close to the lower lip to ensure an unobstructed path in the midline for the Trachlight. The device is then switched on and the ETT-TL is inserted into the oropharynx and positioned in the midline, such that the distal (bent portion) ETT is resting gently against the posterior oropharynx in the midline. The operator's vision is not transitioned to the anterior neck until it is certain that the ETT-TL is in this midline position, resting against the posterior oropharynx. The device is then rocked on the fulcrum created by the bend in the tube, allowing the distal end of the tube to traverse an imaginary arc and enter the glottis. The natural inclination is to push the device as is done with conventional intubation. This approach will only serve to push the ETT-TL into the esophagus.

The jaw lift helps elevate the epiglottis and enhance the passage of the ETT-TL under the epiglottis into the glottic opening. When the tip of the ETT-TL enters the glottic opening, a well-defined circumscribed glow can be seen at the anterior neck slightly below the laryngeal prominence. Retracting the rigid stylet 10 cm makes the distal portion of the ETT-TL more pliable and facilitates its advance into the trachea. The tip of the ETT is advanced until the glow appears in the sternal notch. At this point, the tip of the ETT is approximately midway between the vocal cords and carina. Now the ETT connector is released from the locking device on the Trachlight, and the device is removed from the ETT (Fig. 11-3). In certain lighting conditions, or with particularly dark-skinned or thick-necked patients, it may be desirable to test the transillumination before proceeding through the glottis. After the Trachlight has been placed against the posterior oropharynx as previously described, the ETT-TL is then rocked (not pushed) gently to the right pyriform recess, and the intensity of the transilluminated glow through the neck is noted. The intensity of this glow will approximate that found in the midline with successful placement of the device in

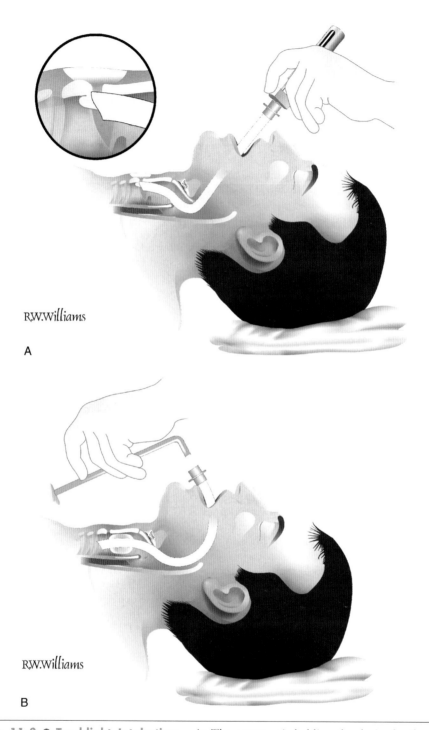

Figure 11-3 ● Trachlight Intubation. **A:** The operator is holding the device by the handle rather than holding the ETT-TL, a technical detail that most prefer. In this figure, the head is more extended than ordinarily recommended. A neutral position is preferred. **B:** Once the ETT-TL have been placed in the trachea, the TL is removed.

the trachea. If necessary, room lights may be dimmed if this test shows that the transillumination might be insufficient in ambient lighting.

TROUBLE SHOOTING

There are several tips that may aid success:

1. Once the ETT-TL is positioned in the hypopharynx with the light on, lift the device ever so slightly toward the ceiling. Imagine that this pulls the ETT up against the undersurface of the epiglottis, enhancing the chance that the device will be rocked anteriorly into the trachea as opposed to more posteriorly into the esophagus.
2. With the device lifted, slightly rotate the handle to the right and left observing the glow in the anterior neck. At some point in many patients, one is able to see the length of the trachea transilluminated (a cone of light), providing a guide as to which direction to rock.
3. Transillumination in dark-skinned persons and those with thick necks may be addressed by dimming the room lights as mentioned previously; in those with thick tissue overlying the anterior neck, it can be thinned by having an assistant retract it downward and to the sides (Fig. 11-4).
4. Load the ETT onto the device "backward" such that the natural curvature of the ETT tends to flip the ETT posteriorly when the rigid stylet is retracted prior to advancement into the trachea. This minimizes the tendency of the tip of the ETT to become impinged on the cricoid ring in the cricothyroid space preventing insertion.
5. Employing an Endotrol ETT (Mallincrodt) for nasal intubation over a Trachlight is helpful if the ETT-TL repeatedly slips into the esophagus.

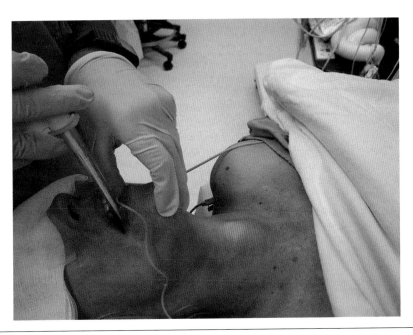

Figure 11-4 ● This figure demonstrates an assistant thinning out the tissues in the front of the neck with the lights dimmed. These maneuvers enhance transillumination in individuals with excessive tissue in the anterior neck (e.g., the obese).

6. In the event advancement of the ETT-TL into the trachea is impossible and one is unsure whether one is impinged against a laryngeal (e.g., arytenoid cartilage, vocal cord) or infralaryngeal structure (e.g., cricoid ring), a series of maneuvers may assist in gaining success after an initial slight withdrawal of the ETT-TL to reduce impingement:
   a. Rotate the ETT-TL to the right and to the left.
   b. Lift the head performing flexion initially, and then extension.
   c. Inflate the cuff of the ETT to "center" the ETT-TL in the airway, advance gently until resistance is felt, and then deflate the balloon and continue advancement.
7. Repeated failure may indicate that the anatomy of the upper airway is not normal or that there is distortion that was unappreciated on airway examination. In these cases, the airway manager is advised to resort to direct (e.g., laryngoscopy) or indirect vision (e.g., GlideScope, fiberoptic stylet, fiberscope) techniques.

COMPLICATIONS

Success rates in the hands of experienced users are consistent with or exceed those associated with conventional laryngoscopy. Limited experience with this device has not identified isolated or persistent complications. The complications would be expected to be similar to those for conventional intubation, but less common because the technique is less traumatic and does not require insertion of a laryngoscope.

However, as might be anticipated, as a nonvisual technique some specific risks have been identified:

- Transient or permanent arytenoid cartilage dislocation
- Bulb detachment
- Invagination of the epiglottis into the glottic opening during insertion

EVIDENCE

1. **Is this technique easier to learn than the standard laryngoscopic intubation technique?** This technique produces a higher success rate than conventional laryngoscopy with a shorter time to intubation when wielded by skilled intubators. It takes about 10 intubations to become familiar with Trachlight intubation and about 20 to become facile (1). Most have found that this technique is easier to teach and has a higher level of skill retention than conventional laryngoscopy (2,3), although one study found the opposite (4).
2. **Does this technique have advantages over conventional laryngoscopic intubation?** The evidence as to whether lighted stylet intubation produces less autonomic stimulation than conventional laryngoscopy is conflicting, although the weight of evidence suggests that this is indeed the case (5–9). The device does appear to produce less trauma to the airway than conventional laryngoscopy. A recent study identified that intubation with a Trachlight produced less autonomic stimulation that that produced with a GlideScope (10).
3. **Is this device useful in the setting of a difficult airway?** There is evidence that the device is useful in managing difficult airways, particularly anterior airways (11–13).
4. **Does Sellick's maneuver interfere with one's ability to successfully employ this device in an RSI situation?** It has been suggested that cricoid pressure may adversely affect the success rate with this device (14), although the weight of evidence suggests that this is not the case (11,12).

5. **Can this device be used with other airway management devices?** The device can be coupled with other intubating techniques, such as nasal intubation (15–17), intubation through a laryngeal mask (18) and an intubating laryngeal mask (Fastrach) (19), and with conventional laryngoscopy (20), to facilitate successful tracheal intubation.

6. **Can it be used to perform nasal intubation as well?** Yes. Most experts recommend that the rigid internal stylet be removed to facilitate nasal intubation, although some leave it in. This technique changes a blind nasal intubation to one that is transillumination assisted. In addition to mounting the nasotracheal tube on the Trachlight, it has been shown that neutral head position and ETT cuff inflation improve success rates (21).

REFERENCES

1. Hung OR, Pytka S, Morris I, et al. Clinical trial of a new lightwand (Trachlight) to intubate the trachea. *Anesthesiology* 1995;83:509–514.

2. Hung OR, Murphy MF. Lightwands, lighted stylets and blind techniques of intubation. In: Sandler AN, Doyle DJ, eds. The difficult airway. *Anaesthesia Clinics NA*, vol 13, Toronto, Ontario, Canada: WB Saunders; 1995:477–491.

3. Hung OR, Stewart RD. Lightwand intubation: I. A new intubating device. *Can J Anaesth* 1995;42:820–825.

4. Soh CR, Kong CF, Kong CS, et al. Tracheal intubation by novice staff: the direct vision laryngoscope or the lighted stylet (Trachlight)? *Emerg Med J* 2002;19:292–294.

5. Hung OR, Pytka S, Murphy MF, et al. Comparative hemodynamic changes following laryngoscopic or lightwand intubation. *Anesthesiology* 1993;79:A497.

6. Kanaide M, Fukusaki M, Tamura S, et al. Hemodynamic and catecholamine responses during tracheal intubation using a lightwand device (Trachlight) in elderly patients with hypertension. *J Anesth* 2003;17:161–165.

7. Kihara S, Brimacombe J, Yaguchi Y, et al. Hemodynamic responses among three tracheal intubation devices in normotensive and hypertensive patients. *Anesth Analg* 2003;96:890–895.

8. Hirabayashi Y, Hiruta M, Kawakami T, et al. Effects of lightwand (Trachlight) compared with direct laryngoscopy on circulatory responses to tracheal intubation. *Br J Anaesth* 1998;81:253–255.

9. Takahashi S, Mizutani T, Miyabe M, et al. Hemodynamic responses to tracheal intubation with the laryngoscope versus lightwand intubating device (Trachlight) in adults with normal airway. *Anesth Analg* 2002;95:480–484.

10. Huang WT, Huang CY, Chung YT. Clinical comparisons between GlideScope video laryngoscope and Trachlight in simulated cervical spine instability. *J Clin Anesth* 2007;19:110–114.

11. Hung OR, Stevens SC, Pytka S, et al. Clinical trial of a new lightwand device for intubation in patients with difficult airways. *Anesthesiology* 1993;79:A498.

12. Hung OR, Pytka S, Morris I, et al. Lightwand intubation: II. Clinical trial of a new lightwand to intubate patients with difficult airways. *Can J Anaesth* 1995;42:826–830.

13. Latto IP. Management of difficult intubation. In: Latto IP, Rosen M, eds. *Difficulties in tracheal intubation*. London: Bailliere Tindall; 1987:99–141.

14. Hodgson RE, Goplan PD, Burrows RC, et al. Effect of cricoid pressure on the success of endotracheal intubation with a lightwand. *Anesthesiology* 2001;94:259–262.

15. Yamamura H, Yamamoto T, Kamiyama M. Device for blind nasal intubation. *Anesthesiology* 1959;20:221.

16. Hung OR. Nasal intubation with the Trachlight. *Can J Anaesth* 1999;46:908.

17. Agro F, Brimacombe J, Marchionni L, et al. Nasal intubation with the Trachlight. *Can J Anaesth* 1999;46:907–908.

18. Agro F, Brimacombe J, Carassiti M, et al. Use of a lighted stylet for intubation via the laryngeal mask airway. *Can J Anaesth* 1998;45:556–560.

19. Fan KH, Hung OR, Agro F. A comparative study of tracheal intubation using an intubating laryngeal mask (Fastrach) alone or together with a lightwand (Trachlight). *J Clin Anesth* 2000;12:581–585.

20. Agro F, Benumof JL, Carassiti M, et al. Efficacy of a combined technique using the Trachlight together with direct laryngoscopy under simulated difficult airway conditions in 350 anesthetized patients. *Can J Anaesth* 2002;49:525–526.

21. Chung YT, Sun MS, Wu HS. Blind nasotracheal intubation is facilitated by neutral head position and endotracheal tube cuff inflation in spontaneously breathing patients. *Can J Anaesth* 2003;50:511–513.

12

Flexible Fiberoptic Intubation

Michael F. Murphy and Peter M. C. DeBlieux

DESCRIPTION

Endotracheal intubation over a fiberoptic bronchoscope has emerged as an invaluable technique in airway management, particularly in patients for whom standard laryngoscopy and orotracheal intubation have failed or are anticipated to be difficult or impossible. No discussion of difficult or emergency airway management is complete without a review of the use of fiberoptic devices to perform diagnostic procedures in the upper airway and endotracheal intubation.

Although fiberoptic bronchoscopes are becoming more widely available in emergency departments (EDs), and published studies have described their use in the ED, few emergency practitioners have extensive experience with them for diagnostic procedures in the upper airway, and fewer still have done fiberoptic intubations.

INDICATIONS AND CONTRAINDICATIONS

Indications for fiberoptic endoscopy in emergency airway management include the following:

- Intubation of the patient who is predicted to be a difficult intubation. The most frequent candidates are those with supraglottic causes of upper airway obstruction such as angioedema, oropharyngeal abscess or hematoma, or Ludwig's angina, or those with slowly progressive laryngeal lesions such as lingual and laryngeal cancers.
- Direct vision laryngoscopy and intubation is recommended for patients with laryngeal trauma and tracheal disruption. The fiberscope meets this indication.
- Cervical spine immobility required, particularly if the airway is predicted to be difficult.
- Anatomical abnormalities, such as patients with restricted mouth opening or severely hypoplastic mandibles, or the morbidly obese.
- Failed intubation in the "*can't* intubate, *can* oxygenate" scenario, when continuing deterioration of the airway is not anticipated.

Contraindications to fiberoptic intubation are mostly relative and may include the following:

- Excessive blood and secretions in the upper airway, which have the great potential to obscure the view and reduce the success rate with the fiberoptic technique. Some experienced bronchoscopists use the fiberscope like a Trachlight (see Chapter 11) in situations such as these, using transillumination to indicate entry into the trachea and only then looking through the scope to verify the position of the fiberscope in the trachea.
- High-grade upper-airway obstruction (due to foreign bodies or other lesions), where the procedure may precipitate total airway obstruction. If a patient has a high-grade supraglottic airway obstruction, the delays and risks of precipitating complete airway obstruction or laryngospasm argue strongly against fiberoptic intubation and in favor of cricothyrotomy.
- Inadequate oxygenation by bag and mask does not permit fiberoptic intubation because of the time required ("*can't* intubate, *can't* oxygenate").

TECHNIQUE

Overview

Fiberoptic intubation is a technical challenge that requires initial training, and then skill maintenance activities to maintain speed and success. Manual dexterity in manipulating the fiberscope is essential to performing fiberoptic intubation in a timely fashion. This skill is best learned by attending fiberoptic intubation workshops with expert instruction, and then practicing on intubation manikins or high-fidelity human patient simulators before one attempts to intubate a patient. This is particularly true of patients with difficult airways. The manufacturers of fiberscopes can usually provide training videos, product support personnel, and manikins to support this endeavor.

The requisite psychomotor skills cannot be developed without practice, and lack of training, practice, and experience constitute the most common cause of failed fiberoptic intubation. A reasonable level of dexterity in bronchoscopic manipulation can be achieved within 3 to 4 hours of independent practice using an intubation model. Recent studies have shown that the technique can also be learned in real-life situations by the performance of upper airway endoscopy when diagnostic opportunities, such as searching for foreign bodies and evaluating the causes of hoarseness, severe sore throat, and other upper airway conditions, present themselves. As is the case with many of the specialized airway techniques, semiemergent intubations, such as overdose victims without anticipated difficult airways and those who are easily ventilated with normal oxygen saturation, may be appropriate candidates for fiberoptic intubation. Because success depends on familiarity and skill in using the device, gaining experience in routine cases is invaluable before one is required to perform a difficult fiberoptic intubation in a crisis.

Preparation

Although the emergency difficult or failed airway situation often does not permit lengthy preparation and a methodical approach, maximal success with this technique requires both psychological and pharmacological patient preparation. When the procedure is to be done "awake" (see Chapter 8), optimizing the chances for success includes the following:

- Educate the patient as to what to expect.
- Administer an antisialogogue, such as glycopyrrolate 0.01 mg/kg, at least 20 minutes in advance of the procedure to minimize obscuring secretions and to maximize the effect of topically applied local anesthesia.
- Achieve profound local anesthesia of the airway. A fiberoptic intubation requires as much sedation and topical anesthesia as is necessary for awake direct laryngoscopy.
- Administer adequate sedation (see Chapter 8).

Scope Selection

Instrument selection for the ED is an important issue. Affordable and durable scopes are easily available from a variety of manufacturers. Selection of a manufacturer may be guided by existing service contracts in your specific institution. These instruments, although expensive, find several uses in the ED to justify such an expenditure:

- Endotracheal intubation, both nasal and oral
- Diagnostic laryngoscopy
- Oropharyngeal foreign body location and extraction
- Pulmonary toilette, particularly when intensive care unit patients are "held over" in the ED

The scope should be of sufficient caliber and stiffness to guide the passage of an endotracheal tube (ETT) over itself through the angles of the airway without kinking and resist being flipped out of the trachea, while maintaining flexibility and ease of manipulation. Most fiberscope manufacturers produce intubation-specific devices that have the added stiffness of the fiber bundle to allow ETTs to be guided into the trachea over the scope. This feature allows scopes that are small enough (3 to 4 mm tip diameter) to be painlessly and atraumatically passed through a topically anesthetized nose for diagnostic work to also be used for fiberoptic intubation. Neonatal and pediatric fiberscopes (2 to 3 mm tip diameter) are also available.

The fiberoptic bundle should be long enough (600 mm) to allow bronchoscopy and airway toilette in the ED. Standard bronchoscopes are 600 mm in length. Some manufacturers produce 400-mm intubating fiberscopes that are not long enough for pulmonary care. A separate channel for the injection of local anesthetic or saline and suctioning is essential, although the smaller neonatal and pediatric fiberscopes may not have them owing to their small size. A formerly recommended practice, the insufflation of oxygen through the suction apparatus to maintain saturations and blow secretions out of the way, is now contraindicated following several cases of gastric insufflation, perforation, and death. A new generation of fiberoptic scopes with battery-powered, portable, self-contained light sources promises to be much more compact and may be preferable for ED applications.

Care of the Instrument

Some general precautions to prevent damage to the scope and its relatively delicate fiberoptic bundles are as follows:

- Do not drop the scope.
- Use a bite-block (e.g., oral airway) to protect the scope. Most oral fiberoptic intubation guides incorporate this feature (e.g., the Berman intubating/pharyngeal airway, also called the "Berman breakaway airway") and are invaluable aids to successful oral fiberoptic intubation (Fig. 12-1).
- Avoid acute bending or kinking of the fiber bundle, especially when sliding the ETT over the scope into the trachea.
- If rotation of the ETT during intubation is necessary, rotate both the ETT and the scope to avoid damage to the fibers.
- Lubricate the ETT by spraying local anesthetic agent or other water-soluble material down the tube to allow easy removal of the scope after the ETT is in place. Lubricating the scope makes it slippery and difficult to manipulate.

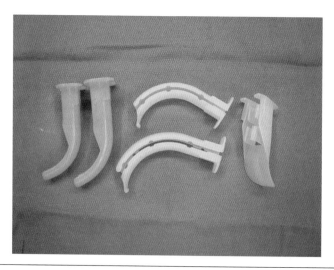

Figure 12-1 ● Three Oral Fiberoptic Intubation Aids are on The Market: the Williams (*left*), the Berman intubating/pharyngeal airway (*center*), and the Ovassapian guide (*right*). The Williams and the Berman serve a "bite-block" function.

- Clean the device, including the working channel, immediately after use. The best routine is to suction 1 L of saline through the device immediately after use. Manufacturers and endoscopy units will provide instructions for acceptable cleaning routines.
- Do not flex the tip against undue resistance to manipulate the direction of an ETT or use it to move tissue out of the way.

Technique of Fiberoptic Intubation

The fiberscope has two main components: a body (handpiece) housing the controls and accessories and a fiber bundle (Fig. 12-2). Scope tip control is simple: flexion forward and backward is achieved with the thumb toggle on the body of the fiberscope, whereas rotation clockwise and counterclockwise is done by rotating the wrist of the hand that is holding the body of the fiberscope (not the entire upper body).

The vast majority of EDs will not have a video-capable system, so this description assumes the operator is holding the eyepiece to his or her eye. When looking through the eyepiece of the fiberscope, select visual targets as you advance the scope using the hand holding the fiber bundle to pull the hand holding the body of the scope along. Move toward these targets slowly but steadily using small manipulations forward and back (toggle) and left and right (wrist flexion and extension) to keep successive targets in the center of the visual image. The hand-eye coordination needed for successful fiberoptic intubation has been likened to the kind of hand-eye coordination used to play a video game.

Preparation for the task depends on how much time is available. Generally, most things should be in a state of instantaneous readiness on the difficult and failed airway cart:

1. Gather all your equipment (usually preassembled on a tray):
   a. Topical airway anesthesia supplies and equipment, including three 5-mL syringes loaded with 4% lidocaine to inject into the airway through the scope as needed
   b. Fiberscope, ETTs, airways, bite-blocks
   c. Tonsil suction
   d. Lubricant and silicone liquid drops (prevents fogging)
   e. Additional airway management equipment as indicated in case of patient deterioration and need for rapid intervention

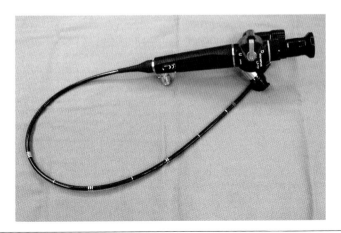

Figure 12-2 ● Body of a Fiberoptic Bronchoscope.

2. Obtain an able and knowledgeable assistant.
3. Prepare the patient:
   a. Antisialogogue, such as glycopyrrolate 0.01 mg/kg intramuscularly or intravenously
   b. Vasoconstrictor for the nose (if nasal route chosen)
   c. Local airway anesthesia
   d. Sedation as appropriate
   e. Preoxygenate the patient as for rapid sequence intubation (see Chapter 3) as much as is possible
4. Lubricate the tube and slide it over the scope up to the handpiece. Press the ETT connector to the handpiece firmly to hold it in place or tape it there. Lubricating the scope makes it slippery and too hard to manipulate.
5. Put a drop of silicone liquid on the tip of the scope or place the tip of the fiber bundle in a bottle of warmed saline (usually available in the warming cabinets of most EDs) for 1 minute to prevent fogging.
6. Insert a bite-block if the oral route is chosen, or, preferably, use an intubating guide such as a Berman intubating/pharyngeal airway. If a Berman guide is used, mount the ETT in the guide, ensuring that the tip of the ETT is at the end of the tubular portion of the airway before inserting the guide into the mouth, and then insert the fiberscope through the ETT.
7. Stand up straight, either at the head of, the side of, or facing the patient. Operator positioning is mostly a matter of personal preference and patient tolerance.
8. *Oral technique:* Stay in the midline, stay in the midline, stay in the midline! The best way is to place the long or ring finger in the middle of the upper lip to maintain a reference point and hold the fiber bundle with the index finger and thumb. Gentle traction on the tongue by an assistant using a gauze bandage helps open the airway and prevent the patient from using the tongue to obstruct access to the airway. Custom made airways, such as the Berman intubating/pharyngeal airway, are helpful in keeping the scope in the midline and obviate the need for the tongue traction maneuver. If such an adjunct is used, insert the ETT into the airway and then insert the scope through the airway/ETT combination, obviating the need to jam or tape the ETT connector onto the scope handpiece.

   Nasal technique: Soften the nasotracheal tube by placing the ETT in a bottle of warmed saline or sterile water from the warming closet for 3 to 5 minutes before inserting the ETT through the nostril. It is helpful to dilate the chosen anesthetized nostril by gently and slowly inserting increasingly large nasopharyngeal airways or a lubricated and gloved small finger into the nostril as far as possible immediately before inserting the ETT. Advance the lubricated nasal tube to the nasopharynx, and then pass the scope through the tube.
9. Hold the body of the fiberscope in the same hand as your dominant eye. This allows one to turn slightly to the side when using the scope, an important detail in keeping the fiber bundle of the scope straight during the procedure for reasons described later. Some advocate holding the body of the scope in the left hand to facilitate clearance of the light source cable and suction tubing, which exit the body of the scope on its left side (Fig. 12-2). Use your thumb to toggle the tip control lever up and down. The index finger can be used to depress and activate the suction feature. Flexing and extending the wrist moves the tip of the fiber bundle left and right, although the fiber bundle must be held straight with mild tension between the two hands to optimize this maneuver. Slackness in the fiber bundle will not permit wrist motion to rotate its tip. The nondominant hand advances, withdraws, and manipulates the fiber bundle, and maintains a midline oral position if the oral route is chosen. The operator should move the hands and arms, not the whole torso, to manipulate the fiber bundle into the airway.
10. The assistant should have tonsil suction available to aspirate oral secretions and blood. The working channel of the scope may provide insufficient suction to clear

the volume of secretions that may be present during the procedure. If the tip becomes soiled or fogged and obscures clear vision, bouncing the tip gently against the mucosa may be sufficient to clear it.

11. Get your bearings. At the head of the bed, the base of the tongue is up; beside or in front of the patient, it is down. Advance slowly while flexing the tip up to pass over the back of the tongue. The epiglottis comes into view. Keep it above you. You will see the white cords opening and closing with respiration.

12. It may be difficult to coordinate it, but attempt to advance the scope through the vocal cords during inspiration when they are open. You may need to inject 5 mL of 4% lidocaine through the working channel onto the larynx to obtund the cough or closure reflex and permit entry into the trachea.

13. If you get lost, withdraw to the oropharynx and find a landmark.

14. Once the tip of the fiber bundle is through the vocal cords, advance the scope almost to the carina. Then slowly advance the ETT over the scope into the trachea, being careful not to kink the scope. A laryngoscope may be useful to straighten out the angle of approach to the glottis. Gentle rotation of the scope/tube unit through 180 degrees may be necessary if the ETT catches on the cords. Newer ETT tip designs may facilitate passage of the ETT through the cords (e.g., Parker tube).

15. If coughing is a persistent problem, inject 5 mL of lidocaine 4% aqueous through the scope.

16. After the ETT has been successfully passed into the trachea, the scope can be used to correctly position the ETT in the midportion of the trachea. Push the tip of the scope through the ETT until it is just distal to the end of the ETT and flex it gently forward. Grasp both the fiberscope and the ETT, and move them together until light transilluminates the sternal notch. The light is shining forward immediately beyond the tip of the ETT, so this corresponds to the midtracheal position.

COMPLICATIONS

Patient complications with this technique are uncommon and include mucosal damage to the airway and epistaxis. As with all techniques, damage to the vocal apparatus is possible but rare. The most frequent complication is damage to the scope from biting, twisting, kinking, or dropping. In the past, it was taught that oxygen ought to be insufflated down the working channel of the scope to blow secretions out of the way and provide an element of oxygenation for the patient. This practice has been associated with gastric insufflation and rupture leading to death, and thus is no longer recommended.

EVIDENCE

Intubating over a fiberoptic bronchoscope, nasally and orally, is a well-established technique for managing difficult airways (1–4). It has been demonstrated that the technique is easily learned and the skill maintained (5), and that nonhuman models are useful in teaching the manipulative skills that are key to successful intubation (6). It is recognized as a skill important to the training of residents in emergency medicine (7). Levitan et al. (8) surveyed academic EDs in 1999, attempting to determine what alternative airway management devices were available for difficult airway management. Sixty-four percent of them had fiberoptic bronchoscopes. Several studies have demonstrated a success rate for ED fiberoptic intubation by emergency physicians in the 70% to 99% range, depending on training and frequency of use (9–13). Both fiberoptic nasal (adults and children) and oral intubation in the ED have been described in the literature (14,15). Emergency fiberoptic intubation has been used in blunt and penetrating head and neck trauma, laryngeal malignancies, tracheal stenosis, and other difficult airway situations (16–20). As mentioned previously, the practice of insufflating oxygen down the working channel of the scope has been associated with gastric insufflation and rupture leading to death (21) and is no longer recommended (22).

Finally, no discussion of fiberoptic intubation would be complete without at least mentioning the uncommon but real risk of sudden and total airway obstruction in patients undergoing topical anesthesia for awake fiberoptic intubation (23–26) (see Chapter 8). This factor simply serves to reinforce the need for preparedness for any eventuality when one is managing an airway in an emergency.

REFERENCES

1. Morris IR. Fiberoptic intubation. *Can J Anesth* 1994;41:996–1008.

2. Messeter MD, Pettersson KI. Endotracheal intubation with the fiberoptic bronchoscope. *Anaesthesia* 1980;35:294–298.

3. Dellinger RP. Fiberoptic bronchoscopy in adult airway management. *Crit Care Med* 1990;18:882–887.

4. Patel VU. Oral and nasal fiberoptic intubation with a single lumen tube. *Anesthesiol Clin North America* 1991;9:83–95.

5. Ovassapian A, Yelich SJ. Learning fiberoptic intubation. *Anesthesiol Clin North America* 1991;9:175–185.

6. Naik VN, Matsumoto ED, Houston PL, et al. Fiberoptic orotracheal intubation on anesthetized patients. *Anesthesiology* 2001;95:343–348.

7. Gallagher EJ, Coffey J, Lombardi G, et al. Emergency procedures important to the training of emergency medicine residents: who performs them in the emergency department? *Acad Emerg Med* 1995;2:630–633.

8. Levitan RM, Kush S, Hollander JE. Devices for difficult airway management in academic emergency departments: results of a national survey. *Ann Emerg Med* 1999;33:694–698.

9. Afilalo M, Guttman A, Stern E, et al. Fiberoptic intubation in the emergency department: a case series. *J Emerg Med* 1993;11:387–391.

10. Mlinek EJ, Clinton JE, Plummer D, et al. Fiberoptic intubation in the emergency department. *Ann Emerg Med* 1990;19:359–362.

11. Schafermeyer RW. Fiberoptic laryngoscopy in the emergency department. *Am J Emerg Med* 1984;2:160–163.

12. Blanda M, Gallo UE. Emergency airway management. *Emerg Med Clin North Am* 2003;21:1–26.

13. Hamilton PH, Kang JJ. Emergency airway management. *Mt Sinai J Med* 1997;64:292–301.

14. Delaney KA, Hessler R. Emergency flexible fiberoptic nasotracheal intubation: a report of 60 cases. *Ann Emerg Med* 1988;17:919–926.

15. Rucker RW, Silva WJ, Worcester CC. Fiberoptic bronchoscopic nasotracheal intubation in children. *Chest* 1979;76:56–58.

16. Mulder DS, Wallace DH, Woolhouse FM. The use of the fiberoptic bronchoscope to facilitate endotracheal intubation following head and neck trauma. *J Trauma* 1975;15:638–640.

17. Wei WI, Siu KF, Lau WF, et al. Emergency endotracheal intubation under fiberoptic endoscopic guidance for malignant laryngeal obstruction. *Otolaryngol Head Neck Surg* 1988;98:10–13.

18. Wei WI, Siu KF, Lau WF, et al. Emergency endotracheal intubation under fiberoptic endoscopic guidance for stenosis of the trachea. *Surg Gynecol Obstet* 1987;165:547–548.

19. Mandavia DP, Qualls S, Rokos I. Emergency airway management in penetrating neck injury. *Ann Emerg Med* 2000;35:221–225.

20. Edens ET, Sia RL. Flexible fiberoptic endoscopy in difficult intubations. *Ann Otol Rhinol Laryngol* 1981;90:307–309.

21. Hershey MD, Hannenberg AA. Gastric distention and rupture from oxygen insufflation during fiberoptic intubation. *Anesthesiology* 1996;85:1479–1480.

22. Ovassapian A, Mesnick PS, Hannenberg AA, et al. Oxygen insufflation through the fiberscope to assist intubation is not recommended. *Anesthesiology* 1997;87:183–184.

23. Ho AM, Chung DC, To EW, et al. Total airway obstruction during local anesthesia in a non-sedated patient with a compromised airway. *Can J Anaesth* 2004;51:838–841.

24. Shaw IC, Welchew EA, Harrison BJ, et al. Complete airway obstruction during awake fibreoptic intubation. *Anaesthesia* 1997;52:582–585.

25. McGuire G, el-Beheiry H. Complete upper airway obstruction during awake fibreoptic intubation in patients with unstable cervical spine fractures. *Can J Anaesth* 1999;46:176–178.

26. Donlon JV Jr. Anesthetic management of patients with compromised airways. *Anesth Rev* 1980;7:22–31.

13

Fiberoptic Stylets and Guides

Calvin A. Brown III and Michael F. Murphy

INTRODUCTION

Rigid and semirigid fiberoptic stylets are novel intubating devices that permit visualization of the glottis indirectly (in contrast to the direct line of sight of direct laryngoscopy) through an image transmitted to an eyepiece via a fiberoptic bundle. Unlike flexible fiberoptic devices, the fiberoptics in rigid and semirigid devices are enclosed in a preformed curved steel stylet designed to navigate around the tongue and hypopharynx to visualize laryngeal structures, often with minimal mouth opening or neck mobility. These devices eliminate the need to straighten the angles of the upper airway to provide the direct line of sight that is required for direct laryngoscopy, thus allowing the clinician to "see around the corner." This carries significant advantages; anatomical features such as an anterior larynx, cervical spine immobility, and limited mouth opening become less of an issue. Rigid stylets have nonmalleable curved metal sheaths, the shape of which cannot be altered, whereas semirigid devices, although not flexible, can be manipulated slightly to fit the particular airway geometry of each patient.

Semirigid stylets include the Shikani optical stylet (SOS) and the Levitan/"First Pass Success" (FPS) scope (Clarus Medical, Minneapolis, MN). Rigid stylets include the Bonfils Retromolar Intubation Fiberscope (Karl Stortz Endoscopy, Tuttlingen, Germany) and the Airway RIFL (Rigid Intubating Fiberoptic Laryngoscope; AI Medical Devices, Inc., Williamstown, MI). New intubating stylets, all similar in shape and principle, are appearing on the market at regular intervals.

Although these devices are not yet a routine part of emergency airway management, they have shown significant potential as alternative devices for the difficult airway or as rescue devices for the failed airway. Their clear advantages over direct laryngoscopy suggest that they will come into increasing use, even for "routine" emergency airways. They also may serve an expanding role in airway training because most devices can be fitted with eyepiece adapters that transmit the image to a video monitor.

The prototypical intubating stylet is the SOS; therefore, more time is devoted to its description, proper use, advantages, and contraindications. The other devices are similar in their core design and application, and are therefore described in less detail, highlighting specific features and differences.

SEMIRIGID STYLETS

Shikani Optical Stylet

The SOS is a semirigid stylet containing fiberoptic bundles for light and vision transmission (Fig. 13-1). The stylet, rounded distally at about 70 to 80 degrees, ends proximally in a high-resolution, fixed-focus eyepiece. The adult stylet can accommodate endotracheal tubes (ETTs) of 5.5 mm internal diameter (ID) or larger. A pediatric version is available and accommodates tubes of 3.0 to 5.0 mm ID. A bright halogen light is supplied from an attachable power pack, which holds four AA batteries, but the stylet is also compatible with Green-specification fiberoptic laryngoscope handles or remote light sources via fiberoptic cable. A video camera can be applied proximally to the eyepiece for teaching purposes. A push-button power switch can be found on the top of the battery pack. An adjustable tube stop is mounted on the stylet to hold the ETT in the desired position. The tube stop incorporates an oxygen port, permitting insufflation of oxygen if indicated. The malleable distal section of the stylet can be adjusted by hand, increasing or decreasing the angle of the bend to conform to the patient's anatomy.

To prepare the SOS, an ETT is loaded on the stylet, with the distal end of the stylet positioned just proximal to the ETT tip, and stabilized in this position by adjusting the tube stop proximally. Prior to insertion, the stylet tip should be warmed with either warmed saline or a warm blanket. Antifog solution should be applied. The device is held by the fingertips and thumb of the dominant hand, with the battery pack cradled in the web space between the

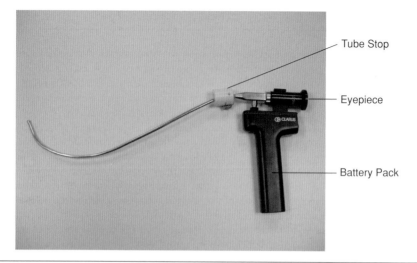

Tube Stop

Eyepiece

Battery Pack

Figure 13-1 ● Shikani Optical Stylet.

thumb and index finger and the pads of all other fingers resting on the anterior part of the eyepiece and proximal stylet (Fig. 13-2). Despite its appearance, the battery pack is not designed to be used as a handle. The ETT-stylet combination is then inserted into the mouth in the midline and advanced into the hypopharynx under direct vision. The entire stylet is oriented in the midline and advanced along its curve gently around the base of the tongue. A firm jaw lift/tongue pull during insertion will help maintain visual orientation through the scope. The operator should begin to visualize glottic structures through the eyepiece as the tip navigates the base of the tongue. The epiglottis should quickly come into view. Guide the stylet under the epiglottis to visualize the laryngeal inlet. A common error is to advance the fiberoptic tip too far into the hypopharynx as its inserted, giving a view of the posterior aspect of the hypopharynx, valleculae, or upper esophagus. To avoid this, ensure the primary motion of the scope is initially rotation around the tongue and not advancement into the hypopharynx. As with other intubating stylets, the instrument can be used in conjunction with direct laryngoscopy. For example, when an unanticipated grade III direct laryngoscopy (epiglottis only) occurs, the ETT-SOS stylet

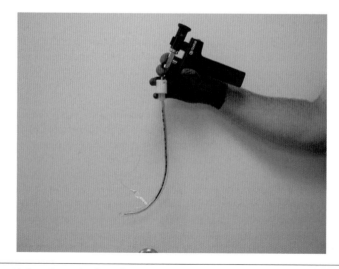

Figure 13-2 ● Shikani Optical Stylet—in Hand.

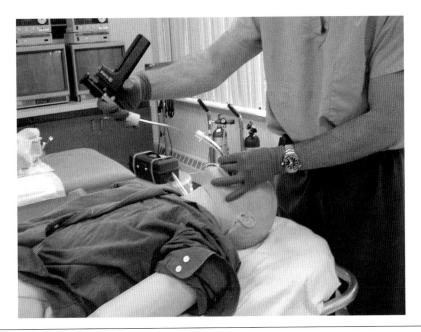

Figure 13-3 ● Removal of a Shikani Optical Stylet.

combination can be inserted under the epiglottis during direct laryngoscopy, and the glottic opening can then be sought through the eyepiece. With either technique, the ETT-stylet is advanced through the cords under visual guidance, and then the ETT is held in place as the stylet is pulled back with a large circular motion toward the patient's chest, facilitating removal (Fig. 13-3). Tube placement confirmation is with end-tidal carbon dioxide (CO_2), auscultation, and chest radiography, as for any other methods of intubation.

The SOS is advertised as being useful for the management of difficult and routine airways, with the video capability facilitating airway management teaching. In the teaching setting, coupling the device with a video system can greatly enhance success by eliminating any potential disorientation associated with the rocking motion of the scope.

The primary limitation of the SOS is its ability to maintain clear vision in the context of a tendency to fog and in the presence of secretions or blood. Fogging is largely eliminated by warming the lens and applying antifog solution, as described previously. Although secretions, vomitus, or blood can obscure the distal lens of the scope, two key design elements come into play:

1. The patient is typically supine, and, with the jaw thrust and tongue pull, most of the manipulation of the scope is occurring anterior to the location of the pooled liquids.
2. If the lens becomes obscured and cannot be cleared, it is quickly and easily removed, wiped, and reinserted in a matter of seconds.

Occasionally, the glottis cannot be visualized using the scope, and, in such cases, adjustment of the scope's curvature (usually increasing the angle, but sometimes decreasing it) provides an improved "line of sight."

Levitan/FPS Scope

The Levitan/FPS scope is a small, semirigid fiberoptic stylet intended to be used in concert with a standard laryngoscope. Its preformed shape is similar to other intubating stylets but with a gentler curve (approximately 45 degrees); however, it can be modified to meet the unique geometry of each patient's airway (Fig. 13-4). It has a handle with a small battery pack that

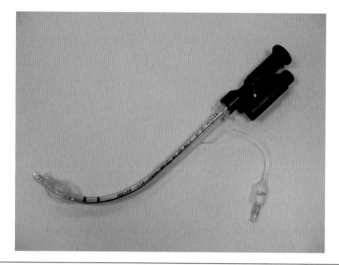

Figure 13-4 ● Levitan FPS Scope.

powers a light-emitting diode to provide illumination. A screw-down cap, rather than a push button, is used to activate the light source. The eyepiece is at the proximal end of the stylet, near the top of the battery pack. The mechanics of the Levitan/FPS are similar to the SOS with one important difference: the Levitan/FPS is *intended* to be used with a standard laryngoscope. An ETT should be cut to 26 cm because the stylet is shorter than the ETT, and then preloaded over the stylet. It is held in place by inserting the ETT connector into a round, nonadjustable tube stop at the top of the scope. As with all intubating fiberoptic stylets, the distal end of the stylet is positioned within 0.5 cm of the ETT tip because positioning more proximally in the ETT defeats the wide-angle view characteristics of the lens and results in severe "tunnel vision."

Unlike the SOS, the oxygen port is on the distal part of the handle and not attached to the adjustable tube stop. A flow of 5 to 10 L/minute is intended to clear secretions and avoid hypoxia during laryngoscopy and tube placement. However, this practice has led to gastric insufflation and perforation during flexible fiberoptic–assisted intubation and should be used with caution.

The Levitan/FPS scope is intended to be of particular benefit in patients with Cormack-Lehane view grade 3 on direct laryngoscopy. If a poor view is obtained by direct laryngoscopy, the operator positions the Levitan/FPS scope with mounted ETT so the tip of the scope is under the proximal tip of the epiglottis. The operator then looks through the eyepiece to visualize the laryngeal inlet (Fig. 13-5). When vocal cords are seen, the entire apparatus is advanced into the trachea. The laryngoscope is then removed. The stylet is removed from the well-immobilized tube in a fashion similar to that described previously for the SOS. Tube confirmation is done in the standard fashion with immediate end-tidal CO_2 detection and auscultation, followed by chest radiography. In the event that laryngoscopy identifies a grade 4 view, the loss of the epiglottis as a landmark greatly impairs the effectiveness of the scope. In such cases, the scope might be used to search for the epiglottis, which, if found, might allow repositioning of the direct laryngoscope to achieve a grade 3 view.

RIGID STYLETS

Bonfils Retromolar Intubating Fiberscope

The Bonfils fiberoptic stylet uses high-grade fiberoptic bundles for light and vision transmission in a manner analogous to that of the SOS (Fig. 13-6). Unlike the SOS, which is inserted

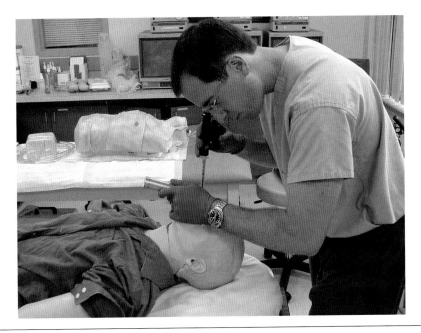

Figure 13-5 ● **Levitan in Use with Laryngoscope.**

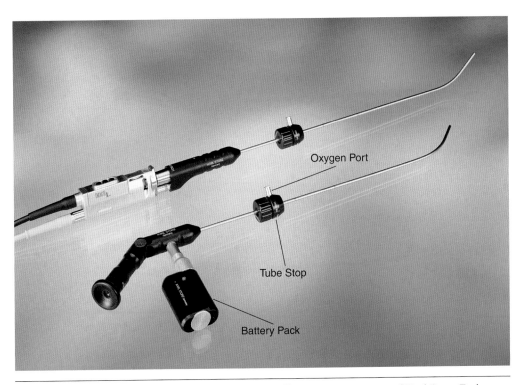

Figure 13-6 ● **Bonfils Retromolar Intubation Fiberscope.** Courtesy of Karl Storz Endoscopy © 2008.

in the midline of the mouth, the Bonfils is intended to use a paraglossal or retromolar approach, capitalizing on the proximity of the glottis to the third (most posterior) molar. The rationale for this approach is discussed in Chapter 6. The stylet incorporates a distal bend to approximately 45 degrees and ends proximally in an eyepiece, which unlike the SOS is moveable, permitting easier use. This confers a substantial technical advantage for the Bonfils over the SOS. A small tube holder device on the shaft of the stylet enables the loaded ETT to be mounted at a position of the clinician's choice. The continuous insufflation of oxygen reduces fogging during use, but an antifog solution is advised. The earlier caveat applies regarding the risk of gastric insufflation and perforation by oxygen insufflation. The Bonfils is intended to be used by itself, but it can also be used in conjunction with direct laryngoscopy.

A small combination battery pack and light source affixes near the proximal end of the stylet, making the device light and easily manipulated. A conventional external fiberoptic light source cable can be used in place of the self-contained pack, if desired. A standard video adapter can be attached to the eyepiece, as for the SOS, and is particularly helpful for learning how to use the Bonfils.

The Bonfils has been used extensively in Europe and in a few North American sites for both routine intubations and difficult airways, but, as with the SOS and Levitan/FPS, there is insufficient literature to draw conclusions about its performance in large series, and there are no published head-to-head comparisons with other devices.

Airway RIFL

The Airway RIFL is a hybrid intubating device with a rigid stylet that ends in a flexible tip that can be dynamically and continuously adjusted by a proximal trigger up to a 135-degree angle (Fig. 13-7). Similar to other devices, a fiberoptic bundle transmits an image to the eyepiece. The manufacturer's literature states that it is intended for use in difficult airways and awake intubations, and can be used both with and without direct laryngoscopy. It uses a bright LED light source and can accommodate ETT size 6.5 and higher. There is no pediatric model. The RIFL is cleaned with STERIS or Cidex OPA. At the time of this

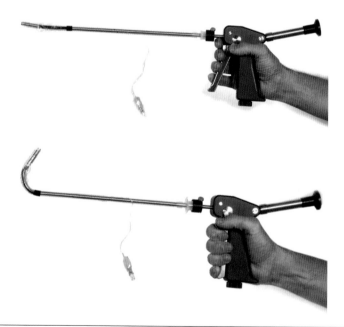

Figure 13-7 ● **Airway RIFL**—straight (*top*) and tip bent (*bottom*).

writing, the RIFL is approved and commercially available. It is currently being field-tested and is under trial with the U.S. Army, but to date no literature or significant real-life experience exists.

SUMMARY

Intubating fiberoptic stylets and video-assisted laryngoscopy (see Chapter 14) represent the vanguard of emergency airway management. The clear design advantages offered by these thin, curved, and often malleable introducers have the potential to make both routine and difficult intubations more successful and safer for patients. The primary advantage is the elimination of the need to create a straight line of sight from outside the patient's mouth to the glottic aperture, the major barrier to successful direct laryngoscopy. By positioning the "viewing port" at the distal end of a stylet, these fiberoptic intubating stylets offer a terrific advantage over direct laryngoscopy, allowing the operator to "steer" the distal end of the ETT through the cords. Considerable work needs to be done to fully evaluate these devices in the emergency arena; however, it seems reasonable that some, if not all, of the benefit seen in anesthesia literature would apply to patients requiring emergency airway management.

EVIDENCE

1. **Do we have any proof that the SOS is superior to direct laryngoscopy?** There are no emergency-based studies evaluating the performance of optical stylets in emergency airway management. Existing studies are relatively small reports in the anesthesia literature using healthy elective surgical patients. Shikani (1) first described its use in the management of difficult airways in adults and children undergoing elective otolaryngologic surgery. Agro et al. (2) did a performance assessment with the SOS in 20 healthy preoperative surgical patients and successfully intubated 14 out of 20 patients on the first attempt. The remaining 6 were successfully intubated on subsequent attempts. They also observed negligible affects on hemodynamics, a property that could be beneficial in emergency patients with head injury. Only one case report describes its use in emergency airway management, where it was successfully used to intubate an obese patient with chronic obstructive pulmonary disease (3). Many versions of fiberoptic stylets exist; the literature to date suggests they are useful adjuncts and perform superiorly to direct laryngoscopy in both real and simulated difficult airway scenarios (4,5). Their use has been described in pediatric difficult airways as well (6,7). Their role in trauma patients, although not described in the literature, may also expand because intubating stylets appear to cause less C-spine motion than direct laryngoscopy (8).

2. **Are there any studies supporting the use of the Levitan/FPS stylet?** Similar to other fiberoptic devices, there is little literature describing use of the Levitan/FPS scope in emergency airway management, although it has been suggested that it can and should be used in both difficult and routine intubations (9). More data are required before a firm recommendation can be made. Overall, the role of fiberoptic intubating stylets in emergency airway management has yet to be defined.

3. **What is known about the Bonfils Retromolar Intubating Fiberscope?** Several small studies have been published in the past few years on the Bonfils fiberscope and its performance in elective surgical patients. One recent European case series reported on six prehospital intubations, the majority being difficult intubations, with all six patients successfully intubated on the first attempt (10). The Bonfils appears to be highly successful in routine airways as well. Haligan and Charters (11) published a report of 60 healthy preoperative patients and found an intubation success rate of

more than 98%. A study of its use in predicted difficult airways identified equivalent success to the intubating laryngeal mask airway (LMA), with the Bonfils-assisted intubations being significantly more rapidly achieved than those using the LMA (12). Overall intubation times range from 30 to 60 seconds across several studies. Like other intubating stylets, the Bonfils may find an expanding role in trauma airway management because similar findings of reduced cervical spine motion during intubation have been reported (13). It also appears to be a successful rescue device following multiple failed direct laryngoscopic attempts by anesthetists (14).

4. **Are there any published studies involving the Airway RIFL?** At the time of this writing, there are no studies of the Airway RIFL.

REFERENCES

1. Shikani AH. New "seeing" stylet-scope and method for the management of the difficult airway. *Otolaryngol Head Neck Surg* 1999;120:113–116.

2. Agro F, Cataldo R, Carassiti M, et al. The seeing stylet: a new device for tracheal intubation. *Resuscitation* 2000;44:177–180.

3. Kovacs G, Law AJ, Petrie D. Awake fiberoptic intubation using an optical stylet in an anticipated difficult airway. *Ann Emerg Med* 2007;49(1):81–83.

4. Liem EB, Bjoraker DG, Gravenstein D. New options for airway management: intubating fibreoptic stylets. *Br J Anaesth* 2003;91:408–411.

5. Biro P, Weiss M, Gerber A, et al. Comparison of a new video-optical intubation stylet versus the conventional malleable stylet in simulated difficult tracheal intubation. *Anaesthesia* 2000;55:886–889.

6. Pfitzner L, Cooper MG, Ho D. The Shikani seeing stylet for difficult intubation in children: initial experience. *Anaesth Intensive Care* 2002;30:462–466.

7. Shukry M, Hanson RD, Koveleskie JR. Management of the difficult pediatric airway with Shikani optical stylet. *Paediatr Anaesth* 2005;15(4):342–345.

8. Turkstra TP, Pelz DM, Shaikh AA, et al. Cervical spine motion: a fluoroscopic comparison of Shikani optical stylet vs. Macintosh laryngoscope. *Can J Anaesth* 2007;54(6):441–447.

9. Levitan RM. Design rationale and intended use of a short optical stylet for routine fiberoptic augmentation of emergency laryngoscopy. *Am J Emerg Med* 2006;24(4):490–495.

10. Byhahn C, Meininger D, Walcher F, et al. Prehospital emergency endotracheal intubation using the Bonfils intubation fiberscope. *Eur J Emerg Med* 2007;14(1):43–46.

11. Halligan M, Charters P. A clinical evaluation of the Bonfils intubation fibrescope. *Anaesthesia* 2003;58(11):1087–1091.

12. Bein B, Worthmann F, Scholz J, et al. A comparison of the intubating LMA and the Bonfils intubating fiberscope in patients with predicted difficult airways. *Anaesthesia* 2004;59(7):668–674.

13. Wahlen BM, Gereck E. Three-dimensional cervical spine movement during intubation using the MacIntosh and Bullard laryngoscopes, the Bonfils fibrescope and the intubating LMA. *Eur J Anaesthesiol* 2004;21(11):907–913.

14. Bein B, Yan M, Tonner PH, et al. Tracheal intubation using the Bonfils intubation fiberscope after failed direct laryngoscopy. *Anaesthesia* 2004;59(12):1207–1209.

14

Video Laryngoscopy

John C. Sakles and Calvin A. Brown III

INTRODUCTION

When tracheal intubation was invented more than 100 years ago, it was performed blindly using the fingers to palpate the laryngeal inlet and guide the tube into the trachea. Shortly thereafter, laryngoscopes were invented, allowing for direct visualization of the larynx. These laryngoscopes were essentially metal spatulas with a light bulb on the tip. The blade lifted the tongue out of the way, and the light bulb illuminated the glottic structures. The straight blade, or Miller blade, was introduced by Robert Miller in 1941, and 2 years later, Sir Macintosh introduced the curved or Mac blade. Interestingly, little has changed, and modern-day intubations are still largely performed with Miller and Mac blades. There have been minor developments in laryngoscopes throughout the years, but their core design remains unaltered. Over the past few years, the most significant change in the field of intubation is video laryngoscopy. This technology involves placement of a micro-video camera on the laryngoscope blade to transmit glottic images to an external monitor, allowing the operator to perform tracheal intubation while watching the video screen instead of looking directly through the mouth. Video laryngoscopy has several important advantages over traditional direct laryngoscopy. First, video laryngoscopy magnifies the view of the airway and allows the operator to see the airway in greater detail, thereby increasing the chance of successful intubation. Second, the anterior angulation of the blade and placement of the video camera allow the operator to see structures that would be difficult or impossible to see under direct vision. Furthermore, video laryngoscopy can enhance education by allowing other health care providers to visualize the anatomy the operator is viewing. The use of the video laryngoscope also makes it possible to record the procedure to provide an excellent teaching resource and documentation for the medical record. There have been several video laryngoscopes introduced over the past few years. This chapter reviews the most important video laryngoscopes currently available on the market.

DEVICES

GlideScope Video Laryngoscope

Device Components

GlideScope System

The GlideScope Video Laryngoscope (GVL) consists of a video laryngoscope with a micro-video camera encased within a modified MacIntosh blade, a rechargeable 7-in. video liquid crystal display (LCD) monitor, and a video cable that transmits the image between the two. There are three system configurations for the GVL system and two mounting options. The monitor can be mounted on a five-legged mobile stand or attached to an intravenous line pole with a C-clamp. The third configuration is to purchase the GVL within a hard shell case with foam compartments housing the monitor, cable, and room for all three blades (Fig. 14-1A). This configuration is ideal for mobile or remote field emergency applications.

The laryngoscope portion of the GVL consists of a combined handle and laryngoscope blade that are made from durable medical-grade plastic. The video camera is placed in a recess midway along the undersurface of the laryngoscope blade, protecting it from contamination from bodily secretions. In addition, the GVL incorporates an antifog mechanism that heats the lens around the video camera, thereby eliminating fogging during laryngoscopy. There are three blade sizes for the GVL: large, midsize, and small. The large blade corresponds to an adult size blade and can be used for most adults, including those who are morbidly obese. The medium-size blade is similar to a pediatric blade and can be used to intubate toddlers up to small adults. The small blade is considered a neonatal blade

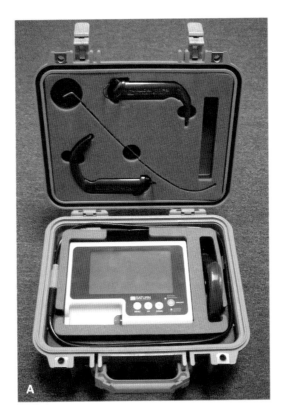

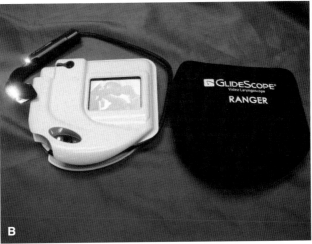

Figure 14-1 ● **A:** The GlideScope Video Laryngoscope system in the hard shell case configuration. The battery-operated monitor is held securely in place with the foam protective insert. Three blades are present in the set: large, midsize, and small. **B:** The GlideScope Ranger with its protective neoprene case. The cord wraps around the device, and the blade locks in place on the left-hand side. The blade and cord detach from the monitor and can be sent for sterilization. The "working light" on the handle is helpful when using the device in low light conditions such as in the prehospital setting.

and is for use in newborns to toddlers 1 or 2 years of age. Because the GVL does not incorporate an endotracheal tube (ETT) guide or stylet connected to the device, ETTs of any size can be used.

The laryngoscope attaches to a 7-in. LCD monitor via a video cable that also carries power to two light-emitting diodes (LEDs) mounted alongside the video camera to provide illumination. The monitor has a video-out port that requires a proprietary cable to connect to the RCA video input, allowing the image to be transmitted to another monitor or recording device. The monitor can be rotated to the optimal viewing angle, and the cradle rests on a mobile telescoping pole that allows easy adjustment of the height of the monitor. The unit is powered by standard alternating current (AC) or backup rechargeable lithium battery. The battery can provide 90 minutes of continuous use and has a low battery indicator light to warn the operator that the unit must be plugged in.

The GVL's solid design makes it well suited for emergent use in suboptimal conditions where the device is likely to be handled roughly.

GlideScope Cobalt

The GlideScope Cobalt is a disposable one-time use version of the original design. The Cobalt consists of a flexible video baton housing the micro-video camera that inserts into a disposable clear plastic blade, called the Stat, which serves to protect the video system. The Cobalt connects to the same color video LCD monitor as the original GlideScope, and is used in identical fashion as the original GlideScope. Currently, there are two blade sizes available, a large blade for adult patients and a small blade for small adult and pediatric patients. The Cobalt blade is angled slightly more anterior than the original design. The Cobalt can be used with the standard GlideScope video monitor; however, it cannot be used with the portable Ranger unit. The primary advantage of the Cobalt is its single-use design—eliminating the logistical problems, costs, and downtime associated with sterilization of the traditional GlideScope.

GlideScope Ranger

The GlideScope Ranger is a rugged, portable, battery-operated GlideScope unit designed for field use (Fig. 14-1B). It uses a transreflective (TFT) 3.5-inch screen, allowing the operator to see the airway anatomy even while viewing the monitor outdoors in bright sunlight. The Ranger's blade, although somewhat smaller than the original blade, has been designed with a 60-degree viewing angle suitable for visualizing anterior airways. It also incorporates a similar antifogging system to maintain a clear view of the airway at all times. The video camera is positioned approximately halfway along the blade to protect the lens from contamination, including secretions, blood, and vomitus. The rechargeable lithium polymer battery provides 90 minutes of use. The GlideScope Ranger is contained within a soft-sided case with belt attachments for ease of use and mobility. The manufacturer recently has developed the Cobalt Ranger, which will incorporate the Cobalt design within the Ranger system. Two blade sizes are available for the Cobalt Ranger, a small blade and a large blade.

Use of Device

The GlideScope can be used for routine intubations and can also be considered an alternative airway device for difficult or failed airways. The device's distal angulation makes it ideally suited to visualize and intubate an anterior larynx where direct laryngoscopy has proven unsuccessful. Because it does not require direct visualization of the larynx through the mouth, it is useful when cervical mobility or mouth opening is limited. Patients in whom it is desirable to minimize movement of the neck are excellent candidates because little force is needed to expose the glottis with the laryngoscope blade. The GlideScope performs well in the presence of secretions, blood, and vomitus, and thus is a good choice in these circumstances.

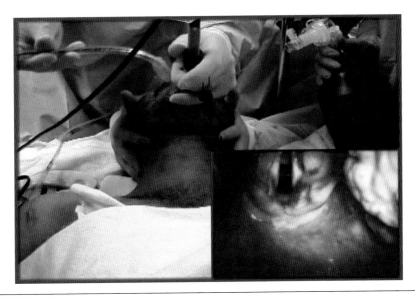

Figure 14-2 ● Intubation being Performed in the Emergency Department Using the Standard GlideScope. Note that the operator has the GlideScope placed directly in the midline and is inserting the tube from the right side of the mouth. The inset photo demonstrates what the operator sees on the GlideScope monitor. Note that the larynx appears in the upper half of the view. This is by design so the operator can see and direct the "approach" of the tube to the airway. A small amount of blood is present on the interarytenoid notch and right vocal cord.

The GlideScope is used in the following manner to perform tracheal intubation (Fig. 14-2). The handle is grasped with the left hand, in the same fashion as a conventional laryngoscope, and the tip of the laryngoscope blade is gently inserted between the teeth under direct vision. The critical point here is to start out in the midline of the tongue and to ensure that the device remains in the midline of the mouth and upper airway. There is no sweeping of the tongue to the left as is done with conventional laryngoscopy. It is difficult to identify landmarks if the blade is off midline. As soon as the tip of the laryngoscope blade passes the teeth, the operator should direct his or her attention to the video monitor and use the landmarks on the video screen to navigate to the glottic aperture. Typically, the uvula will be seen if the blade is correctly situated in the midline. The operator should then continue to walk the blade down the tongue and past the uvula, with a slight elevating motion until the epiglottis is seen. At that point, it is best to continue advancing the blade into the vallecula, with some gentle upward force, to lift the epiglottis out of the way. The blade should ultimately be seated in the vallecula, much in the same way that a Macintosh blade would be. If the glottic view is insufficient, often a gentle tilt of the handle will expose it fully, in contrast to the lifting motion with a conventional laryngoscope. If the glottic aperture still cannot be exposed, the blade can be withdrawn a bit, placed under the epiglottis, and used like a Miller blade to physically displace the epiglottis up and out of the way. The problem with doing this is that this tends to tilt the larynx more sharply, making advancement of the tube into the trachea technically more challenging. Identifying and exposing the glottis is the easy part of using the GlideScope. The challenging part is directing the ETT toward the image of the glottis displayed on the video screen. This is technically more challenging for two reasons. First, the GlideScope video camera is directed at an angle of 50 to 60 degrees, and thus, the angle of attack of the tube is quite steep. The second issue is that using the screen to navigate to the glottis requires some stereoscopic skill and hand-eye coordination that may not come naturally to all operators. The critical factor in getting the tube to enter the trachea is configuring the ETT into a shape that conforms to that of the GlideScope blade before inserting it into the patient's mouth, and for the operator to look directly into the mouth when inserting the tube, until the distal tip of the tube is felt to be in proximity with the distal end of the laryngoscope blade, at which time the eyes are redirected to the video screen to guide the tube through the glottis. There are several options for bending the tube to facilitate insertion. The manufacturer recommends simply bending the ETT to conform to the shape of the GlideScope blade: a gentle curve of 60 degrees. The manufacturer has recently developed a preformed rigid ETT stylet that provides the appropriate curve and angle for the ETT to allow proper placement at the glottic opening. An alternative approach is to bend the tube at a right angle just proximal to the cuff, similar to the configuration of the tube when using the Trachlight (see Chapter 11). The tube is then inserted into the right corner of the mouth and rotated upward, at which point the tip of the tube should be pointing at the glottis. Gentle forward rotation of the tube on the apex of the bend will then allow the operator to align the tip of the tube perfectly with the glottic entrance. Advancement of the tube then allows the tip to pass through the cords under video visualization. At this point, because of the extreme angulation, it is often difficult to continue advancing the tube into the trachea, and thus, it is helpful to withdraw the stylet several centimeters, or even completely, while maintaining gentle steady forward pressure on the tube. In addition, if the GlideScope is withdrawn about 2 cm, the larynx drops down, lessening the angle of attack and thus greatly facilitating further advancement of the tube. As with conventional laryngoscopy, the ETT can sometimes become engaged on the arytenoids, so the manufacturer has developed a GlideRite ETT with a soft tapered tip to facilitate entry of the tube through the glottic inlet. This tube can be used with the GlideScope or any other device.

The only absolute contraindication to use of the GlideScope is restricted mouth opening of less than 16 mm because this is the width of the widest portion of the blade.

The GlideScope laryngoscope blade must be cleaned and disinfected after each use. Gross contaminants and large debris can be scrubbed off with a surgical scrub brush or enzymatically removed with a proteolytic compound such as Enzyme or Medzyme. For sterilization of the blade, Steris, Sterrad, ethylene oxide, pasteurization, or glutaraldehyde are all acceptable and safe. The electrical connector cap should be placed over the contact port on the laryngoscope handle to prevent corrosion of the contacts. The only method of sterilization that is absolutely contraindicated is autoclaving, which involves exposure of the device to very high temperatures that will damage the video camera element. In fact, the laryngoscope blade has a silver temperature indicator that turns black if the device is exposed to temperatures exceeding 80°C.

GlideScope Ranger/Cobalt

The use of the GlideScope Ranger system is identical to the original version, except the slightly increased blade angulation requires less lifting force during laryngoscopy.

Intubation is performed with the GlideScope Cobalt system, as with the other GlideScope units. The major difference between this and the original version is the development of a disposable blade that attaches to a newly designed flexible video baton. The disposable blade, called a Stat, is easily slid over the flexible baton and locks in place with a plastic notched mechanism. This combination provides a similar view to the original GlideScope, and the user can follow the previous recommendations for use. After the intubation is complete, the Stat can be pulled off the video baton and discarded, and another intubation can be immediately performed by simply sliding on a new disposable Stat blade. This design provides a more rapid turnaround time than sterilization. If necessary, the video baton can be cleaned and sterilized similar to other GlideScope units by using a nonautoclavable method such as Sterrad or Steris.

Summary

The GlideScope is a rugged, well-designed device with many features that are compatible with emergency intubation. There are multiple configurations and blade sizes that allow the devices to be used in a variety of clinical situations. Due to its anterior video angulation, superb antifog capabilities, and capacity to maintain an adequate view despite secretions, the GlideScope is one of the most useful videoscopes for emergency intubations.

Karl Storz Video Laryngoscope Intubating System

Device Components

The C-MAC video laryngoscope is a completely new system from Karl Storz in 2008, which replaces the original Storz video laryngoscope (VL), and incorporates numerous improvements. The original VL consists of a fiberoptic and video system integrated into a series of traditional laryngoscope blade styles and sizes. The light provided by this system is more than 100 times greater than the illumination provided by a conventional battery powered Macintosh laryngoscope, but the system is prone to fogging and requires application of an antifog solution to the fiberoptic lens before use. The laryngoscope connects to a conventional fiberoptic light source and video processing unit or to a unified telepak display unit with a flip up eight inch color monitor. The new C-MAC system abandons fiberoptic and conventional video in favor of a CMOS micro video camera, which provides an enhanced field of view and resists fogging, thus requiring no antifog solution. The device incorporates a video recording system, a unique feature among video laryngoscopes that supports both teaching and quality management. The C-MAC is powered by a rechargeable lithium battery, permitting 90 minutes of operation without a power source. A 7 inch video screen with a single cable and straightforward controls greatly simplifies operation over the old VL system (Fig. 14-3). Both the original VL and the new C-MAC are based on specially modified conventional laryngoscope blades, so they do not require a specially curved stylet as is used with the Glidescope. The

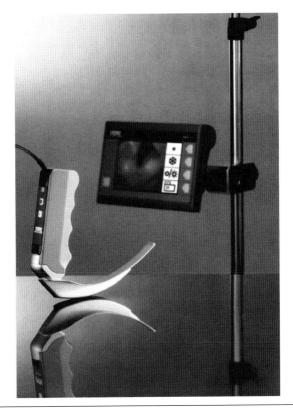

Figure 14-3 ● **The new C-MAC video laryngoscopy system.** The blade incorporates a CMOS image sensor and light system, which conveys the image to the screen via a single cable. Courtesy of Karl Storz Endoscopy.

distally placed video source significantly improves the glottic view when compared to direct laryngoscopy, but for particularly difficult "anterior" airways, it may not be as good as the more sharply angulated blade on the Glidescope. On the other hand, for most airways, tube insertion should be easier with the VL or C-MAC than with the Glidescope because the stylet is shaped as for conventional laryngoscopy, thus permitting more direct insertion and avoiding the impingement on the anterior trachea that occurs with the Glidescope.

As is the case for other video laryngoscopes, the C-MAC blades cannot be autoclaved because this will damage the micro video camera. However, most other types of sterilization, such as Steris, Sterad, and Cidex, are acceptable.

Use of Device

After the C-MAC or VL is brought to the bedside and connected to the monitor, the light intensity is adjusted as desired (continuous range for the VL, three discrete intensity selections for the C-MAC.) A drop of antifog solution is applied to the fiberoptic lens of the VL, but this is not required for the C-MAC. The blade is inserted like a traditional Miller or Macintosh blade with the exception that the traditional tongue sweep is not needed. The operator views the uvula on the screen and follows the midline until the epiglottis comes into view. Then the blade is used in a traditional fashion with blade placement either within the vallecula with anterior lift or under the epiglottis, both providing visualization of the glottic inlet (Fig. 14-4). The angle of attack is less acute than with the GlideScope, and the tube is curved in a similar shape that used for conventional direct laryngoscopy.

Summary

The Storz C-MAC is a dramatic improvement over the prior VL system, with enhancements, including a CMOS video sensor, elimination of fiberoptics, avoidance of fogging, much more simple assembly and operation, portability, and a significantly lower price. The original VL has numerous blade sizes and styles ranging down to a Miller 0, which are easily interchangeable, and a similar array of blades is anticipated for the C-MAC system.

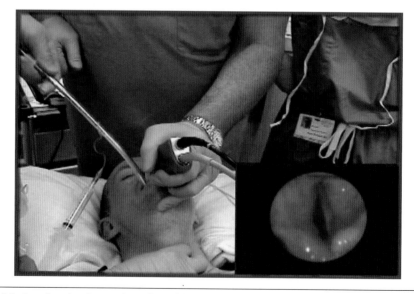

Figure 14-4 ● Intubation using the older style VL. The glottic image is shown in the lower right. Note the traditional curve of the endotracheal tube, as it is being aligned for insertion. Courtesy of Karl Storz Endoscopy.

McGrath Video Laryngoscope Series 5

Device Components

The McGrath video laryngoscope (MVL) (Fig. 14-5) consists of three main parts. First, the handle of the video laryngoscope is made of latex free medical-grade rubber and stainless steel, housing a single AA battery to power the device and an attached 1.7-inch color LCD monitor. The power button is placed at the top of the handle. Second, the camera module incorporates a light source and a micro-video camera that illuminates the hypopharynx and provides a view of the glottis. The last component is a disposable laryngoscope blade made of medical-grade optical polymer that attaches to the camera stick module and can allow one to manipulate and displace the tongue. The blade can be adjusted into three different positions, creating the desired length to facilitate intubation for various anatomical and patient differences. However, there is not a locking mechanism for the three blade positions, and thus, the potential exists for the blade to slip on tension during intubation. A locking pin keeps the blade from disengaging completely from the handle. The MVL does not incorporate antifog technology, nor does the device incorporate a channel guide within the blade, so any ETT size can be used using a standard stylet.

The LCD screen attaches to the proximal portion of the handle module and can be adjusted for an optimal viewing angle. Placement of the screen at the top of the handle improves operator comfort by allowing visualization of the device and patient simultaneously.

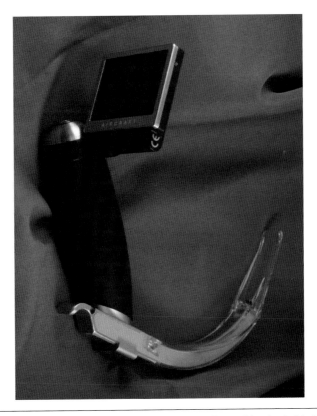

Figure 14-5 ● McGrath Video Laryngoscope. The disposable plastic blade is engaged on the camera stick. The camera stick is in the midposition. Sliding the camera stick forward one notch will lengthen the blade, allowing it to be used for larger patients, while retracting it one notch will shorten it, allowing it to be used for smaller patients. The video monitor is attached to the upper aspect of the handle and can be rotated to the optimal position for viewing.

The LCD screen can be rotated to a variety of positions to optimize clarity and can be rotated along the axis of the handle so the device can lay completely flat. The camera, display, and light are powered by a single AA 1.5-V battery providing approximately 60 minutes of operating time. A battery warning indicator begins to flash when little operating time remains. The MVL does not incorporate an auto-off feature, so the device will completely exhaust the battery if left on.

The MVL is constructed of durable materials and demonstrates a solid feel in the operator's hand. Because it is essentially a conventional laryngoscope with a small screen attached, it is extremely portable. A protective carrying case is not included with the MVL, increasing the risk of damage during transport.

Use of Device

There is little setup needed for the MVL, and once a disposable blade is placed on the camera stick and the device turned on, it is ready for use (Fig. 14-6). The MVL is inserted into the patient's oropharynx much like a traditional laryngoscope; however, rather than sweeping the tongue to the left, the blade is introduced along the midline. The tip of the blade is then guided into the vallecula and used to lift the tongue anteriorly, similar to a conventional Macintosh blade. The device functions best using a curved blade approach; however, a straight blade technique can be used if needed. The latter technique distorts the anatomical landmarks, however, and is not the recommended technique described by the manufacturer. Once a clear view of the airway, appears on the LCD, the operator uses a standard ETT with a malleable stylet to intubate the trachea while visualizing the process on the video screen. The manufacturer recommends the ETT be bent into a hockey stick shape at a point roughly 5 cm from the tip of the tube. This facilitates advancement of the tip of the tube through the glottic inlet. The MVL is smaller and more portable than the GlideScope and Storz VL, thereby facilitating ease of use; however, this portability increases the risk for theft, loss, and damage.

After intubation, the disposable blade is removed and discarded while the handle is cleaned with an antiseptic towelette. The disposable blade does not protect the handle or

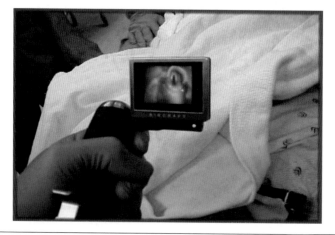

Figure 14-6 ● Intubation Using the McGrath Video Laryngoscope. As with other video laryngoscopes, the device is inserted in the midline and can be used with either a straight blade approach or a curved blade approach. The picture shows the view of the glottis as seen with a curved blade approach, which tends to cause less distortion of the laryngeal anatomy and facilitates tube passage. This view was the initial view attained during laryngoscopy. As the blade was left in the patient's mouth during laryngoscopy, the lens became increasingly fogged, making visualization of the structures much more difficult. It is highly recommended that antifog solution be applied to the tip of the blade prior to insertion.

proximal portion of the device; therefore, it is susceptible to contamination, and the rubber handle can be somewhat difficult to clean and sterilize. The device cannot undergo Steris or Sterrad sterilization procedures.

Summary

The McGrath is a compact, easy-to-use, intuitive device that is the most similar to direct laryngoscopy. The device feels comfortable in the operator's hand and does not require a lot of education or setup time. Therefore, the learning curve is short. The blade is narrower than the other devices, and for patients with large tongues, this can hinder the operator's view. Without the application of antifogging solution, the blade fogs quickly in emergency situations. The delicate nature of the device and lack of an included case make it less suitable for prehospital use.

Pentax Airway Scope, AWS-S100

Device Components

The Pentax airway scope (PAS) consists of two components (Fig. 14-7). The first, an unconventional handle with a more linear design that encompasses a monitor screen, power

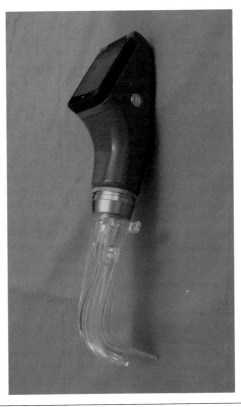

Figure 14-7 ● Pentax Airway Scope.   The disposable blade is attached to the rigid handle. On the side of the blade, the tube guide that holds the endotracheal tube in place can be seen. The video monitor is on the upper posterior aspect of the handle and can flip up for easier viewing or for viewing when intubating the patient face to face. The little plastic disc on the side of the handle screws off to allow access to the video-out port. An optional disposable clear plastic sleeve can be placed on the handle to protect it from gross contamination by body fluids.

button, battery compartment, video-out port, locking connection ring for the disposable blade, and a flexible cable that houses the light source and CCD micro-video camera. The PAS has a disposable sleeve that covers and protects the reusable handle from contamination. The second component is a polycarbonate Lexan disposable blade that incorporates an ETT channel and 12F suction port. The blade does not feature an antifog mechanism; however, the Lexan plastic technology used in the blade reportedly resists fogging and contamination. As of this writing, only a single adult-size blade is available that will accept ETT sizes between 6.0 and 8.5 mm internal diameter. The ETT is preloaded alongside the disposable blade with clips that hold the tube in place. The PAS has a green reticle that can be displayed on the LCD screen to guide the user into the correct position for ETT placement. The 2.4-inch color LCD monitor is attached to the handle and can be tilted into various positions to allow easier viewing. The PAS has video output capabilities, allowing the image to be transmitted to an external video monitor or recording device. The PAS is powered by two AA 1.5-V batteries that provide approximately 60 minutes of continuous operation. A low battery indicator flashes to alert the operator when 5 minutes of battery life remain. The PAS has a protective soft carrying case with preformed foam compartments to house the scope, video cables, and extra batteries. The case does not include space to carry blades.

The PAS is solidly built of strong orange plastic and stainless steel, and has an ergonomic fit within the operator's hand. The laryngoscope is portable and can easily be transported.

The PAS is anticipated to become available in the United States in 2008.

Use of Device

There is virtually no setup for the PAS. A disposable blade is locked onto the video cable, the plastic sheath is secured, and the device is turned on and ready for use (Fig. 14-8). The operator may select whether he or she wants the reticle displayed on the LCD by pressing the

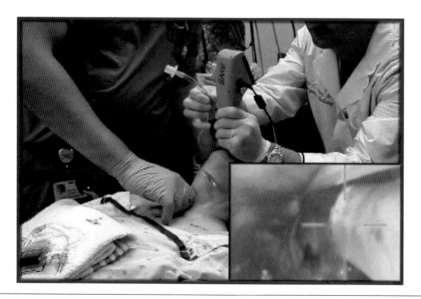

Figure 14-8 ● Intubation Using the Pentax Airway Scope. The operator is guiding the tube into the airway by advancing it through the tube guide. No stylet is necessary. The inset photo shows the view of the glottis seen on the attached monitor by the operator. The scope must be positioned so the green reticle is centered over the glottic inlet. Here, the reticle is to the right of the glottic inlet. Also, the tip of the blade must lift the epiglottis out of the way so the tube can pass unobstructed into the airway.

on-off button. Antifog solution is recommended for use because the Lexan plastic resists fogging but does not eliminate it. The device is advanced midline along the posterior pharyngeal wall, resulting in elevation of the epiglottis. If the epiglottis is visualized, a Miller or straight blade technique must be used for successful intubation. The reticle is "aimed" at the vocal cords for appropriate position. The reduction in ETT maneuverability requires the PAS to be positioned correctly in front of the glottic inlet and decreases the operator flexibility to manipulate the ETT. Therefore, the operator does not use a stylet or provide manual control over the distal portion of the ETT. The ETT is advanced from the channel through the vocal cords. The PAS has the option of recording the intubation via the video output port. This feature allows one to record the entire intubation procedure for later viewing and teaching purposes. The PAS can be rinsed in water without submersion and wiped clean. The protective sheath and disposable blade make the PAS easy to clean and quickly ready for another intubation.

Summary

The PAS is a well-built device video laryngoscope with outstanding optics. However, the lack of an antifog mechanism can impair the quality of the image and make successful intubation more difficult. A more significant problem with the design of the PAS is the requirement to "dip" the scope along the posterior pharynx to elevate the epiglottis. Therefore, if any secretions such as blood or vomitus are present within this location, the scope becomes contaminated and the operator has complete loss of view, making intubation impossible. Unfortunately, this is not an infrequent scenario for emergency intubations.

Res-Q-Scope II

Device Components and Setup

The Res-Q-Scope II (RQS) contains a main video unit with an attached 2.75-inch LCD monitor that is completely mobile to allow for optimal viewing angles (Fig. 14-9). The device

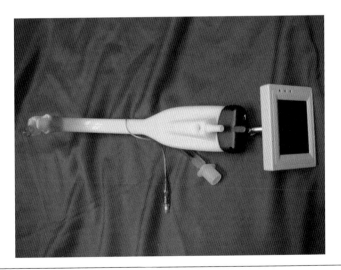

Figure 14-9 ● The Res-Q-Scope II.   The video monitor attaches to the top of the device and can be flipped or rotated to virtually any position for optimal viewing by the operator. The tube guide is on the posterior aspect of the laryngoscope blade, and an endotracheal tube can be seen within it. As can be seen, the proximal portion of the tube is directed laterally, and the scope is removed from the mouth after intubation while extracting the tube laterally. A video-out port is present on the top of the main unit (blue piece).

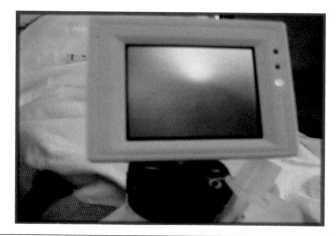

Figure 14-10 ● Intubation Using the Res-Q-Scope II. Note that the distal placement of the video camera results in an extreme close-up of the airway. Poor illumination, coupled with a low-quality video camera, and low-resolution screen results in an unacceptably poor image of the airway. Lack of an antifog feature further degrades the visibility of the airway. The glare at the top of the screen is from the focused light source of the device and is not artifact.

is powered by a rechargeable lithium battery pack. A separate backup emergency power source using four AA batteries is included with the device. A low battery indicator light is displayed on the main video unit. The second piece of the RQS is a disposable laryngoscope blade that contains a channel to preload the ETT and an oxygen/suction port. The blade is currently available in one adult size that will accept ETT sizes between 6.0 and 8.5 mm internal diameter. The preloaded ETT is directly inferior to the camera position and is advanced superiorly into the glottic opening. The device contains a video outport for recording. The blade connects to the main video unit via a standard nine-prong VGA connection.

The RQS comes with a durable metal case that houses the device extra battery pack, video cables, and two blades. However, the RQS is less sturdy overall than other devices.

Use of Device

The RQS requires little setup time. A disposable blade is connected to the main body of the RQS; however, on occasion, the blade can be difficult to connect, and some minor manipulations must be made for adequate connection. The RQS does not have antifog capabilities, and antifog solution cannot be used because there is no protective cover for the video lens. Therefore, the device is very prone to fogging during intubation. The device is turned on, and instead of insertion via midline, the device is inserted perpendicular to the axial plane at the lateral border of the mouth, and then rotated 90 degrees while advancing the scope into the hypopharynx (Fig. 14-10). If a midline insertion is needed, it will be difficult given the bulk of the device, and the anterior chest wall can impede the insertion of the RQS due to its length. The light source of the RQS is suboptimal, providing weak illumination and a poor view of the anatomical structures. The device should be inserted along the posterior pharyngeal wall and used to lift the epiglottis, providing a view of the glottic inlet. The ETT is advanced from the underside of the RQS and through the vocal cords. However, given the superior direction of the ETT advancement, the view of the glottic inlet can be impeded during intubation. After intubation, the disposable blade can be discarded, and the RQS body wiped with an antiseptic towelette.

Summary

The RQS is an inexpensive alternative to the more costly video laryngoscopes previously mentioned. However, despite the cost savings, the functionality of the RQS, including the optical quality, illumination, and significant lens contamination and fogging, is unacceptable. Therefore, based on the aforementioned limitations and problems with this scope, it cannot be recommended for emergency airway management.

CONCLUSION

Video laryngoscopy is progressing at a rapid pace, and the technique generally provides a superior glottic view with less effort than with direct laryngoscopy. Video laryngoscopy is an invaluable tool both in routine emergency airway management and as a first-line adjunct for difficult airways. The video-assisted laryngoscopes will outperform conventional laryngoscopy in those patients with reduced mouth opening, cervical spine immobility, and head and facial trauma. Several models have disposable versions that greatly reduce cleaning time and the potential spread of infectious agents. We have also discovered additional areas where these devices are particularly helpful: confirmation of ETT placement for patients in whom tube location is in question, visualization of upper airway obstructions and foreign material, and aiding in difficult tube exchanges. Most important, all video-assisted laryngoscopes allow real-time feedback for assistance or airway management education. The instructor can provide advice for successful intubation while allowing the operator to maintain control of the scope.

Direct laryngoscopy for the purpose of endotracheal intubation was introduced into clinical medicine almost 70 years ago. Since then, little has changed in its application and performance. The development of video laryngoscopes over the past few years, typified by the GVL, is the most innovative advancement in the field of laryngoscopy and intubation made to date. It is likely video laryngoscopy will soon supplant conventional direct laryngoscopy for emergency airway management.

EVIDENCE

1. **What is known about the GlideScope in clinical practice?** The GVL is the most extensively studied device since the advent of this technology. Several studies have looked at its performance both in routine intubations and in difficult airway scenarios. Agro et al. (1) compared the glottic exposure achieved with the GlideScope to the view obtained with a Macintosh blade in 15 patients with cervical immobilization. They found that the GlideScope improved the Cormack-Lehane (C-L) view of the glottis by one grade in 14 out of 15 patients. In one patient, who was a grade III airway, the GlideScope did not improve the view of the glottis so the patient was intubated with the aid of a bougie. The glottic views in this series of patients were poor during conventional laryngoscopy, when compared to a routine operating room (OR) population or to previous intubation studies, suggesting a difficult airway cohort, although the author did not report this. For example, using a standard Macintosh blade, 1 patient was a grade 4, 9 patients were grade 3, 5 patients were grade 2, and no patients were grade 1. Thus, in this small series, the vocal cords could be identified in only 5 out of 15 patients (33%), compared with 95% in routine OR series. In an abstract by Sakles et al. (2), the GlideScope (GVL) was compared to two fiberoptic airway devices, the UpsherScope (US) and the Shikani optical stylet (SOS; see Chapter 13). Emergency medicine residents with no

prior experience with these devices were asked to intubate manikins, and the success rate for each device and the time needed to perform the intubation was evaluated. The GVL was successful 100% of the time and, on average, required one attempt and 65 seconds to perform the intubation. The US had a success rate of 71% and, on average, required 1.4 attempts and 65 seconds. The SOS was successful in only 43% of the cases and, on average, required 2.2 attempts and 128 seconds. Sun et al. (3) performed the only randomized clinical trial comparing the GlideScope to direct laryngoscopy. Two hundred healthy preoperative patients were randomly assigned to laryngoscopy with either a conventional Macintosh 3 blade or GlideScope. All patients were initially assigned a C-L grade by a separate anesthetist using a Mac 3. In most patients with C-L grade >1 (28/41), the laryngoscopic view was improved using the GlideScope, and nearly all patients with a C-L grade 3 or higher view had improvement in glottic exposure. However, time to ETT placement took an average of 16 seconds longer in the GlideScope group. In 2005, Cooper et al. (4) published a multicenter trial with 728 consecutive patients evaluated with both direct laryngoscopy and the GlideScope. Nearly all patients (99%) had a C-L grade of 1 or 2 using the GlideScope, which significantly improved a poor direct laryngoscopic view in the majority of cases. Intubation success was 96%, and failed intubations occurred despite adequate visualization, again suggesting that difficulty with ETT manipulation can impair intubation success. A 90-degree angle placed proximal to the cuff has been suggested as the optimal ETT shape to help facilitate tracheal intubation (5,6). A smaller performance assessment in 50 preoperative surgical patients again showed laryngoscopic superiority of one to two C-L grades using the GlideScope compared to direct laryngoscopy (7). In simulated difficult airway scenarios, the GlideScope also seems to perform equal to or better than direct laryngoscopy. A recent manikin study evaluated 30 anesthetists using a MacIntosh laryngoscope versus the GlideScope in three simulated difficult airways: cervical rigidity, pharyngeal obstruction, and tongue edema (8). Although numbers were small, the GlideScope was superior to direct laryngoscopy in the pharyngeal obstruction scenario. There was no significant advantage in the other settings. Other smaller studies have shown similar results with the GlideScope significantly outperforming conventional Macintosh laryngoscopes both in preoperative patients and in selected difficult airways such as ankylosing spondylitis (9,10). Overall, the GlideScope appears to be superior to direct laryngoscopy in providing optimal visualization of the laryngeal inlet and vocal cords in both routine and difficult airways. The data suggest a slightly longer time to tube placement; however, an ETT configuration that includes a 90-degree angle may expedite intubation. Specialized, preformed ETTs with angled tips and easily retractable stylets are now available. Due to their more recent introduction, there are no published studies yet evaluating the GlideScope Ranger or the GlideScope Cobalt. Currently, data are being gathered with respect to the GlideScope's use in emergency airway management as part of the National Emergency Airway Registry Project (NEAR).

2. **What are the advantages of the Karl Storz Video Laryngoscope Intubating System?**
Two recent studies have evaluated the VL compared to direct laryngoscopy and the GlideScope, respectively. Kaplan et al. (11) published a large prospective multicenter trial of 865 patients undergoing general anesthesia with paralysis. The operator would obtain the best view with direct visualization then record the best view using the video monitor. Intubation was then performed using the video monitor. Visualization was considered easy when a C-L grade 1 or 2 was obtained by either method and was significantly easier using the video monitor when compared to direct visualization. In addition, maneuvers such as external laryngeal manipulation and BURP (Backward, Upward, Rightward Pressure) were less often needed for adequate visualization with video assistance. In addition to improving glottic exposure, the video

laryngoscope will likely become an effective teaching tool for airway managers in training (12). There are no published studies to date evaluating this tool in emergency department populations, but the NEAR V–EVAL (Emergency Video-Assisted Laryngoscopy) study is currently underway.

3. **Are there any studies related to use of the McGrath Video Laryngoscope?** Only one study has evaluated the MVL. Shippey et al. (13) described their initial experience in 75 preoperative patients, all with normal airway anatomy. This small prospective single-center study recorded intubation success rates, laryngoscopic view, and time to ETT placement, and found that in nearly all patients (99%), a C-L grade 1 or 2 was obtained with an average time of 6.3 seconds needed for optimal visualization. Overall success rate was 98%. Although this preliminarily shows promise for the MVL, more study is needed before a firm recommendation can be made.

4. **What is the experience with the Pentax Airway Scope?** There is little published about this device. Suzuki et al. (14) published their experience with 100 patients undergoing elective surgery and compared the C-L grade obtained with the Macintosh laryngoscope with that of the PAS. They were able to obtain grade 1 views on every patient using the PAS and in 65% of patients using a conventional laryngoscope. Any recommendation about this device is premature, and its performance in difficult or emergency airway situations has not been adequately studied.

5. **Are there any data supporting the use of the Res-Q-Scope?** No studies are published as of this writing.

REFERENCES

1. Agro F, Barzoi G, Montecchia F. Tracheal intubation using a Macintosh laryngoscope or GlideScope in 15 patients with cervical spine immobilization [letter]. *Br J Anaesth* 2003;90: 705–706.

2. Sakles JC, Tolby N, VanderHeyden TC, et al. *Ability of emergency medicine residents to use alternative optical airway devices.* Paper presented at the Western Meeting of the Society for Academic Emergency Medicine; April 2003; Phoenix, AZ.

3. Sun DA, Warriner CB, Parsons DG, et al. The GlideScope video laryngoscope: randomized clinical trial in 200 patients. *Br J Anaesth* 2005;94(3):381–384.

4. Cooper RM, Pacey JA, Bishop MJ, et al. Early clinical experience with a new video laryngoscope (GlideScope) in 728 patients. *Can J Anaesth* 2005;52(2):191–198.

5. Dupanovic M, Diachun CA, Isaacson SA, et al. Intubation the GlideScope videolaryngoscope using the "gearstick technique." *Can J Anaesth* 2006;53(2):213–214.

6. Jones PM, Turkstra TP, Armstrong KP, et al. Effect of stylet angulation and endotracheal tube camber on time to intubation with the GlideScope. *Can J Anaesth* 2007;54(1):21–27.

7. Rai MR, Dering A, Verghese C. The GlideScope system: a clinical assessment of performance. *Anaesthesia* 2005;60(1):60–64.

8. Benjamin FJ, Boon D, French RA. An evaluation of the GlideScope, a new video laryngoscope for difficult airways: a manikin study. *Eur J Anaesthesiol* 2006;23(6):517–521.

9. Hsiao WT, Lin YH, Wu HS, et al. Does a new video laryngoscope (GlideScope) provide better glottic exposure? *Acta Anaesthesiol Taiwan* 2005;43(3):147–151.

10. Lai HY, Chen IH, Chen A, et al. The use of the GlideScope for tracheal intubation in patients with ankylosing spondylitis. *Br J Anaesth* 2007;98(3):408–409.

11. Kaplan MB, Hagberg CA, Ward DS, et al. Comparison of direct and video-assisted views of the larynx during routine intubations. *J Clin Anesth* 2006;18(5):357–362.

12. Kaplan MB, Ward DS, Berci G. A new video laryngoscope—an aid to intubation and teaching. *J Clin Anesth* 2002;14(8):620–626.

13. Shippey B, Ray D, McKeown D. Case series: the McGrath videolaryngoscope—an initial clinical evaluation. *Can J Anaesth* 2007;54(4):307–313.

14. Suzuki A, Toyama Y, Katsumi N, et al. Pentax-AWS improves laryngeal view compared with MacIntosh blade during laryngoscopy and facilitates easier intubation. *Masui* 2007;56(4): 464–468.

15

Optically Enhanced Laryngoscopy

John C. Sakles and Ross B. Rodgers

INTRODUCTION

Most intubating laryngoscopes that achieve an image of the glottic entrance without requiring direct line of sight use video or fiberoptic technology. These technologies are expensive and thus raise the overall cost of the device. Combinations of mirrors, prisms, or lenses, which allow one to "see around the corner" of the airway, can transmit the glottic image to the operator's eye at a much lower expense. This chapter reviews two recently released optically enhanced laryngoscopes.

DEVICES

Airtraq

Device Components

The Airtraq optical laryngoscope is a single-unit, plastic, disposable laryngoscope that does not require a direct line of sight of the glottic structures for intubation (Fig. 15-1). The Airtraq uses a series of mirrors, prisms, and lenses to provide the operator a magnified and enhanced image of the airway through an optical channel. The Airtraq has an endotracheal tube (ETT) channel alongside the optical channel where the operator preloads the ETT prior to intubation. The device is currently available in two sizes, small and regular, and a pediatric size is under development. The small Airtraq requires 16 mm of mouth opening and accommodates ETT sizes from 6.0 to 7.5 mm, and the regular Airtraq requires 18 mm of mouth opening and accommodates ETT sizes from 7.0 to 8.5 mm internal diameter. The device is powered by three disposable AAA batteries that provide approximately 90 minutes of operating time. The Airtraq is turned on by pressing a button located on top of the device. The illumination is derived from a low-heat light-emitting diode (LED), and the device contains a heat monitoring unit that prevents the Airtraq from reaching temperatures that could harm the patient. The rubber eyepiece, which is connected to the optical channel, can be removed to allow attachment of an optional video composite system that can

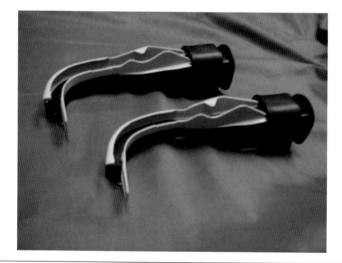

Figure 15-1 ● **Airtraq Optical Laryngoscope.** Note the black rubber eyepiece atop the viewing channel and grey endotracheal tube guide (*top*: small size, *bottom*: regular size).

transmit the optical image via video cable or wirelessly using a 2.4-GHz receiver to an external monitor. The shelf-life of the Airtraq is approximately 2 years. The device cannot be cleaned or sterilized and will not function properly if either is attempted.

Use of Device

The Airtraq requires little setup time and is self-contained within its protective packaging. The Airtraq's antifogging mechanism requires the device be turned on for approximately 30 seconds to maximize this benefit. The LED will flash when the device is turned on and become constant when the heating element has reached the appropriate antifog temperature and the device is therefore ready for use. The ETT should be lightly lubricated and preloaded into the ETT channel. Also, the anterior surface of the Airtraq blade, which will come in contact with the tongue, can be lubricated to help facilitate passing the device around the tongue. The Airtraq should be placed into the mouth using a midline approach. Gentle traction is applied to the tongue, if necessary, to ensure that the tongue is not pushed into the hypopharynx. As the Airtraq is advanced, the operator visualizes the epiglottis through the optical channel and continues to move the device forward into the vallecula. At this time, the Airtraq is lifted in the vertical plane to elevate the epiglottis and align the vocal cords within the center of the optical field (Fig. 15-2). The ETT is slowly advanced through the vocal cords, and then disengaged from the device and the Airtraq is removed. If the ETT is obstructed by the epiglottis or arytenoids, the entire device must be manipulated to better align the ETT position with the glottic entrance. The Airtraq can be pulled back slightly and rotated within the horizontal plane to help align the glottic structures. Alternatively, the epiglottis can be lifted directly by the Airtraq blade via a straight blade approach to appropriately align the glottic structures. However, this technique can somewhat distort the anatomy and is not the recommended approach.

If the proprietary composite video system is used, then the rubber optical eyepiece is removed and the video adaptor is snapped onto the Airtraq prior to insertion. The operator then visualizes the entire procedure on the external monitor. This approach allows the operator to maintain a safe distance from the patient and provides a larger view of the anatomical structures.

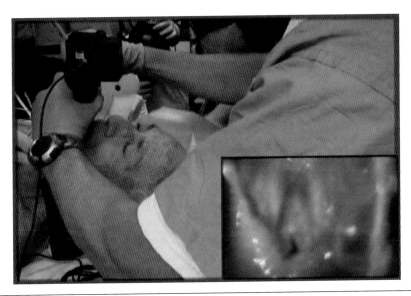

Figure 15-2 ● Clinical use of Airtraq optical laryngoscope using optional video camera adaptor with glottic view inset in the right lower corner. As can be seen, the endotracheal tube is approaching the vocal cords from the right side of the image.

Summary

The Airtraq is an inexpensive and lightweight device that provides an alternative approach to emergency airway management. The quality of the optics is substantially less than the video laryngoscopes but provides a clear and reasonable image of the glottis. The operator must learn to manipulate the device instead of the ETT for proper intubation. This technique may feel somewhat uncomfortable to the operator who is used to adjusting the ETT instead of the device for proper ETT placement. The antifog technology provides adequate clarity during the intubation process and is an added benefit for a low-cost device. The camera attachment greatly enhances the image and allows the operator to remain at a safe distance from the patient. Overall, the Airtraq is reasonably easy to learn and use within the emergency setting.

TruView EVO

Device Components

The TruView EVO consists of a conventional laryngoscope handle that houses two C batteries and an attached laryngoscope blade with several unique features (Fig. 15-3). First, the EVO blade has a straight proximal portion with a steep angulation of the distal end. On the straight portion of the blade, there is a channel that houses the view tube, which consists of a prism and lens providing 42 degrees of light refraction. The design of the eyepiece allows the operator to view the glottic structures at a distance of 2 feet from the device. At this distance, the image seen by the operator is actual size. In addition, the eyepiece will accept all universal 32-mm endoscopic camera heads. This feature allows the operator to perform the intubation while viewing the procedure on an external monitor. This configuration also allows others to view the intubation and can be used for instruction during the procedure, or the intubation can be recorded for teaching after the intubation. The manufacturer also distributes a digital camera with a 2.5-in. LCD and video capabilities that attaches directly to the view tube eyepiece. The

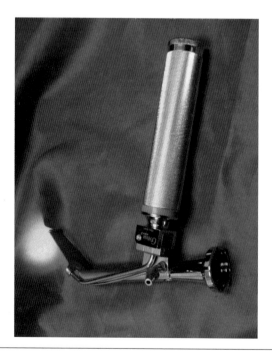

Figure 15-3 • TruView EVO optical laryngoscope connected to a standard green-line fiberoptic handle.

EVO blade incorporates an oxygen port that can be attached to standard medical tubing, and oxygen can be delivered at 10 L/minute. The flow of oxygen is directed in front of the distal portion of the optical system to potentially help keep the lens clear of contamination and reduce fogging. In addition, insufflation of oxygen can allow the operator slightly more time for intubation by reducing patient hypoxia. Currently, there are two sizes of the EVO, adult and small adult. Each is designed to attach to a conventional laryngoscope handle or a fiberoptic greenline handle. The manufacturer also offers the OptiShape stylet, which can be used to facilitate correct direction of the ETT during intubation.

Use of Device

The setup time for the EVO is minimal. The view tube is secured to the blade with the view tube button located in the up position. Antifog solution can be applied to the distal portion of the view tube lens to minimize fogging. Oxygen tubing is connected to the oxygen port, and oxygen flow is set to 10 L/minute. The operator then conforms the ETT with stylet to a shape comparable to that of the EVO blade. Alternatively, the operator can use the OptiShape, a specially designed stylet that exactly corresponds to the EVO blade. The OptiShape has a locking device to prevent the stylet from advancing past the ETT. As opposed to standard laryngoscopy, the operator places the EVO blade into the patient's mouth using a midline approach. The blade should be inserted until the handle is approximately 2 to 3 cm from the patient's lips. Very little or no neck extension is required. The operator then looks through the eyepiece at a comfortable standing position. In most circumstances, the glottic structures are visualized; however, adjustments may be required to obtain the best possible view for intubation. Due to the limited field of view and the necessity for perfect alignment of the operator's line of sight with the eyepiece, it may be difficult to gain visualization of the glottic inlet. Connecting the device to a standard camera adaptor and external video monitor alleviates the previous difficulty, but results in a smaller glottic image (Fig. 15-4). The ETT is then inserted at the right corner of the patient's mouth

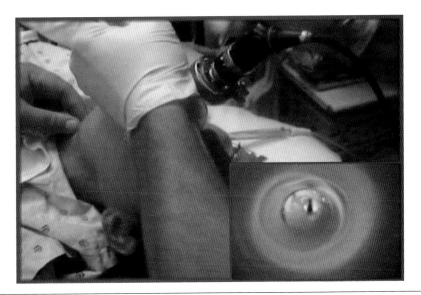

Figure 15-4 ● Clinical use of TruView EVO with optional camera attachment and oxygen delivery at 10 L per minute. The insert in the right lower corner shows the glottic inlet surrounded by reflection within the metal eyepiece. Notice the V-shaped clearing of the upper portion of the lens provided by the oxygen flow that is surrounded by fogging. This view is similar to that shown when the operator looks through the optical channel.

in the horizontal plane and rotated 90 degrees toward the midline during advancement into the hypopharynx, bringing the tip of the ETT into view at the laryngeal inlet. The ETT is then advanced through the vocal cords, and the device is removed from the patient's mouth.

Summary

The TruView EVO is a newly developed and promising optical laryngoscope that allows the operator to see and intubate the larynx with less applied vertical force and without having a direct line of sight. Although the device appears similar to a standard laryngoscope, the technique is quite different due to the requirement of standing away from the patient and directing the ETT toward structures that are visualized through the viewing port, rather than directly in the line of sight. The decreased field of view may also increase the difficulty to navigate toward the glottic structures. Overall, the EVO provides an alternative to direct laryngoscopy, especially for patients with a known anterior airway or cervical spine injury, by allowing the operator to perform intubation without direct line of sight.

CONCLUSION

These two devices both capitalize on optics to improve glottic view without requiring a direct line of sight from outside the patient's mouth, and so share many of the advantages of the more expensive video and fiberoptic systems. Although the two devices appear to perform well in limited testing, there are no published studies of their use in emergency or difficult airway situations. As we acquire further knowledge and experience related to these devices, their strengths, limitations, and role in emergency airway management will become better elucidated.

EVIDENCE

1. **Is the Airtraq device easy to learn?** There are currently no literature-based evaluations for the Airtraq device for emergency patients. Studies in elective anesthesia patients show significant promise, however. In a study of 60 elective anesthesia patients, the Airtraq was compared to direct laryngoscopy using a MacIntosh blade. All patients in the Airtraq group and all but one in the MacIntosh group were intubated on the first attempt, but the intubations were scored as more difficult in the MacIntosh group. Time to intubation did not differ between the groups. Anesthetists rated the Airtraq easier to use than the MacIntosh laryngoscope (mean scores of 1.2 vs. 2.0 on a 0–10 visual analog scale) (1). The same investigators, in a subsequent study, evaluated the Airtraq versus the MacIntosh laryngoscope in 40 elective surgical patients with manual inline stabilization (2). The Airtraq provided superior laryngeal views and shorter intubation times, and was rated as easier to use by anesthesiologists who had used both instruments.
2. **What is the role of the EVO in emergency intubations?** There are currently no literature-based evaluations for the TruView EVO for emergency patients. There are several studies for routine intubations and case series of patients with difficult airways within a controlled setting. Further research is needed to evaluate the utility of this device for intubation of emergency department patients.

REFERENCES

1. Maharaj CH, O'Croinin D, Curley G, et al. A comparison of tracheal intubation using the Airtraq or the Macintosh laryngoscope in routine airway management: a randomised, controlled clinical trial. *Anaesthesia* 2006;61:1093–1099.
2. Maharaj CH, Buckley E, Harte BH, et al. Endotracheal intubation in patients with cervical spine immobilization: a comparison of Macintosh and Airtraq laryngoscopes. *Anesthesiology* 2007;107:53–59.

16

Surgical Airway Techniques

Robert J. Vissers and Aaron E. Bair

INTRODUCTION

Surgical airway management is defined as the creation of an airway by an invasive technique. All other methods of airway management use existing anatomical portals of access to the trachea (i.e., nasopharynx, oropharynx). Surgical airway management involves the creation of an opening to the trachea by surgical means. This opening is then used to provide ventilation and oxygenation. There is some confusion engendered by use of the term *surgical airway management*. In some discussions, surgical airway management includes both cricothyrotomy and needle cricothyrotomy with percutaneous transtracheal ventilation (PTV). Other discussions limit surgical airway management to cricothyrotomy, and consider PTV to be simply another airway management technique. For the purposes of discussion in this chapter, surgical airway management is deemed to include cricothyrotomy, PTV, and placement of a surgical airway using a cricothyrotome, which is a device intended to place a surgical airway percutaneously, usually in one or two steps, without performance of formal cricothyrotomy. The cricothyrotomes may be considered as an alternative to cricothyrotomy; however, cricothyrotomes that place an uncuffed tube do not protect the airway.

PTV through a catheter is rarely, if ever, done in adults. It does not protect the airway and is grossly inferior to cricothyrotomy in terms of both airway protection and gas exchange. In adults, cricothyrotomy by open or Seldinger technique is preferred. PTV should be reserved for children younger than 12 years, whose anatomy is not conducive to cricothyrotomy. The faculty of The Difficult Airway Course: Emergency recently designed a kit that offers the instruments and equipment to perform either the Seldinger percutaneous cricothyrotomy or an open cricothyrotomy, using a cuffed tube for both methods (Melker Universal Emergency Cricothyrotomy Catheter Set, Cook Critical Care, Bloomington, IN; Fig. 16-1). Each main surgical airway technique is described in detail in the sections that follow.

Description

Cricothyrotomy is the establishment of a surgical opening in the airway through the cricothyroid membrane and placement of a cuffed tracheostomy tube or endotracheal tube (ETT).

A cricothyrotome is a kit or device that is intended to establish a surgical airway without resorting to formal cricothyrotomy. These kits use two basic approaches. One approach relies on the Seldinger technique, in which the airway is accessed via a small needle through which a flexible guide wire is passed. The airway device, with a dilator, is then passed over this guide wire and into the airway in a manner analogous with that of central line placement by the Seldinger technique. The other technique relies on the direct percutaneous placement of an airway device without the use of a Seldinger technique. There have been no clinical studies to date demonstrating the superiority of one approach over another or of any of these devices over formal surgical cricothyrotomy. However, certain attributes of the devices make them intuitively more, or less, hazardous for insertion (see the *Evidence* section).

Indications and Contraindications

The primary indication for cricothyrotomy is when a failed airway has occurred (see Chapter 2) and the patient cannot be adequately ventilated or oxygenated with a bag and mask, or the patient is adequately oxygenated, but there is not another available device (e.g., fiberoptic scope, lighted stylet, intubating laryngeal mask airway [LMA]) that is believed likely to successfully secure the airway. A second indication is a method of primary airway management in patients for whom intubation is contraindicated or believed to be impossible. Thus, cricothyrotomy should be thought of as a rescue technique in most circumstances, and only infrequently will it be used as the primary method of airway management. An example of a circumstance in which cricothyrotomy is the primary method of airway management is the patient with severe

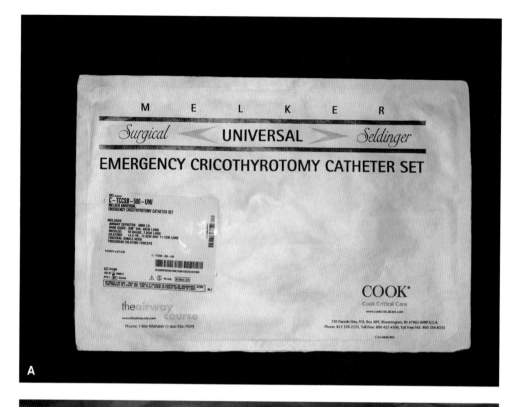

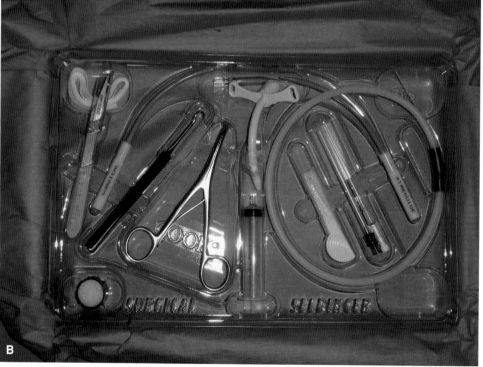

Figure 16-1 ● **A:** Melker Universal Emergency Cricothyrotomy Catheter Set (Cook Critical Care, Bloomington, IN). **B:** Opened set containing cuffed tracheostomy tube, as well as equipment for both open surgical and Seldinger techniques.

lower facial trauma in whom access through the mouth or nose would be too time consuming or impossible. This patient requires immediate airway management because of the risk of aspiration of blood and secretions, and cricothyrotomy is indicated.

The primary hurdle to performing cricothyrotomy is simply recognizing when it is necessary to proceed with surgical airway management, and abandoning further attempts at laryngoscopy, or the use of an alternative device. Rapid sequence intubation (RSI), augmented by a variety of noninvasive airway management methods, is so successful that cricothyrotomy is often viewed as a method of last resort, to be undertaken only after multiple noninvasive attempts or techniques have failed. However, the relentless, unsuccessful, pursuit of a noninvasive airway, along with the resultant delay in the initiation of a surgical airway, can readily result in hypoxic disaster. This fact is particularly true in the "*can't intubate, can't oxygenate*" (CICO) circumstance, when surgical airway management is immediately indicated and must not be delayed for attempts using other devices.

Once the decision to initiate surgical airway management has been made, there are a few fundamental considerations:

a. Will accessing the cricothyroid membrane be *effective*? In other words, will an incision at the level of the cricothyroid membrane bypass the obstruction and solve the problem? If the obstructing lesion is significantly distal to the cricothyroid membrane, performing a cricothyrotomy is a critical waste of time (see Chapter 36).

b. Will the patient's anatomy or pathological process make cricothyrotomy *difficult* to perform? Placement of the initial skin incision is based on palpating the pertinent anatomy. If adiposity, burns, trauma, or infection make this procedure difficult, then the strategy should be adjusted accordingly. A mnemonic for difficult cricothyrotomy (SHORT) is shown in Box 16-1 and is discussed in Chapter 7.

c. Which *type* of invasive technique will most readily be used (i.e., open surgical or percutaneous)? This consideration takes into account provider preference based on previous experience and equipment availability.

Contraindications to surgical airway management are few and, with one exception, are relative. That one exception is young age. Children have a small, pliable, mobile larynx and cricoid cartilage, making cricothyrotomy extremely difficult. For children younger than 12 years, unless they are teenage or adult size, PTV should be used as the surgical airway management technique of choice (see Chapters 21 and 22). Relative contraindications include preexisting laryngeal or tracheal pathology such as tumor, infections, or abscess in the area in which the procedure will be performed; hematoma or other anatomical destruction of the landmarks that would render the procedure difficult or impossible; coagulopathy; and lack of operator expertise. Cricothyrotomy has been performed successfully after systemic thrombolytic therapy. Cricothyrotomy has a high success rate when performed in the emergency department (ED) setting. The presence of an anatomical barrier, in particular, should prompt consideration of alternative techniques that might result in a successful airway. However, in cases in which no alternative method of airway management is likely to be successful or timely enough, cricothyrotomy should be performed without hesitation. The same principles apply for both the cricothyrotome and for PTV.

BOX 16-1 SHORT Mnemonic for Difficult Cricothyrotomy

Surgery (history of neck surgery, presence of surgical scar)
Hematoma
Obesity
Radiation (history or evidence of radiation therapy)
Trauma (direct laryngeal trauma with disrupted landmarks)

PTV is not contraindicated in small children and, in fact, is the surgical airway method of choice for children younger than 12 years. The cricothyrotomes have not been demonstrated to improve success rates or time or to decrease complication rates when compared with surgical cricothyrotomy. As with formal cricothyrotomy, experience, skill, knowledge of anatomy, and adherence to proper technique are essential for success when a cricothyrotome is used.

TECHNIQUE

Anatomy and Landmarks

The cricothyroid membrane is the anatomical site of access in the emergent surgical airway, regardless of the technique used. It has several advantages over the trachea in the emergent setting. The cricothyroid membrane is more anterior than the lower trachea, and there is less soft tissue between the membrane and the skin. There is less vascularity and less chance of significant bleeding.

The cricothyroid membrane is identified by first locating the laryngeal prominence (notch) of the thyroid cartilage. Approximately one fingerbreadth below the laryngeal prominence, the membrane may be palpated in the midline of the anterior neck, as a soft depression between the inferior aspect of the thyroid cartilage above and the hard cricoid ring below. The relevant anatomy may be easier to appreciate in males because of the more prominent thyroid notch. The thyrohyoid space, which lies above the laryngeal prominence, and the hyoid bone, which resides high in the neck, should also be identified. This will prevent the misidentification of the thyrohyoid membrane as the cricothyroid membrane, which would lead to misplacement of the tracheostomy tube above the vocal cords. In children, the cricothyroid membrane is disproportionately smaller because of a greater overlap of the thyroid cartilage over the cricoid cartilage. For this reason, cricothyrotomy is not recommended in children age 12 years or younger.

Unfortunately, the same anatomical or physiological abnormalities (i.e., trauma, morbid obesity, congenital anomalies) that necessitated the surgical airway may also hinder easy palpation of landmarks. One way of estimating the location of the cricothyroid membrane is by placing four fingers on the neck, oriented longitudinally, with the small finger in the sternal notch. The membrane is approximately located under the index finger and can serve as a point at which the initial incision is made. Except as described later in the technique for the rapid four-step cricothyrotomy, a vertical skin incision is preferred, and particularly so if anatomical landmarks are not readily apparent. Palpation through this vertical incision can then confirm the location of the cricothyroid membrane. Alternatively, identification may be assisted by using a locator needle, attached to a syringe containing saline or lidocaine. Aspiration of air bubbles suggests entry into the airway, but it will not distinguish between the cricothyroid membrane and a lower tracheal placement.

The No-drop Technique

The cricothyrotomy instrument set should be simple, consisting of only the equipment necessary to complete the procedure. A sample listing of recommended contents of a cricothyrotomy tray is shown in Box 16-2. Commercial kits are now available that also contain the instruments required for a cricothyrotomy (Fig. 16-1).
   (1) *Identify the landmarks.* The cricothyroid membrane is identified using the landmarks described previously (Fig. 16-2).
   (2) *Prepare the neck.* If time permits, apply appropriate antiseptic solution. Local anesthesia is desirable if the patient is conscious. Infiltration of the skin and subcutaneous tissue of the anterior neck with 1% lidocaine solution will provide adequate anesthesia. If time permits and the patient is conscious and responsive, anesthetize the airway by

---

BOX 16-2 Recommended Contents of Cricothyrotomy Tray

Trousseau dilator
Tracheal hook
Scalpel with no. 11 blade
Cuffed, nonfenestrated, no. 4 tracheostomy tube
Optional equipment: several 4 × 4 gauze sponges, two small hemostats, and surgical
  drapes

---

injecting lidocaine by transcricothyroid membrane puncture (see Chapter 8). The patient
will cough briefly, but the airway will be reasonably anesthetized and further cough
reflexes suppressed.

(3) *Immobilize the larynx.* Throughout the procedure, the larynx must be immobilized
(Fig. 16-3). This is best done by placing the thumb and long finger on opposite sides
of the superior laryngeal horns, the posterior superior aspect of the laryngeal cartilage. With the thumb and long finger thus placed, the index finger is ideally positioned anteriorly to relocate and reidentify the cricothyroid membrane at any time
during the procedure.

(4) *Incise the skin.* A 2-cm vertical midline skin incision should be used (Fig. 16-4). Care
should be taken to avoid cutting the deeper structures of the neck. The cricothyroid

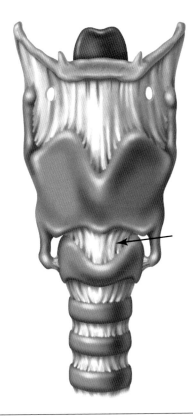

Figure 16-2 ● Anatomy of the Larynx.   The cricothyroid membrane (*arrow*) is bordered above
by the thyroid cartilage and below by the cricoid cartilage.

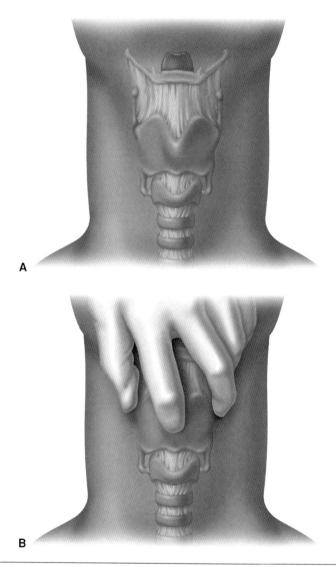

A

B

Figure 16-3 ● **A:** Surface anatomy of the airway. **B:** The thumb and long finger immobilize the superior cornua of the larynx; the index finger is used to palpate the cricothyroid membrane.

membrane is separated from the outside world only by skin, subcutaneous tissue, and anterior cervical fascia. An overly vigorous incision risks damage to the larynx, cricoid cartilage, and the trachea.

(5) *Reidentify the membrane.* With the thumb and long finger maintaining immobilization of the larynx, the index finger can now palpate the anterior larynx, the cricothyroid membrane, and the cricoid cartilage without any interposed skin or subcutaneous tissue (Fig. 16-5). The landmarks thus confirmed, the index finger can be left in the wound by placing it on the inferior aspect of the anterior larynx, thus providing a clear indicator of the superior extent of the cricothyroid membrane.

(6) *Incise the membrane.* The cricothyroid membrane should be incised in a horizontal direction, with an incision at least 1 cm long (Fig. 16-6A). It is recommended to try to incise the lower half of the membrane rather than the upper half because of the

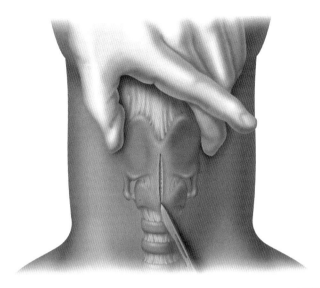

Figure 16-4 ● With the index finger moved to the side but continued firm immobilization of the larynx, a vertical midline skin incision is made, down to the depth of the laryngeal structures.

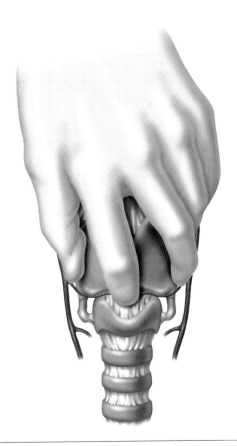

Figure 16-5 ● With skin incised, the index finger can now directly palpate the cricothyroid membrane.

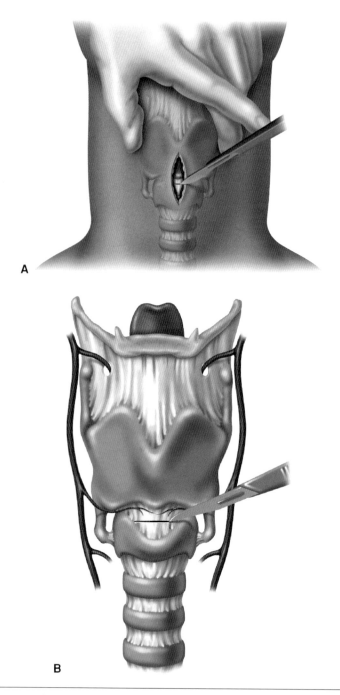

Figure 16-6 ● **A:** A horizontal membrane incision is made near the inferior edge of the cricothyroid membrane. The index finger may be swung aside or may remain in the wound, palpating the inferior edge of the thyroid cartilage, to guide the scalpel to the membrane. **B:** A low cricothyroid incision avoids the superior cricothyroid vessels, which run transversely near the top of the membrane.

relatively cephalad location of the superior cricothyroid artery and vein; however, this may be unrealistic in the emergent setting (Fig. 16-6B).

(7) *Insert the tracheal hook.* The tracheal hook is rotated so that it is oriented in the transverse plane, passed through the incision, and then rotated again so the hook is oriented in a cephalad direction. The hook is then applied to the inferior aspect of the thyroid cartilage, and gentle upward and cephalad traction is applied to bring the airway immediately out to the skin incision (Fig. 16-7). If an assistant is available, this hook may be passed to the assistant to maintain immobilization of the larynx.

(8) *Insert the Trousseau dilator.* The Trousseau dilator may be inserted in one of two ways. One method is to insert the dilator well in through the incision, directing the blades

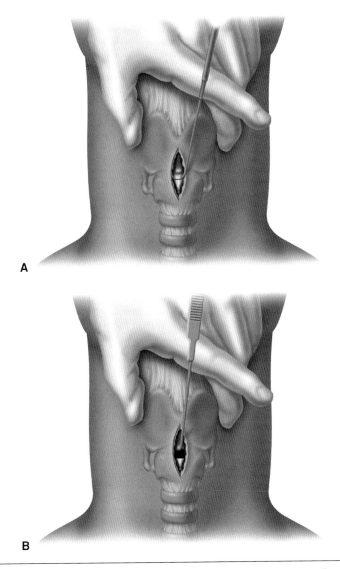

A

B

Figure 16-7 ● **A:** The tracheal hook is oriented transversely during insertion. **B** and **C:** After insertion, cephalad traction is applied to the inferior margin of the thyroid cartilage. (*continued*)

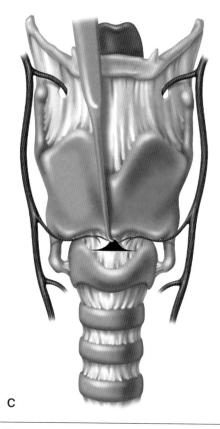

C

Figure 16-7 ● (Continued)

of the dilator longitudinally down the airway. The second method, which is preferred, is to insert the dilator minimally into the anterior wound with the blades oriented superiorly and inferiorly, allowing the dilator to open and enlarge the vertical extent of the cricothyroid membrane incision, which is often the anatomically limiting dimension (Fig. 16-8). When this technique is used, care must be taken not to insert the dilator too deeply into the airway because it will impede subsequent passage of the tracheostomy tube.

(9) *Insert the tracheostomy tube.* The tracheostomy tube, with its inner cannula in situ, is gently inserted through the incision between the blades of the Trousseau dilator. As the tube is advanced gently following its natural curve, the Trousseau dilator is rotated to allow the blades to orient longitudinally in the airway (Fig. 16-9). The tracheostomy tube is advanced until it is firmly seated against the anterior neck. The Trousseau dilator is then carefully removed.

(10) *Inflate the cuff, and confirm tube position.* With the cuff inflated, the tracheostomy tube position can be confirmed by the same methods as the ETT position. Carbon dioxide (CO_2) detection will reliably indicate correct placement of the tube and is mandatory, as for endotracheal intubation. Immediate subcutaneous emphysema with bagging suggests probable paratracheal placement. If doubt remains, rapid insertion of a nasogastric tube through the tracheostomy tube will result in easy passage if the tube is in the trachea and obstruction if the tube has been placed through a false passage into the tissues of the neck. Auscultation of both lungs and

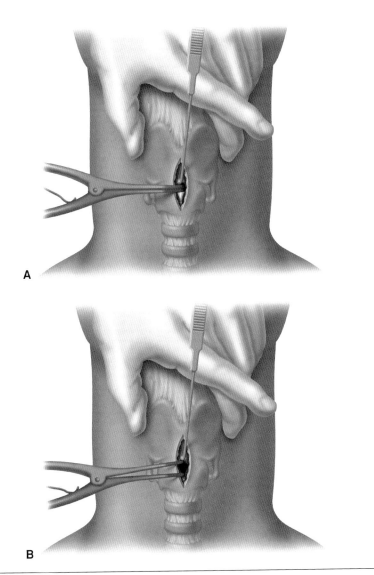

Figure 16-8 ● **A:** The Trousseau dilator is inserted a short distance into the incision. **B:** In this orientation, the dilator enlarges the opening vertically, the crucial dimension.

the epigastric area is also recommended, although esophageal placement of the tracheostomy tube is exceedingly unlikely. Chest radiography should be performed to assist in the assessment of tube placement and to evaluate for the presence of barotrauma.

The Rapid Four-step Technique

This abbreviated cricothyrotomy method has been developed and adopted for training purposes at some centers. As with all techniques, the patient should be maximally oxygenated and, if given sufficient time, the anterior neck may be prepared and locally anesthetized as

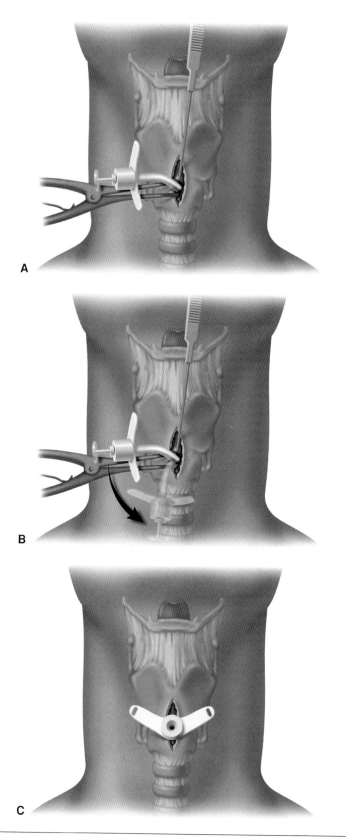

Figure 16-9 ● **A:** Insertion of the tracheostomy tube. **B:** Rotation of the Trousseau dilator to orient the blades longitudinally in the airway facilitates passage of the tracheostomy tube. **C:** Tracheostomy tube fully inserted; instruments removed.

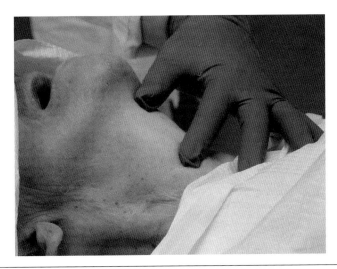

Figure 16-10 ● Palpation: the operator's thumb is on the hyoid bone, while the cricothyroid membrane is identified using the index finger.

for the no-drop method. From a *position at the head of the bed*, the rapid four-step technique for cricothyrotomy proceeds sequentially:

(1) *Palpate and identify landmarks.* The cricothyroid membrane should be identified as described previously (Fig. 16-10). If the key landmarks are unable to be identified by palpation through the soft tissue, then a vertical skin incision is required to permit accurate identification.

(2) *Make skin incision.* Once the pertinent palpable anatomy is identified, the cricothyroid membrane is incised. If the anatomy is fully appreciated through the intact skin, and there is no uncertainty about landmarks or location, then incise the skin and cricothyroid membrane simultaneously with a single horizontal incision of approximately 1.5 cm in length (Fig. 16-11A). For this type of incision, a no. 20 scalpel yields an incision that requires little widening, once used to puncture the skin and cricothyroid membrane. If the anatomy is not readily and unambiguously identified through the skin, then an initial vertical incision should be created to allow more precise palpation of the anatomy and identification of the cricothyroid membrane. In either situation, the cricothyroid membrane is incised with the no. 20 blade that is maintained in the airway, while a tracheal hook (preferably a blunt hook) is placed parallel to the scalpel on the caudad side of the blade (Fig. 16-11B). The hook is then rotated to orient it in a caudad direction to put gentle traction on the cricoid ring. The scalpel is then removed from the airway. At no time during this procedure is the incision left without instrument control of the airway. This detail is particularly important in a scenario where the patient still has the ability to respond or swallow. The newly created stoma could be irretrievably lost if the airway is uncontrolled and moves relative to the skin incision. In addition, as is the case for the no-drop method, this is a technique that relies exclusively on palpation of key structures. Bleeding will inevitably obscure visualization of the anatomy. No time should be wasted using suction or gauze or manipulating the overhead lighting.

(3) *Apply traction.* The tracheal hook that has been rotated caudally and is controlling the cricoid ring is now used to lift the airway toward the skin incision. This action provides modest stoma dilation. The direction of hook pull is reminiscent of the up and

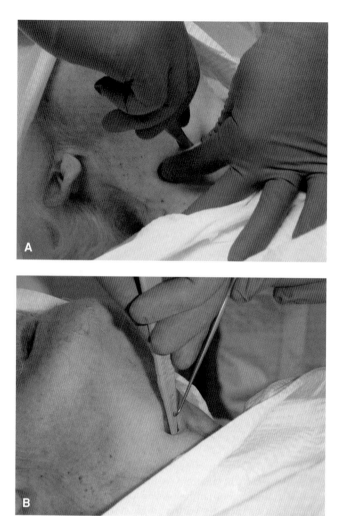

Figure 16-11 ● Incision: **A:** A horizontal incision is initiated while stabilizing the larynx. **B:** Before removing the scalpel from the airway, a hook is placed on the caudal side of the scalpel, parallel to the blade.

away direction used with laryngoscopy (Fig. 16-12). The amount of traction force required for easy intubation (18 newtons or 4.05 pounds force) is significantly lower than the force that is associated with breakage of the cricoid ring (54 newtons or 12.14 pounds force). Use of the hook in this direction generally provides sufficient widening of the incision, and a Trousseau dilator is usually not required. The technique of pulling the airway upward in this way also minimizes the possibility of intubating the pretracheal potential space.

(4) *Intubate.* With adequate control of the airway using the hook placed on the cricoid ring, tracheostomy tube is readily placed into the airway and secured (Fig. 16-13). Confirmation techniques proceed as described in the no-drop technique.

Complications

Because of the common adoption of RSI, cricothyrotomy is infrequently performed in EDs, so reports of complications are difficult to evaluate. In the National Emergency Airway Reg-

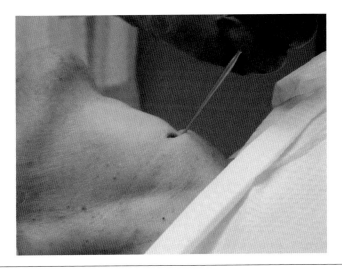

Figure 16-12 ● **Traction:** the hook is applied to the cricoid ring and lifted.

istry (NEAR II) study, less than 1% of more than 7,700 ED intubations involved cricothyrotomy.

The most important complication for the patient in the context of surgical airway management is when delayed decision making after initial intubation failure leads to prolonged, ineffective intubation attempts that result in hypoxic injury. Failure to rapidly place the tracheotomy tube into the trachea or misplacement of the tube into the soft tissues of the neck is more a failure of technique than a complication and must be recognized immediately, as is the case with any misplaced ETT. Complications such as pneumothorax, significant hemorrhage requiring operative intervention, laryngeal or tracheal injury, and long-term complications, such as subglottic stenosis or permanent voice change, are relatively infrequent and usually minor. The potential for these complications to occur in no way outweighs the need to establish the airway. In general, the incidence of all complications, immediate and

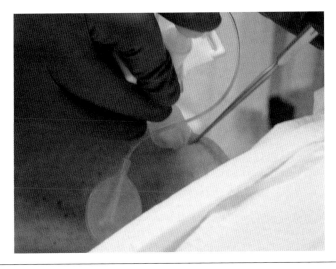

Figure 16-13 ● **Intubation:** the tracheostomy tube is passed into the incision as the hook stabilizes the cricoid ring.

> **BOX 16-3** Complications of Surgical Airway Management
>
> Hemorrhage
> Pneumomediastinum
> Laryngeal/tracheal injury
> Cricoid ring laceration
> Barotrauma (transtracheal jet ventilation)
> Infection
> Voice change
> Subglottic stenosis

delayed, and major or minor, is approximately 20%. Most of these complications are minor, particularly when compared to the consequences of a persistently failed airway. Box 16-3 lists complications of surgical airway management.

Cricothyrotome Technique

Seldinger Technique

Numerous commercial cricothyrotome devices are available. The Melker Universal Emergency Cricothyrotomy Catheter Set uses a modified Seldinger technique to assist in the placement of a tracheal airway (Figs. 16-1 and 16-14A). This method is similar to the one commonly used in the placement of central venous catheters and offers some familiarity to the operator uncomfortable with or inexperienced in the surgical cricothyrotomy technique described previously. Devices that incorporate an inflatable cuff are recommended (Fig. 16-14B).

(1) *Identify landmarks.* The cricothyroid membrane is identified by the method described previously. The nondominant hand is used to control the larynx and maintain identification of the landmarks.

(2) *Prepare neck.* Antiseptic solution is applied to the anterior neck, and, if time permits, infiltration of the site with 1% lidocaine with epinephrine is recommended.

(3) *Insert locator needle.* The locator needle (18-gauge) is then inserted into the cricothyroid membrane in a slightly caudal direction (Fig. 16-14C). The needle is attached to a syringe and advanced with the dominant hand, while negative pressure is maintained on the syringe. The sudden aspiration of air indicates placement of the needle into the tracheal lumen.

(4) *Insert guide wire.* The syringe is then removed from the needle. A soft-tipped guide wire is inserted through the needle into the trachea in a caudal direction (Fig. 16-14D). The needle is then removed, leaving the wire in place. Control of the wire must be maintained at all times.

(5) *Incise skin.* A small skin incision is then made adjacent to the wire. This facilitates passage of the airway device through the skin (Fig. 16-14E). Alternatively, the skin incision may be made vertically over the membrane before insertion of the needle and guide wire.

(6) *Insert the airway and dilator.* The airway catheter (3–6 mm internal diameter [ID]) with an internal dilator in place is inserted over the wire into the trachea (Fig. 16-14F). If resistance is met, the skin incision should be deepened and a gentle twisting motion applied to the airway device (Fig. 16-14G). When the airway device is firmly seated in the trachea, the wire and dilator are removed together (Fig. 16-14H).

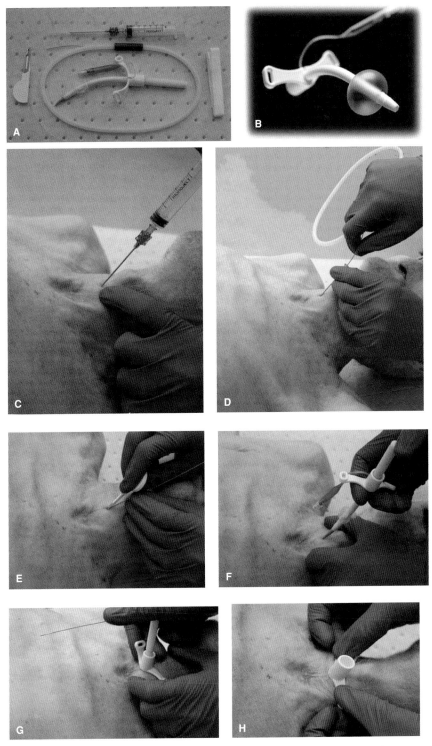

Figure 16-14 ● **A:** Kit contents. **B:** Cuffed tube. **C:** Needle insertion. **D:** Wire placement through needle. **E:** Small incision. **F:** Airway with dilator inserted with wire guidance. **G:** Airway inserted to the hub using a gentle twisting motion. **H:** Wire and dilator removed as one. (Melker Universal Cricothyrotomy Kit, Cook Critical Care, Bloomington, IN.)

(7) *Confirm tube location.* If the device has a cuff, inflate it at this time. Tube location can then be confirmed as for surgical cricothyrotomy, including mandatory end-tidal CO_2 detection. The devices are radiopaque on radiographs. The airway must then be secured properly.

Direct Airway Placement Devices

Several direct airway devices (e.g., Nu-Trake, Pertrach) are commercially available. These generally involve multiple steps in the insertion, using a large device that functions as both introducer and airway. The details of the operation of these devices may be obtained from the manufacturer and are provided as inserts with the kits. These devices offer no clear advantage in technique, are rarely (if ever) as easily placed as is claimed, and are considered more likely to cause traumatic complications during their insertion than those that use a Seldinger technique, primarily because of the cutting characteristics of the airway device. In particular, cricothyrotomes recommended for children should be approached with extreme caution and are not recommended.

Percutaneous Transtracheal Jet Ventilation Technique

Needle cricothyrotomy with percutaneous transtracheal jet ventilation (TTJV) is a surgical airway that may be used to temporize in the CICO situation, particularly in children. Although TTJV is rarely performed in the emergency setting, it is a simple, relatively effective means of supporting oxygenation. Advantages of this technique over cricothyrotomy may include speed, a simpler technique, and less bleeding. It can also provide an alternative for operators unable to perform a cricothyrotomy. Age is not a contraindication to TTJV, which is the surgical airway of choice for children younger than 12 years (see Chapters 20–22).

Several other aspects of this technique that differ from cricothyrotomy are important to consider. To provide ventilation, supraglottic patency must be maintained to allow for exhalation. In the case of complete upper-airway obstruction, air stacking from TTJV will cause barotrauma; therefore, cricothyrotomy is preferable. Another significant difference is that the catheter in TTJV does not provide airway protection. Also, suctioning cannot adequately be performed through the percutaneous catheter. TTJV has been associated with a significant incidence of barotrauma and is less commonly used as a rescue device, particularly with the widespread use of other devices such as the LMA. TTJV is therefore best considered a temporizing means of rescue oxygenation until a more definitive airway can be obtained.

a. **Procedure**

(1) *Identify the landmarks.* The anatomy and landmarks used in needle cricothyrotomy are identical to those described previously for a surgical cricothyrotomy. If there are no contraindications, the head of the patient should be extended. Placing a towel under the shoulders may facilitate cervical hyperextension. The area overlying the cricothyroid membrane should be prepared with an antiseptic solution and, if time permits, anesthetized with 1% lidocaine and epinephrine.

(2) *Immobilize the larynx.* Use the thumb and the middle fingers of the nondominant hand to stabilize the larynx and cricoid cartilage while the index finger palpates the cricothyroid membrane. It is essential to maintain control of the larynx throughout the procedure.

(3) *Insert transtracheal needle.* A large-bore intravenous (IV) catheter (12–16 gauge) is attached to a 20-mL syringe, which may be empty or partially filled with a clear liquid. A 15-degree angle can be created by bending the needle/catheter combination 2.5 cm from the distal end of the IV catheter, or a commercially available catheter can be employed (Fig. 16-15A). A commercial catheter may be preferred because it is reinforced with wire coils to prevent kinking (Fig. 16-16). The dominant hand holds the syringe with the needle directed caudally in the long axis of the trachea at a 30-degree angle to the skin (Fig. 16-15B). While maintaining negative pressure on

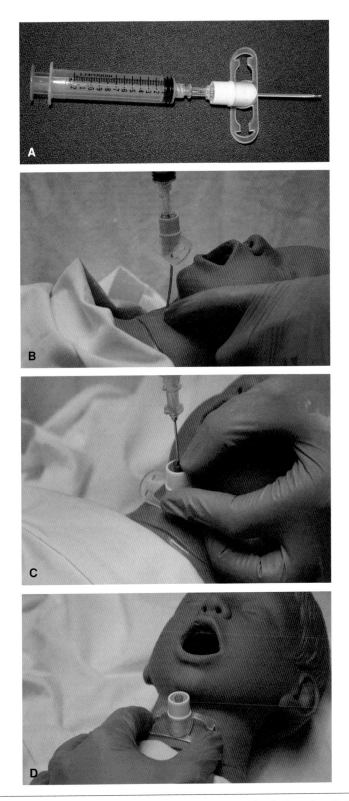

Figure 16-15 ● **A:** Nonkinking catheter for jet ventilation. **B:** Needle insertion. **C:** Removal of needle. **D:** Tracheotomy catheter placed. (*continued*)

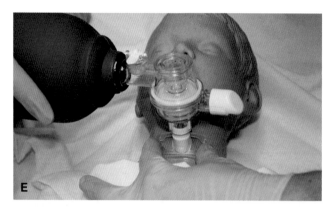

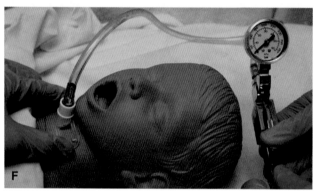

Figure 16-15 ● **(Continued)** **E:** Oxygenation with bag. **F:** Oxygenation with jet ventilator. (Acutronic, Germany).

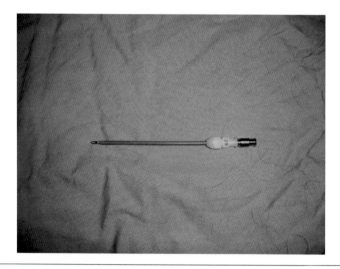

Figure 16-16 ● Nonkinkable wire-coiled transtracheal jet ventilation catheter (Cook Critical Care, Bloomington, IN).

the syringe, the needle is inserted through the cricothyroid membrane into the trachea. As soon as the needle enters the trachea, the syringe will easily fill with air. If a liquid is used, bubbles will appear. Any resistance implies that the catheter remains in the tissue. In the awake patient, lidocaine may be used in the syringe and then injected into the tracheal lumen to suppress the cough reflex.

(4) *Advance catheter.* Once entry into the trachea is confirmed, the catheter can be advanced. The needle may be partially or completely withdrawn before advancement; however, the needle should not be advanced with the catheter. A small incision can assist with catheter advancement if there is resistance at the skin (Fig. 16-14C and D).

(5) *Confirm location.* The catheter should be advanced to the hub and controlled by hand at all times. Air should be reaspirated to confirm once again the location of the catheter within the trachea.

(6) *Connect to bag or jet ventilation.* The catheter may be connected to a bag ventilator using a pre-existing adapter, or if there is only a Luer lock present, the adapter from a 3-0 pediatric ETT will fit the Luer lock (Fig. 16-15E). For jet ventilation, the catheter is connected to the female end of the tubing of the jet ventilation system by a Luer lock. The hub should not be secured in place by anything other than a human hand until a definitive airway is established (Fig. 16-15F). Firm, constant pressure must be applied by hand to ensure that proper positioning is maintained and to create a seal at the skin to minimize air leak.

(7) *Perform jet ventilation.* In the adult, the jet ventilation system should be connected to an oxygen source of 50 pounds per square inch (psi) with a continuously adjustable regulator to allow the pressure to be titrated so the lowest effective pressure (often about 30 psi) required to safely deliver a tidal volume is used. In general, inspiration is less than 1 second followed by 3 seconds of expiration. Because the gas flow through a 14-gauge needle at 50 psi is 1,600 mL/second, less than 1 second of inspiratory time is required for an adequate tidal volume in a normally compliant lung. Exhalation depends on the elastic recoil of the lung, which is a relatively low driving pressure. Therefore. the recommended inspiratory-to-expiratory ratio (I:E) is 1:3. It is important to maintain upper-airway patency to allow for exhalation and avoid air trapping and barotrauma. All patients should have an oral and nasal airway placed. For small adults and children, oxygen pressure should be downregulated to less than 20 to 30 psi, if possible. For children younger than 5 years, a bag should be used for ventilation, connected to the catheter using the ETT adapter from a 3.0-mm-ID ETT.

b. **Equipment**

(1) *Transtracheal catheters.* A large-bore IV catheter is acceptable. The proper placement is made easier by placing a small angle 2.5 cm from the tip. Commercially available devices include precurved (Acutronic, Germany) and nonkinkable wire-coiled (Cook Critical Care, Bloomington, IN) catheters (Figs. 16-15A and 16-16). The wire-coiled catheter will not kink when bent; therefore, it provides a more secure airway.

(2) *Transtracheal jet ventilation systems.* The TTJV system consists of a high-pressure oxygen source (usually central wall oxygen pressure of 50 psi), high-pressure oxygen tubing, a regulator to control the driving pressure, an on-off valve to control inspiratory time, high-pressure tubing, and a Luer lock to connect to the catheter (Fig. 16-17).

A regulator to control the driving pressure is optional but recommended. This device is particularly useful where barotrauma is a concern and in pediatrics, where the inspiratory pressures should be reduced to less than 20 to 30 psi, if possible. Although a system can be assembled inexpensively from readily available materials, a commercially made, preassembled system is recommended. The reliability and control inherent in the commercial devices are well worth the marginal increase in cost.

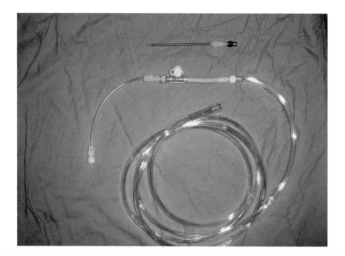

Figure 16-17 • Disposable jet ventilator system with high-pressure oxygen tubing, on-off valve, and PVC tubing with Luer lock. Note that this device does not include a pressure regulator (Cook Critical Care, Bloomington, IN).

A TTJV system can also be connected to a low-flow portable oxygen tank when circumstances require mobility. When the flow is set at the maximal 15 L/minute and no flow is allowed, the pressure temporarily increases to 120 psi. Once flow is released, high flow occurs momentarily and then rapidly decreases to the steady state of 5 to 10 psi. Adequate tidal volumes may be achieved through a 14-gauge catheter in the first 0.5 second. A shorter I:E ratio of 1:1 is recommended.

Another setup using manual ventilation with a self-inflating reservoir bag has been described, using standard equipment found in any ED. Bag ventilation may be connected directly to the percutaneous transtracheal catheter in two ways. The male end of a 15-mm ETT adapter from a 3-mm-ID ETT will fit directly into the catheter. Alternatively, the male end of a plungerless 3-mL syringe will fit into the catheter, and the male end of an 8-mm-ID ETT adapter will then insert into the female end of the empty syringe. Ventilation is temporary at best, and partial arterial CO_2 pressure ($PaCO_2$) will increase at a rate 2 to 4 mm Hg/minute. Even the simple assembly of this system is too time consuming to be done during the event, so it must be preassembled. This arrangement may have particular utility in the pediatric patient younger than 5 years when excessive pressures may be delivered via a TTJV device, even when a regulator to control inspiratory pressures is available. In general, children younger than 5 years should receive TTV via a ventilation bag; ages 5 to 12 years old at less than 30 mm Hg and older than 12 years to adult at 30 to 50 mm Hg. A catheter of less than 3 mm ID will be insufficient to adequately ventilate/oxygenate the adult patient using a bag, and 50 psi pressurized oxygen is required.

  c. **Complications specific to transtracheal jet ventilation**
   • Subcutaneous emphysema
   • Barotrauma
   • Reflex cough with each ventilation (may be aborted with lidocaine)
   • Catheter kinking
   • Obstruction from blood or mucus
   • Esophageal puncture
   • Mucosal damage if nonhumidified gas is used

TIPS AND PEARLS

Surgical airway management is rarely the method of first choice for patients requiring emergency airway management. However, there is a population of patients for whom surgical airway management will literally make the difference between life and death. Therefore, emergency physicians and others who provide care for patients requiring emergency airway management must be proficient with surgical airway management.

There may be little advantage to using a cricothyrotome rather than a formal, surgical cricothyrotomy set. Time of performance of the procedure, complication rates, degree of difficulty, and success rates are all comparable between the two methods. Of the available cricothyrotomes, those that use the Seldinger technique and use a cuffed tube are preferable. Personal preference should also guide selection. A new kit offers all instruments and equipment to perform both the Seldinger-based cricothyrotome insertion and a formal, open, cricothyrotomy by either the standard "no-drop" or rapid four-step technique (Melker Universal Emergency Cricothyrotomy Catheter Set, Cook Critical Care, Bloomington, IN; Fig. 16-1). There is no evidence that any cricothyrotome can be placed in a child younger than 10 to 12 years of age with acceptable success and safety, regardless of the design of the device or the claims of the manufacturer.

PTV is virtually never indicated in the adult patient. In adults, establishment of a more functional surgical airway using a cricothyrotome or by formal cricothyroidotomy is vastly preferable. However, PTV remains a useful temporizing measure. In children younger than 12 years, the opposite is true. In this age group, PTV is the primary surgical airway management method of choice, and cricothyrotomy and cricothyrotomes should be avoided. Despite the extreme infrequency of use of PTV in the ED, it is important to have a PTV set readily available and to be familiar with how to connect and use it. The wire-coiled catheter designed for TTJV is preferable to standard IV catheters because of the tendency for the latter to kink.

Of the methods described in this chapter, only a formal surgical cricothyrotomy and variations of the recently modified Melker set result in the placement of a cuffed tube within the trachea. The other techniques described here must be considered temporary at best. Placement of a tracheostomy tube or ETT through a formal surgical cricothyrotomy incision results in an airway that can be used as a definitive airway for the patient.

The no. 4 cuffed tracheostomy tube, which has an inside diameter of 5 mm, should be used for virtually all cases of adult cricothyrotomy in the ED. The tube is of adequate size to provide ventilation in virtually all circumstances, and its outside dimensions are such that it will almost always be easily inserted. For very large adult men, a no. 6 can be used.

EVIDENCE

1. **Which technique is best?** There is almost no literature that effectively compares different techniques of invasive surgical airway management. The relatively rare performance of an emergency surgical airway, compounded with the urgency of the circumstance, may explain the absence of any controlled clinical trials comparing techniques in the emergency setting. Comorbid injuries or illnesses often preclude long-term assessment of sequelae, and the few studies performed do not compare or identify specific invasive techniques (1). As such, the current level of evidence for or against a particular technique exists as expert consensus based on collective experience, limited descriptive series, or studies in cadaveric and animal models (2–10).

Several studies have directly compared the percutaneous, wire-guided technique to the traditional open, or no-drop, technique in cadavers (11–13). Eisenberger et al. (11), studying the performance of intensive care trainees, and Chan et al. (12), in a similar study of emergency residents and attendings, compared the two techniques in randomized, cross-over studies and found no difference in times to completion between groups. Immediate complications were also similar. Interestingly, the majority of participants in Chan's study stated a preference for the percutaneous, wire-guided technique (12).

2. **Rapid four-step or no-drop technique for open cricothyrotomy?** Each approach has its proponents. The no-drop technique has been in use for decades and has withstood the test of time. The rapid four-step technique (RFST) is proposed to be an improvement over the no-drop technique based on the following:

   a. The rapid four-step technique requires only one person to perform the procedure. Ideally, the no-drop technique requires *two* people (i.e., one operator and one assistant). The assistant is responsible for not dropping the tracheal hook as it stabilizes the trachea. Without an assistant, the operator must maintain the no-drop approach with the Trousseau dilator while inserting the tube; not a desirable circumstance.

   b. The rapid four-step technique can be readily performed from the head of the bed without having to move to the patient's side, where the operator is best positioned for the no-drop technique.

   c. The rapid four-step technique requires only a simple hook and a scalpel, which may be available even in the absence of a formal cricothyrotomy kit. This is a minimal advantage because the standard cricothyrotomy kit is also simple containing only three basic instruments (scalpel, hook, and dilator).

   There are no controlled human trials comparing these approaches; however, case series suggest RFST is an acceptable approach in the emergency setting (10,14,15). In a randomized, cross-over, cadaveric study comparing the two techniques, Holmes et al. (16) found the RFST to be significantly faster (43 seconds vs. 134 seconds, $p <$.001), without a significant difference in immediate complications. In a similar study, Davis et al. (17) also found the RFST to be faster.

   Potential disadvantages of the rapid four-step technique.

   a. The RFST relies on a single, relatively small incision to hasten the placement of the ETT. Although literature exists that supports the routine use of this technique, the location of the initial incision is of critical importance (10,14,15). Most of the reported complications related to the RFST in patients have been related to the initial incision being made too small and then requiring time-consuming revision of the incision (10). If the initial incision is misplaced or initially made too small and subsequently requires revision, then any proposed time-saving advantage is lost.

   b. Concerns over a possible higher incidence of cricoid ring damage and esophageal perforation have been raised, but larger studies are needed to determine whether this possibility is real (16,17). The use of a double hook may significantly reduce the potential for cricoid ring injury (17,18).

   Overall, choice of the RFST versus the no-drop method will be made by the operator on the basis of training, experience, and judgment, and either approach is acceptable, each having some advantages and disadvantages and neither being clearly superior.

3. **Can a procedure done so rarely be taught, retained, and used successfully?** Ultimately, any discussion of the technical merits of a procedure will be irrelevant if hesitancy on the part of the provider results in significant delay in establishing a definitive airway. Fortunately, this potential hesitancy is readily overcome by technical proficiency. Anyone responsible for emergency airway management should choose

an invasive method, learn it, and practice it at regular intervals to maintain proficiency.

Recent articles regarding the popularity and success of RSI have prompted editorials concerned with the current problem of gaining and maintaining competency in invasive airway management (19–21). Retrospective studies suggest a current cricothyrotomy rate of approximately 1% of all emergency airways. The reasons for this low incidence have been attributed to emergency medicine training, the success of RSI, and reduced transport rate for blunt traumatic arrests (19,21). Regardless of the cause, this incidence is believed to be too low to ensure adequate training, yet highlights the probability that all emergency physicians will be called on to perform an invasive airway at some point in their career.

To address this issue, some authors have advocated the performance of invasive airway techniques on the newly dead (22). Many physicians have received cricothyrotomy and endotracheal intubation training on the recently deceased without consent from the family. This practice, however, has raised ethical concerns and is no longer considered an acceptable practice at many institutions. Olsen et al. (23) studied the feasibility of obtaining family consent for teaching cricothyrotomy on the newly dead in the ED. Consent was obtained for postmortem cricothyrotomy in 20 of 51 deaths (39%) in a large teaching hospital over a 7-month period. It is unclear how feasible this approach would be in other settings, but it does represent a potential opportunity to practice in a way that most closely approximates the true anatomy.

To ensure familiarity with the equipment and technique, it is likely that practice must occur outside the clinical setting. Koppel and Reed (24) reported that although 80% of anesthesiology programs instruct their residents on cricothyrotomies, 60% use lectures only, a poor teaching technique for developing proficiency in manual skills. One study attempted to determine the minimum training required to perform cricothyrotomy in 40 seconds or less in a manikin. One hundred and two physicians performed 10 procedures, and by the fifth attempt, 96% plateaued in their success (25).

There are no studies that have identified the optimal interval between training episodes for retention, although one small report suggested increased retention when repeated monthly versus every 3 months (26). Studies in cadavers performed primarily to compare different techniques have also identified a similarly rapid learning curve; however, the time to procedure completion was greater (73–102 seconds) (11,13).

There are no studies examining the clinical correlation of these training techniques; however, the high success rates of emergency cricothyrotomies suggest that retention and application have occurred. Based on the limited available literature, we make the following recommendations regarding the learning and retention of invasive airway techniques:

a. Identify a preferred method of invasive airway management to learn; select one that is immediately available to you.
b. Practice the technique one to two times per year on live animal models, animal tracheas, patient simulators, or manikins, depending on availability.
c. Practice the procedure five times at each training session.
d. When appropriate, consider requesting consent for cricothyrotomy on the newly dead.

Tracheas may be ordered from a slaughter house at relatively low cost, and the technique may be attempted multiple times on each specimen. Simulators represent a significant purchase cost; however, they are useful for training multiple critical skills and are increasingly commonly available at teaching institutions because prices have become much lower. Models specifically for cricothyrotomy training are also available. Live animal models and cadavers are generally used only in formal residency training sessions and specialized procedural courses because of significant expense and limited access.

4. **Why is it important to acquire and maintain surgical airway skills if invasive airways are employed so infrequently?** Although a surgical airway may be viewed as a rare or desperate recourse by some providers, prompt execution can be absolutely lifesaving. Although required infrequently, and mostly in the setting of trauma, it is still performed in about 1% of ED intubations (9,27,28). Hence, it is likely that a physician responsible for emergency airway management will be called on at some point to provide this potentially lifesaving intervention. However, because it is done infrequently it takes occasional practice to remain comfortable with your chosen technique. In addition, it is important to consider, in advance of the actual clinical circumstance, when to perform an invasive airway. The failed and difficult algorithms help in this regard (see Chapter 2). However, as a rule of thumb, when a CICO airway is encountered, cricothyrotomy is immediately indicated.

5. **When is a surgical airway indicated?** The failed airway algorithm (see Chapter 2) suggests that cricothyrotomy should be a considered, even in a "*can't* intubate, *can* oxygenate" situation, when it is clear that alternative approaches have failed or are judged likely to fail. However, it helps to recognize that a given provider attempting laryngoscopy may have a certain "emotional inertia" when it comes to changing strategies. First, one must recognize that a laryngoscopist may not want to recognize that his or her laryngoscopy has failed. In addition, the hesitancy to perform an infrequently used technique may conspire to tempt the provider to have just "one more look." Such perseveration on a single method of intubation can have disastrous results. In all likelihood, the main complication associated with cricothyrotomy, or other invasive airways, is not doing it soon enough.

6. **Is there a role for surgical airways in the prehospital setting?** Although its use is rare, cricothyrotomy has been widely taught and employed in the prehospital environment. The data are limited but suggest that the technique can be employed in this setting; however, there appears to be higher incidence of complications and poor outcomes compared to the hospital setting (29,30). There are less data on the use of percutaneous cricothyrotomes. Cadaveric studies suggest that this technique may be associated with fewer complications than open cricothyrotomy when used by prehospital providers (31). Field studies for percutaneous cricothyrotomes and needle TTJT are very limited and inconclusive. A recent position paper on the use of alternate airways in the out-of-hospital setting, from the National Association of EMS Physicians (32), also concluded that there is insufficient evidence to either support or refute the need for all agencies to have a surgical airway technique available. If cricothyrotomy is to be used in an emergency medical services system, training, skill retention, individual case review, and systemwide quality management are essential. A field cricothyrotomy might be viewed as analogous to a police officer discharging a firearm. Each event is significant and worthy of thoughtful review.

REFERENCES

1. McGill J, Clinton JE, Ruiz E. Cricothyrotomy in the emergency department. *Ann Emerg Med* 1982;11:361–364.

2. Esses BA, Jafek BW. Cricothyrotomy: a decade of experience in Denver. *Ann Otol Rhinol Laryngol* 1987;96:519–524.

3. Walls RM. Cricothyroidotomy. In: Campbell WH, ed. *Emergency Medicine Clinics of North America*. Philadelphia: WB Saunders; 1988;725–736.

4. Elandson MJ, Clinton JE, Ruiz E, et al. Cricothyrotomy in the emergency department revisited. *J Emerg Med* 1989;7:115–118.

5. DeLaurier GA, Hawkins ML, Treat RC, et al. Acute airway management: role of cricothyroidotomy. *Am Surg* 1990;56:12–15.

6. Salvino CK, Dries D, Gamelli R, et al. Emergency cricothyroidotomy in trauma victims. *J Trauma* 1993;34:503–505.

7. Hawkins ML, Shapiro MB, Cue JI, et al. Emergency cricothyroidotomy: a reassessment. *Am Surg* 1995;61:52–55.

8. Bair AE, Filbin MR, Kulkarni RG, et al. Failed intubation in the emergency department: analysis of prevalence, rescue techniques and personnel. *J Emerg Med* 2002;23:131–140.

9. Bair AE, Panacek EA, Wisner DH, et al. Cricothyrotomy: a 5-year experience at one institution. *J Emerg Med* 2003;24:151–156.

10. Isaacs JH. Emergency cricothyrotomy: long-term results. *Am Surg* 2001;67:346–349.

11. Eisenberger P, Laczika K, List M, et al. Comparison of conventional surgical versus Seldinger technique emergency cricothyrotomy performed by inexperienced clinicians. *Anesthesiology* 2000;92:687–690.

12. Chan TC, Vilke GM, Bramwell KJ, et al. Comparison of wire-guided cricothyrotomy versus standard surgical cricothyrotomy technique. *J Emerg Med* 1999;17:957–962.

13. Johnson DR, Dunlap A, McFeely P, et al. Cricothyrotomy performed by prehospital personnel: a comparison of two techniques in a human cadaver model. *Am J Emerg Med* 1993;11:207–209.

14. Brofeldt BT, Panacek EA, Richards JR. An easy cricothyrotomy approach: the rapid four-step technique. *Acad Emerg Med* 1996;3:1060–1063.

15. Brofeldt BT, Osborn ML, Sakles JC, et al. Evaluation of the rapid four-step cricothyrotomy technique: an interim report. *Air Med J* 1998;17:127–130.

16. Holmes JF, Panacek EA, Sakles JC, et al. Comparison of 2 cricothyrotomy techniques: standard method versus rapid 4-step technique. *Ann Emerg Med* 1998;32:442–447.

17. Davis DP, Bramwell KJ, Hamilton RS, et al. Safety and efficacy of the rapid four-step technique for cricothyrotomy using a Bair claw. *J Emerg Med* 2000;19:125–129.

18. Bair AE, Laurin EG, Karchin A, et al. Cricoid ring integrity: implications for emergent cricothyrotomy. *Ann Emerg Med* 2003;41:333–337.

19. Chang RS, Hamilton RJ, Carter WA. Influence of an emergency medicine residency on the role of cricothyrotomy. *Acad Emerg Med* 1996;3:534.

20. Knopp RK, Waeckerle JF, Callaham ML. Rapid sequence intubation revisited. *Ann Emerg Med* 1998;31:398–400.

21. Chang RS, Hamilton RJ, Carter WA. Declining rate of cricothyrotomy in trauma patients with an emergency medicine residency: implications for skills training. *Acad Emerg Med* 1998;5:247–251.

22. Knopp RK. Practicing cricothyrotomy on the newly dead. *Ann Emerg Med* 1995;25:694–695.

23. Olsen J, Spilger S, Windisch T. Feasibility of obtaining family consent for teaching cricothyrotomy on the newly dead in the emergency department. *Ann Emerg Med* 1995;25:660–665.

24. Koppel J, Reed A. Formal instruction in difficult airway management. *Anesthesiology* 1995;83:1343–1346.

25. Wong DT, Prabhu AJ, Coloma M, et al. What is the minimum training required for successful cricothyrotomy? *Anesthesiology* 2003;98:349–353.

26. Prabhu AJ, Correa R, Wong DT, et al. What is the optimal training interval for a cricothyrotomy? *Can J Anesth* 2001;48:A59.

27. Sagarin MJ, Barton ED, Chng YM, et al. Airway management by U.S. and Canadian emergency medicine residents: a multicenter analysis of more than 6,000 endotracheal intubation attempts. *Ann Emerg Med* 2005;46(4):328–336.

28. Sakles JC, Laurin EG, Rantapoa AA, et al. Airway management in the emergency department: a one-year study of 610 tracheal intubations. *Ann Emerg Med* 1998;31(3):325–332.

29. Bulger EM, Copass MK, Maier RV, et al. An analysis of advanced prehospital airway management. *J Emerg Med* 2002;23(2):183–189.

30. Fortune JB, Judkins DG, Scanzaroli D, et al. Efficacy of prehospital surgical cricothyrotomy in trauma patients. *J Trauma* 1997;42(5):832–836.

31. Keane MF, Brinsfield KH, Dyer KS, et al. A laboratory comparison of emergency percutaneous and surgical cricothyrotomy by prehospital personnel. *Prehosp Emerg Care* 2004;8(4):424–426.

32. O'Connor RE. Alternate airways in the out-of-hospital setting. Position statement of the National Association of EMS Physicians. *Prehosp Emerg Care* 2007;11(1):54–55.

17

Pretreatment Agents

David A. Caro and Stephen Bush

INTRODUCTION

Pretreatment refers to the administration of drugs 3 minutes before the paralysis step of rapid sequence intubation (RSI) in order to diminish adverse effects of laryngoscopy and intubation for certain patients. This concept is based on analysis of the effects of airway manipulation on intracranial pressure (ICP), circulating catecholamines, and bronchial reactivity, among others. The timing of pretreatment agents and a brief overview of their use are provided in Chapter 3. This chapter discusses the effects and mitigation of the various pathophysiological effects of intubation.

During intubation, laryngoscopy and tracheal intubation stimulate sympathetic and parasympathetic nerves innervating the hypopharynx, larynx, and trachea, resulting in a number of predictable physiological responses. In adults, systemic catecholamines are released, causing an increase in mean heart rate (approximately 30/minute), an increase in the mean arterial blood pressure (approximately 20–25 mm Hg), and resultant increases in arterial wall shear stress. Bradycardia, particularly in younger (<1 year old) children, can occur as a manifestation of monosynaptic, parasympathetic reflexes. Laryngoscopy and endotracheal intubation can also cause a rise in ICP, believed to be due to increased oxygen demand resulting from a stimulation or arousal response of the cerebral cortex. Respiratory responses include upper airway reflexes leading to coughing or laryngospasm and lower airway bronchospasm leading to an increase in mean airway pressure.

The mechanisms behind these responses are believed to include 9th and 10th cranial nerves, with stimulation of the brainstem and spinal cord resulting in either sympathetic or parasympathetic stimulation. Sympathetic activation releases norepinephrine from adrenergic nerve terminals and epinephrine from the adrenal glands. The subsequent elevation in blood pressure may be exacerbated by activation of the renin-angiotensin system. Parasympathetic activation can result in bronchoconstriction and airway protective reflexes (cough). The impact on patient outcomes is not clear, but these reactions could worsen the various pathophysiological conditions that mandate the intubation or are present as complicating comorbidities.

A wide variety of pharmacological agents have been studied in an attempt to identify agents that can blunt these reflexes in both elective and emergency airway management. Those most commonly discussed in the emergent setting include lidocaine (lignocaine, Xylocaine), ultra–short-acting opioids such as fentanyl (Sublimaze) and its derivatives, atropine, and defasciculating doses of neuromuscular blocking agents. Of these, lidocaine and the ultra–short-acting opioids have had the most evaluation. Although these drugs may be helpful when given prior to intubation in both elective and emergency airway management, data collection in the setting of emergency RSI is difficult, and so few formal studies have examined the ability of the drugs to mitigate responses or improve outcome in the context of emergency RSI. In previous editions of this manual, we recommended the LOAD mnemonic for pretreatment of emergency patients undergoing RSI. This mnemonic was intended to cue the use of lidocaine, opioid (fentanyl), atropine, and defasciculation in appropriate patients. Based on systematic analysis of prior and new evidence, and direct observation of physicians and other providers applying this mnemonic in thousands of simulated adult and pediatric cases as part of The Difficult Airway Course: Emergency and The Difficult Airway Course: Anesthesia, we have substantially updated our recommendations for pretreatment agents for emergency RSI, the agents to be used, and the patient populations to which they apply (Table 17-1).

Lidocaine blunts reflexive rises in ICP during intubation, and mitigates reactive increases in small and medium-size airways resistance in patients with reactive airways disease who are undergoing intubation. Fentanyl and other ultra–short-acting opioids have been reported to blunt reflexive sympathetic stimulation to laryngoscopy in a dose-related fashion. Control of this sympathetic response reduces the magnitude of the rise in ICP, which can occur as a result of blood pressure increases during laryngoscopy and intubation. Similarly, patients at risk from the adverse effects of a sudden rise in blood pressure, myocardial oxygen demand,

TABLE 17-1
Pretreatment Agent Summary

Drug	Dose	Time to Onset	Duration of action	$T_{1/2}$	Elimination	Special Considerations
Lidocaine	1.5 mg/kg IV	Within 45–90 seconds	10–20 minutes	1.5–2 hours	Metabolism: hepatic (90%) Excretion: renal	Category B in pregnancy Readily crosses the blood–brain barrier and the placenta
Fentanyl	1–3 mcg/kg IV	2–3 minutes	30–60 minutes	Initial: rapid redistribution (<5 minutes); total 7 hours	Metabolism: hepatic (90%) and small intestine Excretion: renal	Certain cytochrome P-450 (CYP) isoenzyme 3A4 inhibitors will prolong action (e.g., macrolides, azoles, protease inhibitors)

or cardiac force of contraction may benefit from reduction of this sympathetic discharge. For example, patients with coronary artery disease; neurovascular events, such as intracranial hemorrhage; or major vascular disease, such as aortic dissection, ideally should not be exposed to the effects of a sudden and significant release of catecholamines.

We no longer advocate the routine use of atropine, which was formerly recommended to prevent bradycardia in children 10 years of age or younger receiving succinylcholine. Our current recommendation in this regard is to administer atropine only if necessary to treat bradycardia when it occurs (after excluding hypoxia as a possible cause). Empiric administration of atropine to children under 1 year old who will be receiving succinylcholine is considered a reasonable (optional) practice (see Chapter 20). Similarly, we formerly recommended defasciculation with a small dose of a competitive neuromuscular blocking agent before succinylcholine was given to patients with suspected elevated ICP. Our current recommendation is that defasciculation not be considered a routine part of emergency RSI. In summary, with respect to atropine and defasciculating drugs, we do not believe that there is sufficient evidence to support a continued recommendation for the routine use of either of these agents.

LIDOCAINE

Lidocaine functions by blocking fast sodium channels in neurons, stopping their ability to depolarize and carry signals. It is an amide anesthetic that is metabolized in the liver and excreted in the urine. A single intravenous (IV) dose does not require adjusting in renal failure patients.

IV lidocaine is absolutely contraindicated in patients with amide anesthetic allergy and in patients with severe heart block or bradycardia unless a pacemaker has been placed. Lidocaine can worsen hypovolemic and cardiogenic shock, and is also relatively contraindicated in Wolff-Parkinson-White syndrome. Box 17-1 shows the drugs for which severe drug interactions have been reported with lidocaine.

Adverse effects include rare central nervous system (CNS) toxicity (seizures, coma) and cardiac conduction abnormalities (severe bradycardia, arrhythmias), and cardiogenic shock when used at high doses. There are good quality data to show that IV lidocaine at a dose of 1.5 mg/kg IV can effectively suppress the cough reflex in humans (see *Evidence* section). This mechanism may be important in patients in whom coughing might be detrimental, including patients with elevated ICP or possibly those with suspected cervical spine injury who are undergoing intubation without neuromuscular blockade. Lidocaine has also been used and recommended widely for its potential to mitigate the ICP response to upper airway manipulation, laryngoscopy, and intubation. This recommendation was based predominantly on the results of older studies of patients with elevated ICP undergoing various airway procedures, including tracheal suctioning and laryngoscopy. The data supporting the use of lidocaine to prevent the ICP rise in response to airway manipulation are conflicting. No studies have directly addressed its use in emergency RSI, and none have used patient outcome as a primary end point (see *Evidence* section). However, we continue to recommend the use of lidocaine for patients with elevated ICP, based on the cough suppression effect, the potential to reduce the ICP response during laryngoscopy and intubation, and the fact that the drug and dosing are safe and commonly used, and therefore unlikely to cause patient harm or lead to medication error. Lidocaine also appears to diminish the reflex bronchospasm that may occur with intubation of patients with reactive airways disease. We believe that the evidence is sufficient to continue to recommend the use of lidocaine as a pretreatment agent in patients with reactive airways disease who are undergoing intubation. The new recommendations for the use of lidocaine as a pretreatment agent for emergency RSI are shown in Box 17-2.

FENTANYL AND OTHER ULTRA–SHORT-ACTING OPIOIDS

Given in sufficiently high doses, most sedative/hypnotic agents will attenuate the reflex sympathetic response to laryngoscopy. However, the drug dose required to produce this degree of CNS depression will usually produce significant hypotension.

Fentanyl (Sublimaze) is an opioid receptor agonist that selectively activates the mu-receptor. It is metabolized in the liver and has first-phase redistribution within 5 minutes, but has an elimination half-life of 7 hours. Fentanyl has a time to onset of 2 to 3 minutes and duration of action of approximately 30 to 60 minutes. It is a class C drug in pregnancy. Major side effects include dose-related respiratory depression and hypotension in patients dependent on sympathetic tone.

Fentanyl attenuates the sympathetic response to laryngoscopy with minimal side effects other than dose-related respiratory depression, which is rarely an issue in the doses used for RSI pretreatment. Fentanyl does not release histamine and has no direct effect on the pulmonary response to laryngoscopy. Fentanyl has been shown to have a partial attenuating effect on the reflex sympathetic response to laryngoscopy at doses as low as 2 mcg/kg IV. Relatively more attenuation is seen at 6 mcg/kg IV, and almost complete attenuation is seen at 11 to 15 mcg/kg IV, a rather large dose usually reserved for patients undergoing general anesthesia for cardiac surgery.

For emergency intubation, fentanyl is recommended in a dose of 3 mcg/kg IV 3 minutes before the induction and paralytic agents for patients who might be adversely affected by a systemic release of catecholamines with the resulting transient, but significant, increase in heart rate, blood pressure, and cardiac force of contraction. Patients with increased ICP are presumed to have lost autoregulation, and, consequently, increases in blood pressure may exacerbate the ICP elevation. Patients with intracranial hemorrhage, ischemic heart disease, known or suspected cerebral or aortic aneurysm, or dissection or rupture of a great vessel are similarly at risk from an acute hypertensive response.

Fentanyl should be given as the last of the pretreatment drugs, over a period of 30 to 60 seconds, to minimize the likelihood of significant respiratory depression. Whenever fentanyl is given, the patient should be closely watched for signs of hypoventilation prior to administration of the sedative and paralytic agents. Because fentanyl is being given precisely to reduce sympathetic tone, caution must be used in the hemodynamically compromised patient who is dependent on sympathetic tone to maintain hemodynamic stability (e.g., compensated or decompensated shock). Fentanyl is not recommended in pediatric RSI because the administration would further complicate the resuscitation, and the benefit for children has not been demonstrated.

Muscle wall rigidity is a unique and idiosyncratic response to opioids and is probably related to the dose and speed of opioid administration, the concomitant use of nitrous oxide, and the presence or absence of muscle relaxants. It is not reversible with naloxone (Narcan). It is usually seen with fentanyl doses well in excess of 500 mcg (0.5 mg) and primarily affects the chest and abdominal wall musculature. The rigidity has rarely been reported in conscious patients. It tends to occur very quickly after the patient begins to lose consciousness. Rigidity has not been reported with the use of fentanyl in the emergency department (ED). Rigidity is abolished by the administration of paralyzing doses of succinylcholine once the abnormality is recognized. Fentanyl is used in low doses for emergency RSI, and it is exceedingly unlikely that any muscle rigidity will occur.

Recommendations for the use of fentanyl as a pretreatment agent for emergency RSI are given in Box 17-3. Three important caveats apply to the use of fentanyl as a pretreatment agent during RSI:

1. Avoid fentanyl pretreatment if the patient is in compensated or decompensated shock, or minimally hemodynamically stable and dependent on sympathetic drive.
2. Be prepared for dose-related respiratory depression.
3. Give fentanyl as the final pretreatment agent and administer over 30 to 60 seconds.

BOX 17-3 Recommendations for Fentanyl as a Pretreatment Agent for RSI

- Patients with elevated intracranial pressure (at risk from increasing blood pressure)
- Patients with cardiovascular disease at risk from increased blood pressure and cardiac force of contraction (ischemic coronary disease, aneurysmal disease, great vessel rupture or dissection, intracranial hemorrhage)

OTHER PRETREATMENT AGENTS

A number of other agents have been studied and suggested for pretreatment of a patient undergoing intubation, including atropine, beta-blockers, calcium channel blockers, beta-2 adrenergic agonists, "defasciculating" doses of nondepolarizing neuromuscular blockers prior to succinylcholine, and others. We no longer recommend the routine use of any of these agents for pretreatment for emergency RSI. The beta-2 agonist, albuterol, can mitigate the bronchospastic response to airway manipulation, and is used for this purpose for elective anesthesia in the operating room and for elective bronchoscopy. We do not classify it as a pretreatment agent for emergency RSI because it is universally given to patients with severe asthma, regardless of whether the patient is ultimately intubated. We previously recommended both atropine and a defasciculating dose of a competitive NMBA for selected patients in this manual and as part of The Difficult Airway Course: Emergency and The Difficult Airway Course: Anesthesia. Atropine is an anticholinergic agent that has been recommended and used to prevent reflexive bradycardia in pediatric patients. Our former recommendation was that atropine be given to children 10 years of age or younger who were to undergo intubation using succinylcholine. Recent studies show conflicting results (see *Evidence* section). Proponents of the routine use of atropine argue that pretreatment with atropine outweighs any potential risk because young children can tolerate heart rates of 180 to 200 with little effect. Opponents point out that pediatric resuscitation is difficult and stressful for providers, and that variations in patient size and weight combine with the infrequency of pediatric resuscitation to make decision making and equipment and drug dose selection complex. They argue in favor of eliminating any steps without clear proof of benefit with the goal of keeping the procedure as streamlined and simple as possible to limit the likelihood for error. Atropine has itself been linked to some dysrhythmias in case reports, although the links are admittedly tenuous. On the basis of available evidence and in consideration of the goal of eliminating medical error, we no longer recommend the routine use of atropine during the pretreatment phase of pediatric RSI. It is considered optional as a pretreatment agent for children less than 1 year old who will be receiving succinylcholine (see Chapter 20).

Bradycardia has also been reported in adults receiving a second dose of succinylcholine, and is believed to be due to stimulation of cardiac muscarinic receptors. Whether this uncommonly observed bradycardia is caused directly by succinylcholine, by manipulation of the airway, or by the patient's underlying condition or comorbidity is unknown, but profound bradycardia and cardiac arrest can occur during intubation of critically ill patients. Atropine should be immediately available as a rescue agent when intubation is undertaken.

Pretreatment using a defasciculating dose of a nondepolarizing (competitive) neuromuscular blocking agent 3 minutes before succinylcholine has been recommended (including in previous editions of this manual) for patients with elevated ICP on the basis that this practice reduces the ICP response to succinylcholine. However, there are no high-quality data to support this practice in the emergency setting. Whether succinylcholine truly causes a rise in ICP has been disputed, and the magnitude of the ICP rise, if any, appears small. In addition, there are no hard data to support the contention that a small dose (one tenth of the paralyzing dose) of a competitive NMBA, such as vecuronium or rocuronium, will have any effect on any possible ICP rise from succinylcholine, particularly in the setting of emergency RSI. Therefore, we no longer support the use of a defasciculating agent for this purpose. Debate continues in elective anesthesia regarding the effect of defasciculation on muscle pain and other adverse effects of succinylcholine, but this has no role in decision making related to emergency intubation.

Beta-blockers (e.g., esmolol [Brevibloc]) have been shown to be beneficial in attenuating the sympathetic response to laryngoscopy. They are not effective in attenuating any rise in ICP, except that caused by elevations in blood pressure. Beta-blockers may increase airways resistance, especially in patients with reactive airways disease, and they are negative inotropes, and so are contraindicated in clinical situations in which maximum cardiac out-

---

BOX 17-4 Current Status of the LOAD Recommendations for Pretreatment

---

Lidocaine: no change. Recommended for reactive airways disease, elevated intracranial pressure (ICP)
Opioid (fentanyl): no change. Recommended for elevated ICP, cardiovascular disease
Atropine: no longer recommended (optional in children under 1 year old)
Defasciculation: no longer recommended

---

put is mandatory. Thus, although these agents are capable of blunting the sympathetic response to laryngoscopy, we do not recommend them for use as routine pretreatment agents for emergency RSI. On balance, fentanyl is a more appropriate agent for this purpose. An update on the recommendations that formerly were represented by the mnemonic LOAD is shown in Box 17-4.

SUMMARY AND NEW RECOMMENDATIONS

1. Pretreatment agents are used to attenuate the adverse physiological responses to laryngoscopy and intubation.
2. As is discussed in Chapter 3, there are three classes of patients for whom pretreatment is indicated, and the mnemonic ABC can be used: Asthma (representing reactive airways disease), Brain (representing elevated ICP), and Cardiovascular (representing those at risk from RSRL [i.e., patients with ischemic heart disease, vascular disease (especially cerebrovascular disease), hypertension, and vascular events, such as rupture or dissection of a great vessel]). The two drugs, lidocaine and fentanyl, and their relationship to the ABC conditions, are shown in Figure 17-1.

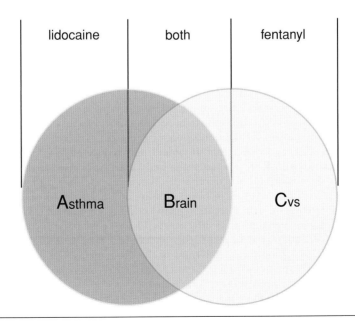

Figure 17-1 ● **The ABC Approach to Pretreatment.**

3. Ideally, any pretreatment agent should be administered 3 minutes before the sedative agent to match peak drug effect with airway manipulation. Even if time is short, there may be some benefit to giving lidocaine pretreatment. Fentanyl, if indicated, can be given after intubation, was not sufficient time to give it as a pretreatment agent.

EVIDENCE

1. **Can lidocaine suppress coughing related to intubation?** Good evidence (multiple randomized, placebo-controlled, double-blinded studies) demonstrates that lidocaine, at a dose of 1.5 mg/kg IV, can suppress cough reflexes when administered 1 to 3 minutes prior to intubation (1–10).

2. **Does lidocaine attenuate the rise in ICP seen with airway manipulation?** Data on the effect of lidocaine on the increase in ICP with intubation is conflicting. A best evidence review of the use of lidocaine in head injury patients undergoing RSI found that there were no studies that directly addressed this precise setting with outcome as the primary end point (11). Another in 2002 found three relevant articles on the subject but concluded that high-quality evidence is lacking (12). Another third systematic review found no strong evidence for lidocaine in either endotracheal suctioning or as a pretreatment for RSI (13). Three randomized, controlled trials show no benefit to lidocaine in blunting ICP rise, the first with 124 subjects, the second with 30, and the third with 9 (14–16). Four randomized, controlled trials report benefits with lidocaine pretreatment; their sizes range from an N of 10 to 30 (17–20). These studies demonstrated lidocaine to be as effective as thiopental at controlling ICP rise due to pain or endotracheal suctioning, without a corresponding drop in mean arterial pressure. There are conflicting data on the topic, with some authors downgrading studies if the airway was suctioned instead of intubated, or if intubation was by standard sequence, rather than rapid sequence, or if the patients had medical causes of elevated ICP, rather than head trauma. On balance, there is suggestive evidence that lidocaine may mitigate the ICP response to airway manipulation, and the drug is commonly used and safe in the doses recommended. We recommend lidocaine for use in patients with elevated ICP until further evidence clarifies this issue.

3. **Does lidocaine attenuate the bronchospastic response to intubation?** This is discussed in the evidence section of Chapter 29. In the absence of a sufficiently sized, properly designed, randomized, double-blind study of the effect of lidocaine in preventing postintubation bronchospasm during RSI, we believe there is sufficient evidence to recommend the routine use of lidocaine pretreatment for patients with reactive airways disease who are undergoing RSI, whether the reactive airways disease is the reason for the intubation, or is present as a comorbidity.

4. **What evidence is there that an opioid may reduce adverse hemodynamic effects associated with RSI?** Hypertension and tachycardia associated with RSI increase the risk of poor outcome in critically ill patients (21,22). 5 μg/kg Fentanyl is effective at reducing changes in blood pressure and heart rate during RSI (23–25) and is more effective than 2 μg/kg fentanyl or 2 mg/kg esmolol (23,26).

   5 μg/kg Fentanyl is as effective as 10 μg/kg fentanyl in reducing changes in hemodynamic variables in patients undergoing cardiac revascularization (27). On balance, weighing the effectiveness of the drug against the likelihood of inducing hypoventilation in the preintubation period, we recommend 3 μg/kg IV of fentanyl, when fentanyl pretreatment is indicated.

5. **What evidence is there that an opioid may reduce any adverse effects RSI may have on the injured brain?** Little data exist, or are likely to be produced, regarding the effects of RSI on the ICP of E patients with head injuries. In intubated patients

with severe head injury, a combination of neuromuscular blocking agent and opioid was more effective in reducing ICP elevation seen with endotracheal suctioning than either drug alone (28). Fentanyl itself has been associated with a rise in ICP in head injured patients in some studies (29,30) but not in others (31).

6. **What evidence is there that an opioid may cause other unwanted effects when used as a pretreatment drug?** High-dose fentanyl (100 μg/kg, or approximately 30 times the dose used in emergency RSI) caused 8% of patients undergoing cardiac surgery to develop extreme thoracic and abdominal rigidity (32).

   There is a single case report of rigidity in a patient who received fentanyl (approximately 2 μg/kg) while taking venlafaxine (33). Fentanyl has been widely used for procedural sedation in doses similar to those used for RSI, and reports of muscle rigidity are absent, even from large series (34,35).

7. **What is the evidence for the use of atropine to prevent bradycardia in pediatric patients undergoing RSI?** No relevant, systematic reviews were identified. Five prospective, randomized, double-blinded studies; one prospective, randomized, non-blinded study; five prospective, randomized case series; and one retrospective review were identified. The five highest-quality studies are all small (N = 20–90). Three studies focus only on neonatal intubations. Of the neonatal studies, only one demonstrated no incidences of bradycardia with atropine alone or with succinylcholine (36), but this study had only 20 subjects. Three others showed drops in heart rate even with atropine (37–39). Two studies (N = 90 and 36) in older children found no episodes of bradycardia but did report minor arrhythmias such as bigeminy, premature atrial contractions, and sinus tachycardia with atropine (40,41). One study (N = 41) in older children reported one episode of bradycardia in a child pretreated with atropine (42). A good quality retrospective review of 143 pediatric intubations with RSI demonstrated 6 episodes of bradycardia, 3 of whom received atropine pretreatment (43). The data continue to be difficult to interpret. Although there exists a potential for bradycardia during intubation of pediatric patients, either with or without succinylcholine, atropine has not been shown to prevent this, and there are no grounds to support the routine use of atropine for pediatric intubation with succinylcholine.

8. **What is the evidence for the use of atropine to prevent bradycardia in patients receiving a second dose of succinylcholine for RSI?** A number of case series in the 1980s reported bradycardic responses to second doses of succinylcholine, presumably due to an acetylcholine "priming" mechanism (44,45). A search for relevant, systematic, evidence-based reviews was unsuccessful. A PubMed search revealed more than 450 articles, of which 10 were relevant. Two studies had subjects who became bradycardic after a second dose of succinylcholine even though they were pretreated with atropine (46,47). Four studies reported no episodes of bradycardia but multiple episodes of tachyarrhythmias, including ventricular tachycardia, with atropine pretreatment (48–51). Only one study (N = 80) demonstrated no bradycardia and no arrhythmias with atropine pretreatment in this setting (52). On balance, the evidence supports the use of atropine to treat symptomatic bradycardia after succinylcholine use, particularly when a second dose of succinylcholine has been given, but does not support the routine dose of atropine in preventative fashion when a second dose of succinylcholine is contemplated.

9. **What evidence is there that RSI with succinylcholine causes a rise in ICP in head injured patients?** No good systematic review was identified. Multiple animal studies demonstrate elevations in ICP when succinylcholine is given (53–57). One well-designed study demonstrates a rise in human ICP with succinylcholine administration (58); others show minimal (59) or no change (60–62) in neurosurgical patients with direct ICP measurements. The increase in ICP from succinylcholine appears to be sufficiently small, and sufficiently variable, as to preclude recommending any particular steps to mitigate it.

10. **What evidence is there that a defasciculating dose of a nondepolarizing muscle relaxant reduces the rise in ICP associated with RSI in head injured patients?**
One good, systematic review demonstrated no good study that addresses this issue directly (63). Various nondepolarizing agents and succinylcholine itself have been demonstrated to have some effect with blunting fasciculations, but any link between this and improved outcome from elevated ICP is lacking. Routine defasciculation is not recommended, even in the presence of elevated ICP (64,65).

ACKNOWLEDGMENT

The authors want to thank Robert E. Schneider, MD, for his significant contribution to prior editions of this chapter.

REFERENCES

1. Vacanti CA, Silbert BS, Vacanti FX. The effects of thiopental sodium on fentanyl-induced muscle rigidity in a human model. *J Clin Anesth* 1991;3(5):395–398.
2. Aouad MT, Sayyid SS, Zalaket MI, et al. Intravenous lidocaine as adjuvant to sevoflurane anesthesia for endotracheal intubation in children. *Anesth Analg* 2003;96(5):1325–1327.
3. Davidson JA, Gillespie JA. Tracheal intubation after induction of anaesthesia with propofol, alfentanil and i.v. lignocaine. *Br J Anaesth* 1993;70(2):163–166.
4. Jakobsen CJ, Ahlburg P, Holdgard HO, et al. Comparison of intravenous and topical lidocaine as a suppressant of coughing after bronchoscopy during general anesthesia. *Acta Anaesthesiol Scand* 1991;35(3):238–241.
5. Lin CS, Sun WZ, Chan WH, et al. Intravenous lidocaine and ephedrine, but not propofol, suppress fentanyl-induced cough. *Can J Anaesth* 2004;51(7):654–659.
6. Nishino T, Hiraga K, Sugimori K. Effects of i.v. lignocaine on airway reflexes elicited by irritation of the tracheal mucosa in humans anaesthetized with enflurane. *Br J Anaesth* 1990;64(6):682–687.
7. Pandey CK, Raza M, Ranjan R, et al. Intravenous lidocaine suppresses fentanyl-induced coughing: a double-blind, prospective, randomized placebo-controlled study. *Anesth Analg* 2004;99(6):1696–1698.
8. Pandey CK, Raza M, Ranjan R, et al. Intravenous lidocaine 0.5 mg.kg-1 effectively suppresses fentanyl-induced cough. *Can J Anaesth* 2005;52(2):172–175.
9. Warner LO, Balch DR, Davidson PJ. Is intravenous lidocaine an effective adjuvant for endotracheal intubation in children undergoing induction of anesthesia with halothane-nitrous oxide? *J Clin Anesth* 1997;9(4):270–274.
10. Yukioka H, Hayashi M, Terai T, et al. Intravenous lidocaine as a suppressant of coughing during tracheal intubation in elderly patients. *Anesth Analg* 1993;77(2):309–312.
11. Robinson N, Clancy M. In patients with head injury undergoing rapid sequence intubation, does pretreatment with intravenous lignocaine/lidocaine lead to an improved neurological outcome? A review of the literature. *Emerg Med J* 2001;18(6):453–457.
12. Butler J, Jackson R. Towards evidence based emergency medicine: best BETs from Manchester Royal Infirmary. Lignocaine premedication before rapid sequence induction in head injuries. *Emerg Med J* 2002;19(6):554.
13. Brooks D, Anderson CM, Carter MA, et al. Clinical practice guidelines for suctioning the airway of the intubated and nonintubated patient. *Can Respir J* 2001;8(3):163–181.

14. Bachofen M. [Suppression of blood pressure increases during intubation: lidocaine or fentanyl?] *Der Anaesthesist* 1988;37(3):156–161.

15. Samaha T, Ravussin P, Claquin C, et al. [Prevention of increase of blood pressure and intracranial pressure during endotracheal intubation in neurosurgery: esmolol versus lidocaine.] *Ann Fr Anesth Reanim* 1996;15(1):36–40.

16. Yano M, Nishiyama H, Yokota H, et al. Effect of lidocaine on ICP response to endotracheal suctioning. *Anesthesiology* 1986;64(5):651–653.

17. Bedford RF, Persing JA, Pobereskin L, et al. Lidocaine or thiopental for rapid control of intracranial hypertension? *Anesth Analg* 1980;59(6):435–437.

18. Donegan MF, Bedford RF. Intravenously administered lidocaine prevents intracranial hypertension during endotracheal suctioning. *Anesthesiology* 1980;52(6):516–518.

19. Grover VK, Reddy GM, Kak VK, et al. Intracranial pressure changes with different doses of lignocaine under general anaesthesia. *Neurol India* 1999;47(2):118–121.

20. White PF, Schlobohm RM, Pitts LH, et al. A randomized study of drugs for preventing increases in intracranial pressure during endotracheal suctioning. *Anesthesiology* 1982;57(3):242–244.

21. Horak J, Weiss S. Emergent management of the airway. New pharmacology and the control of comorbidities in cardiac disease, ischemia, and valvular heart disease. *Crit Care Clin* 2000;16(3):411–427.

22. Reynolds SF, Heffner J. Airway management of the critically ill patient: rapid-sequence intubation. *Chest* 2005;127(4):1397–1412.

23. Chung KS, Sinatra RS, Halevy JD, et al. A comparison of fentanyl, esmolol, and their combination for blunting the haemodynamic responses during rapid-sequence induction. *Can J Anaesth* 1992;39(8):774–779.

24. Cork RC, Weiss JL, Hameroff SR, et al. Fentanyl preloading for rapid-sequence induction of anesthesia. *Anesth Analg* 1984;63(1):60–64.

25. Dahlgren N, Messeter K. Treatment of stress response to laryngoscopy and intubation with fentanyl. *Anaesthesia* 1981;36(11):1022–1026.

26. Hussain A, Sultan S. Efficacy of fentanyl and esmolol in the prevention of haemodynamic response to laryngoscopy and endotracheal intubation. *J Coll Physicians Surg Pak* 2005;15(8):454–457.

27. Weiss-Bloom L, Reich D. Haemodynamic responses to tracheal intubation following etomidate and fentanyl for anaesthetic induction. *Can J Anaesth* 1992;39:780–785.

28. Kerr M, Sereika S, Orndoff P, et al. Effect of neuromuscular blockers and opiates on the cerebrovascular response. *Am J Crit Care* 1998;7(3):205–217.

29. DeNadal M, Susina A, Sahuquillo J, et al. Effects on intracranial pressure of fentanyl in severe head injured patients. *Acta Neurochirugica Suppl* 1998;71:10–12.

30. Sperry R, Bailey P, Reichman M, et al. Fentanyl and sufentanil increase intracranial pressure in head trauma patients. *Anesthesiology* 1992;77(3):416–420.

31. Weinstabl C, Mayer J, Tichling B, et al. Effect of sufentanil on intracranial pressure in neurosurgical patients. *Anaesthesia* 1991;46(10):837–840.

32. Caspi J, Klausner J, Safadi T, et al. Delayed respiratory depression following fentanyl anesthesia for cardiac surgery. *Crit Care Med* 1988;16:238–240.

33. Roy S, Fortier L. Fentanyl-induced rigidity during emergence from general anesthesia potentiated by venlafaxine. *Can J Anaesth* 2003;50:32–35.

34. Roback MG, Wathen JE, Bajaj L, et al. Adverse events associated with procedural sedation and analgesia in a pediatric emergency department: a comparison of common parenteral drugs. *Acad Emerg Med* 2005;12(6):508–513.

35. Sacchetti A, Senula G, Strickland J, et al. Procedural sedation in the community emergency department: initial results of the ProSCED registry. *Acad Emerg Med* 2007;14(1):41–46.

36. Barrington KJ, Finer NN, Etches PC. Succinylcholine and atropine for premedication of the newborn infant before nasotracheal intubation: a randomized, controlled trial. *Crit Care Med* 1989;17(12):1293–1296.

37. Kelly MA, Finer NN. Nasotracheal intubation in the neonate: physiologic responses and effects of atropine and pancuronium. *J Pediatr* 1984;105(2):303–309.

38. Oei J, Hari R, Butha T, et al. Facilitation of neonatal nasotracheal intubation with premedication: a randomized controlled trial. *J Paediatr Child Health* 2002;38(2):146–150.

39. Roberts KD, Leone TA, Edwards WH, et al. Premedication for nonemergent neonatal intubations: a randomized, controlled trial comparing atropine and fentanyl to atropine, fentanyl, and mivacurium. *Pediatrics* 2006;118(4):1583–1591.

40. Desalu I, Kushimo OT, Bode CO. A comparative study of the haemodynamic effects of atropine and glycopyrrolate at induction of anaesthesia in children. *West Afr J Med* 2005;24(2):115–159.

41. Shorten GD, Bissonnette B, Hartley E, et al. It is not necessary to administer more than 10 micrograms.kg-1 of atropine to older children before succinylcholine. *Can J Anaesth* 1995;42(1):8–11.

42. McAuliffe G, Bissonnette B, Boutin C. Should the routine use of atropine before succinylcholine in children be reconsidered? *Can J Anaesth* 1995;42(8):724–729.

43. Fastle RK, Roback MG. Pediatric rapid sequence intubation: incidence of reflex bradycardia and effects of pretreatment with atropine. *Pediatr Emerg Care* 2004;20(10):651–655.

44. McCauley CS, Boller LR. Bradycardic responses to endotracheal suctioning. *Crit Care Med* 1988;16(11):1165–1166.

45. Sorensen M, Engbaek J, Viby-Mogensen J, et al. Bradycardia and cardiac asystole following a single injection of suxamethonium. *Acta Anaesthesiol Scand* 1984;28(2):232–235.

46. Cozanitis DA, Dundee JW, Khan MM. Comparative study of atropine and glycopyrrolate on suxamethonium-induced changes in cardiac rate and rhythm. *Br J Anaesth* 1980;52(3):291–293.

47. Magee DA, Sweet PT, Holland AJ. Effect of atropine on bradydysrhythmia induced by succinylcholine following pretreatment with D-tubocurarine. *Can Anaesth Soc J* 1982;29(6):573–576.

48. Brandt MR, Viby-Mogensen J. Halothane anaesthesia and suxamethonium III. Atropine 30 s before a second dose of suxamethonium during inhalation anaesthesia: effects and side-effects. *Acta Anaesthesiol Scand Suppl* 1978;67:76–83.

49. Greenan J, Dewar M, Jones CJ. Intravenous glycopyrrolate and atropine at induction of anaesthesia: a comparison. *J R Soc Med* 1983;76(5):369–371.

50. Latorre F, Ellmauer S, Dick W. [Atropine in the premedication of patients at risk. Its effect on hemodynamics and salivation during intubation anesthesia using succinylcholine.] *Anaesthesist* 1992;41(2):76–82.

51. Shipton EA, Roelofse JA, Luus HG. Effect of intramuscular atropine and glycopyrrolate on the cardiovascular response to tracheal intubation. *S Afr Med J* 1984;66(14):528–530.

52. Viby-Mogensen J, Wisborg K, Sorensen O. Cardiac effects of atropine and gallamine in patients receiving suxamethonium. *Br J Anaesth* 1980;52(11):1137–1142.

53. Bozeman WP, Idris AH. Intracranial pressure changes during rapid sequence intubation: a swine model. *J Trauma* 2005;58(2):278–283.

54. Lanier WL, Iaizzo PA, Milde JH. Cerebral function and muscle afferent activity following intravenous succinylcholine in dogs anesthetized with halothane: the effects of pretreatment with a defasciculating dose of pancuronium. *Anesthesiology* 1989;71(1):87–95.

55. Ducey JP, Deppe SA, Foley KT. A comparison of the effects of suxamethonium, atracurium and vecuronium on intracranial haemodynamics in swine. *Anaesth Intensive Care* 1989;17(4):448–455.

56. Thiagarajah S, Sophie S, Lear E, et al. Effect of suxamethonium on the ICP of cats with and without thiopentone pretreatment. *Br J Anaesth* 1988;60(2):157–160.

57. Cottrell JE, Hartung J, Giffin JP, et al. Intracranial and hemodynamic changes after succinylcholine administration in cats. *Anesth Analg* 1983;62(11):1006–1009.

58. Stirt JA, Grosslight KR, Bedford RF, et al. "Defasciculation" with metocurine prevents succinylcholine-induced increases in intracranial pressure. *Anesthesiology* 1987;67(1):50–53.

59. Minton MD, Grosslight K, Stirt JA, et al. Increases in intracranial pressure from succinylcholine: prevention by prior nondepolarizing blockade. *Anesthesiology* 1986;65(2):165–169.

60. Brown MM, Parr MJ, Manara AR. The effect of suxamethonium on intracranial pressure and cerebral perfusion pressure in patients with severe head injuries following blunt trauma. *Eur J Anaesthesiol* 1996;13(5):474–477.

61. Kovarik WD, Mayberg TS, Lam AM, et al. Succinylcholine does not change intracranial pressure, cerebral blood flow velocity, or the electroencephalogram in patients with neurologic injury. *Anesth Analg* 1994;78(3):469–473.

62. McLesky C, Cullen B, Kennedy R, et al. Control of cerebral perfusion pressure during induction of anaesthesia in high risk neurosurgical patients. *Anesth Analg* 1974;53:985–992.

63. Clancy M, Halford S, Walls R, et al. In patients with head injuries who undergo rapid sequence intubation using succinylcholine, does pretreatment with a competitive neuromuscular blocking agent improve outcome? A literature review. *Emerg Med J* 2001;18(5):373–375.

64. Martin R, Carrier J, Pirlet M, et al. Rocuronium is the best non-depolarizing relaxant to prevent succinylcholine fasciculations and myalgia. *Can J Anaesth* 1998;45:521–525.

65. Eisenkraft J, Mingus M, Herlich A, et al. A defasciculating dose of d-tubocurarine causes resistance to succinylcholine. *Can J Anaesth* 1990;37(5):538–542.

18

Sedative Induction Agents

David A. Caro and Katren R. Tyler

INTRODUCTION

Agents used to sedate, or "induce," patients for intubation during rapid sequence intubation (RSI) are properly called sedative induction agents because induction of general anesthesia is at the extreme of the spectrum of their sedative actions. In this chapter, we refer to this family of drugs as "induction agents." Induction agents are among the most potent medications used in medicine today. The ideal agent would smoothly and quickly render the patient unconscious, unresponsive, and amnestic in one arm/heart/brain circulation time. Such an agent would also provide analgesia, maintain stable cerebral perfusion pressure and cardiovascular hemodynamics, be immediately reversible, and have few, if any, adverse side effects. Unfortunately, such an induction agent does not exist. Most induction agents meet the first criterion because they are highly lipophilic and, therefore, have a rapid onset within 15 to 30 seconds of intravenous (IV) administration. Their clinical effect is likewise terminated quickly as the drug rapidly redistributes to less well-perfused tissues. All induction agents have the potential to cause myocardial depression and subsequent hypotension. These effects depend on the particular drug; the patient's underlying physiological condition; and the dose, concentration, and speed of injection of the drug. The faster the drug is administered (intravenous [IV] push), the larger the concentration of drug that saturates those organs with the greatest blood flow (i.e., brain, heart) and the more pronounced the effect. Because RSI requires rapid administration of a preselected dose of the induction agent, the choice of drug and the dose must be individualized to capitalize on desired effects, while minimizing those that might adversely affect the patient. Some patients are so unstable that the primary goal is to produce amnesia rather than anesthesia because to produce the latter might lead to severe hypotension and organ hypoperfusion.

The induction agents include ultra–short-acting barbiturates: thiopental (Pentothal) and methohexital (Brevital); benzodiazepines: principally midazolam (Versed); and miscellaneous agents: etomidate (Amidate), ketamine (Ketalar), and propofol (Diprivan). Other agents, such as the opioid analgesic fentanyl (Sublimaze), can function as anesthetic induction agents when used in large doses (e.g., for fentanyl 30 μg/kg, 0.03 mg/kg); however, they are rarely, if ever, used for that purpose during emergency intubation, and so are not discussed here.

General anesthetic agents act via two principal mechanisms: (a) an increase in inhibition via GABA A receptors (e.g., benzodiazepines, barbiturates, propofol, isoflurane, etomidate, enflurane, halothane), and (b) a decreased excitation through NMDA receptors (e.g., ketamine, nitrous oxide, xenon).

The IV induction agents discussed in this chapter share important pharmacokinetic characteristics. As mentioned previously, they are highly lipophilic and, therefore, a standard induction dose of each in a euvolemic, normotensive patient will onset within 30 seconds. The observed clinical duration of each drug is measured in minutes and is due to the drugs' redistribution half-life ($t_{1/2}\alpha$) characterized by redistribution of the drug from the central circulation (brain) to larger, well-perfused tissues, such as fat and muscle. The elimination half-life ($t_{1/2}\beta$, usually measured in hours) is characterized by each drug's re-entry from fat and lean muscle into plasma down a concentration gradient, followed by hepatic metabolism and renal excretion. Generally, it requires four to five elimination half-lives to clear the drug completely from the body.

Because the target organ is the brain, and the desired effect is produced rapidly following bolus injection of the drug, dosing of induction agents in non-obese adults should be based on ideal body weight in kilograms. This dosage can be estimated based on the patient's actual body weight, or a rough approximation can be obtained by subtracting 100 from the patient's height in centimeters; that is, 6 ft 4 inch = 76 inch $\times$ 2.54 cm/ inch = 193 cm – 100 = 93 kg. This approach provides an acceptable estimate of ideal body weight, and the administered induction dose can then be adjusted based on the clinical status of the patient. For obese patients, the situation is more complicated. The high lipophilicity of the induction agents and the increased volume of distribution (V_d) of these drugs in obesity would argue for total body weight dosing (see Chapter 35). Opposing this, however, is the significant cardiovascular depression that would occur if such a large quantity of drug was injected as a single bolus. Balancing these two considerations, and given the paucity of actual pharmacokinetic studies in obese patients, the best advice is probably to administer the induction agents according to lean body weight, where lean body weight is approximated by subtracting the ideal body weight from actual body weight and adding 30% of this difference to the ideal body weight. This is in contrast to succinylcholine, for which studies support dosing by total body weight in both adults and children. Further dosing guidelines are provided in Chapters 20 and 21 for pediatric patients and in Chapter 35 for morbidly obese patients.

Aging affects the pharmacokinetics of induction agents. In the elderly, lean body mass and total body water decrease while total body fat increases, resulting in an increased volume of distribution, an increase in $t_{1/2}\beta$, and an increased duration of drug effect. In addition, the elderly ordinarily have decreased reserve and are much more sensitive to the hemodynamic and respiratory depressant effects of these agents, and consequently, most induction doses should be reduced, generally to approximately one half to three fourths of the dose used in their healthy, younger counterparts.

Ultrashort-acting Barbiturates

	Usual Emergency Induction dose (mg/kg)	Onset (sec)	$t_{1/2}\alpha$ (min)	Duration (min)	$t_{1/2}\beta$ (hr)
Thiopental (Pentothal)	3	<30	2–4	5–10	3–8
Methohexital (Brevital)	1.5	<30	5–6	5–10	2–5

A. *Clinical Pharmacology*

Thiopental is the prototypical barbiturate used for anesthetic induction. Methohexital is a close relative. Both are ultrashort-acting central nervous system (CNS) depressants that induce hypnosis (sleep) but not analgesia. Recovery after a small dose is rapid with some somnolence and retrograde amnesia. Repeated IV doses lead to prolonged anesthesia because fatty tissues act as a reservoir; they accumulate thiopental in concentrations significantly greater than the plasma concentration, and then they release the drug slowly to cause prolonged anesthesia.

Methohexital is two to three times more potent than thiopental, 1.5 mg of methohexital being equal to 4 mg of thiopental. The $t_{1/2}\beta$ for methohexital is shorter than that for thiopental.

At low doses, ultrashort-acting barbiturates decrease GABA dissociation from its receptor, which enhances GABA's neuroinhibitory activity. At higher doses, they can directly stimulate the GABA receptor itself.

Barbiturates are cerebroprotective, causing a dose-dependent decrease in cerebral metabolic oxygen consumption and a parallel decrease in cerebral blood flow (CBF) and intracranial pressure (ICP), provided cerebral perfusion pressure is maintained.

Thiopental and methohexital are largely degraded in the liver. Neither have active metabolites.

B. *Indications and Contraindications*

Thiopental was widely used as a general purpose induction agent in the past, but it has largely been supplanted by etomidate and propofol. Its primary use now is as an induction agent for patients suspected of having increased ICP or status epilepticus because it has significant anticonvulsant activities in addition to the cerebroprotective properties outlined previously.

Thiopental releases histamine, and so is relatively contraindicated in patients with reactive airways disease.

Thiopental and all of the other barbiturates are absolutely contraindicated in patients with acute intermittent porphyria, or variegate porphyria, because they can activate the enzyme responsible for precipitating an acute attack, which can be life threatening.

Thiopental is classified by the U.S. Food and Drug Administration (FDA) as a pregnancy category C, primarily for risk of teratogenesis. Methohexital is an FDA pregnancy category B. Both readily cross the placenta and may cause respiratory depression in neonates.

C. *Dosage and Clinical Use*

The dosing of thiopental depends on the hemodynamic status of the patient and the concomitant use of other agents in RSI. Thiopental is a potent venodilator and myocardial depressant. Consequently, the dose must be decreased in patients with decreased intravascular volume, those with compromised myocardial function, the elderly, and whenever thiopental is used with other drugs that affect sympathetic tone or cardiovascular function. In euvolemic, normotensive adults, the recommended induction dose is 3 to 5 mg/kg IV. For most emergency intubations, the lower dose of this range, that is, 3 mg/kg, achieves excellent sedation and intubating conditions with less tendency to cause the hypotension that often occurs with the 5 mg/kg dose. The onset of methohexital is more rapid and the duration of action shorter than with thiopental. The recommended induction dose in the euvolemic, normotensive patient is 1.5 mg/kg IV.

In the adult patient who is suspected of hypovolemia, myocardial dysfunction, or compromised hemodynamic status, the dose of thiopental should be reduced to 1 to 2 mg/kg IV, and the dose of methohexital decreased to 0.5 to 1 mg/kg IV. Both should be avoided entirely in frankly hypotensive patients for whom other drugs, especially etomidate or ketamine, may preserve greater hemodynamic stability. With the widespread adoption of etomidate, which has significant cardiovascular stability, the ultra–short-acting barbiturates have seen limited use as induction agents for emergent RSI.

D. *Adverse Effects*

As with any induction agent, inadequate dosing leaves the patient more lightly sedated and makes laryngoscopy more difficult, even when neuromuscular blocking agents are used. The principal side effects of thiopental include central respiratory depression, venodilation, and myocardial depression. These latter two may be manifested by hypotension that tends to be greater in both treated and untreated hypertensive patients compared with normotensive patients. Both can be detrimental in many patients in whom optimal preload is required to maintain cardiac output and prevent organ ischemia. Barbiturates cause a dose-related release of histamine that in most situations is not clinically significant, but may cause or exacerbate bronchospasm in patients with reactive airways disease. Ketamine is the preferred induction agent for patients with reactive airways disease. Methohexital causes more excitatory phenomena (twitching, hiccups) than thiopental.

One to two percent of patients will experience pain on injection of thiopental, especially if small veins on the dorsum of the hand are used. Five percent of patients will experience pain on injection with methohexital. Inadvertent intra-arterial injection or subcutaneous extravasation of thiopental can result in chemical endarteritis and distal thrombosis, ischemia, and tissue necrosis due to its highly alkaline pH (>10). If extravasation occurs, 40 to 80 mg of papaverine (Cerespan) in 20 mL normal saline or 10 mL of 1% lidocaine (Xylocaine) should be injected intra-arterially proximal to the site to inhibit smooth muscle spasm. Consider local infiltration of an alpha-adrenergic blocking agent such as phentolamine into the vasospastic area.

Benzodiazepines

	Usual Emergency Induction dose (mg/kg)	Onset (sec)	$t_{1/2}\alpha$ (min)	Duration (min)	$t_{1/2}\beta$ (hr)
Midazolam (Versed)	0.2–0.3	60–90	7–15	15–30	2–6

A. *Clinical Pharmacology*

Although chemically distinct from the barbiturates, the benzodiazepines also exert their effects via the GABA-receptor complex. Benzodiazepines specifically stimulate the benzodiazepine receptor, which in turn modulates GABA, the primary neuroinhibitory transmitter. The benzodiazepines provide amnesia, anxiolysis, central muscle relaxation, sedation, anticonvulsant effects, and hypnosis. Although the benzodiazepines generally have similar pharmacological profiles, they differ in selectivity, which makes their clinical usefulness variable. The benzodiazepines have potent, dose-related amnestic properties, perhaps their greatest asset for emergency indications. The lipophilicity of the benzodiazepines varies widely. Greater lipid solubility confers a more rapid onset of action because of the brain's high lipid content. The three benzodiazepines of interest for emergency applications are midazolam (Versed), diazepam (Valium), and lorazepam (Ativan). Of the three, midazolam is the most lipid soluble and is the only benzodiazepine suitable for use as an induction agent for emergent RSI. That said, midazolam is virtually never used in correct induction doses for emergency intubations and is notoriously underdosed. Furthermore, the time to clinical effectiveness of benzodiazepines, in general, is longer than any of the other induction agents, further mitigating their role in emergent RSI. When IV midazolam is given as an anesthetic induction agent, induction of anesthesia occurs in approximately 1.5 minutes when narcotic premedication has been used and in 2 to 2.5 minutes without narcotic premedication. This slow onset of action is mitigated, to an extent, by the profound amnestic effects of midazolam, but its pharmacokinetic attributes make it a poor induction agent, and it cannot be recommended for this purpose. Midazolam's activity is primarily due to the parent drug. Elimination of the parent drug takes place via hepatic metabolism of midazolam to hydroxylated metabolites that are conjugated and excreted in the urine. The termination of action of midazolam is due to initial redistribution and subsequent hepatic metabolism via microsomal oxidation. Midazolam has one significant active metabolite, 1-hydroxy-midazolam, which may contribute to the net pharmacological activity of midazolam. Clearance of midazolam is reduced in association with old age, congestive heart failure, and liver disease. The elimination half-life of midazolam ($t_{1/2}\beta$) may be prolonged in renal impairment. The benzodiazepines do not release histamine, and allergic reactions are very rare.

B. *Indications and Contraindications*

The primary indications for benzodiazepines are to promote amnesia and sedation. In this regard, the benzodiazepines are unparalleled. Midazolam's primary use in the emergency department and elsewhere in the hospital is for procedural sedation, lorazepam is used primarily for treatment of seizures and alcohol withdrawal, and these agents are used for sedation and anxiolysis in a variety of settings, including postintubation.

Because of their dose-related reduction in systemic vascular resistance and direct myocardial depression, dosage must be adjusted in volume-depleted or hemodynamically compromised patients. Studies have shown that induction doses of midazolam, 0.3 mg/kg, are rarely used, but, even at this dose, midazolam is a poor induction agent for emergency RSI.

All benzodiazepines are FDA pregnancy category D.

C. *Dosage and Clinical Use*

Although midazolam is used as an induction agent in the operating room, we do not recommend its use for emergency RSI. Even in the correct induction dose for hemodynamically stable patients of 0.2 to 0.3 mg/kg IV push, the onset is slow, and not suited to emergency applications. Midazolam should be reserved for sedative applications, and its use in emergency RSI is not advised because superior agents are readily available. Similarly, diazepam and lorazepam are not recommended for emergent RSI because of their slow onset of action.

D. *Adverse Effects*

Except for midazolam, the benzodiazepines are insoluble in water and are usually in solution in propylene glycol. Unless injected into a large vein, pain and venous irritation on injection can be significant.

Miscellaneous Agents

Etomidate (Amidate)

Usual Emergency Induction dose (mg/kg)	Onset (sec)	$t_{1/2}\alpha$ (min)	Duration (min)	$t_{1/2}\beta$ (hr)
0.3	15–45	2–4	3–12	2–5

1. **Clinical Pharmacology**

   Etomidate is an imidazole derivative that is primarily a hypnotic and has no analgesic activity. With the exception of ketamine, etomidate is the most hemodynamically stable of the currently available induction agents. It exerts its effect by enhancing GABA activity at the GABA-receptor complex, inhibiting excitatory stimuli. Etomidate attenuates underlying elevated ICP by decreasing CBF and cerebral metabolic oxygen demand ($CMRO_2$). Its hemodynamic stability preserves cerebral perfusion pressure. Etomidate may not be the most cerebroprotective of the various available induction agents (that attribute probably resides with the barbiturates), but its hemodynamic stability and favorable CNS effects make it an excellent choice for patients with elevated ICP.

   Etomidate does not release histamine and is safe for use in patients with reactive airways disease. However, it lacks the direct bronchodilatory properties of ketamine, which may be a preferable agent in these patients.

2. **Indications and Contraindications**

   Etomidate has become the induction agent of choice for most emergent RSIs because of its rapid onset, its hemodynamic stability, its positive effect on $CMRO_2$ and cerebral perfusion pressure, and its rapid recovery. As with any induction agent, dosage should be adjusted in hemodynamically compromised patients. Etomidate is an FDA pregnancy category C.

   Etomidate is not FDA approved for use in children, but many series report safe and effective use in pediatric patients (see Chapters 20 and 21).

3. **Dosage and Clinical Use**

   In euvolemic and hemodynamically stable patients, the normal induction dose of etomidate is 0.3 mg/kg IV push. In compromised patients, the dose should be reduced commensurate with the patient's clinical status; reduction to 0.2 mg/kg is usually sufficient.

4. **Adverse Effects**

   Pain on injection is common because of the diluent (propylene glycol) and can be somewhat mitigated by having a fast-flowing IV solution running in a large vein. Myoclonic movement during induction is common and has been confused with seizure activity. It is of no clinical consequence and generally terminates promptly as the neuromuscular blocking agent takes effect.

The most significant and controversial side effect of etomidate is its reversible blockade of 11-beta-hydroxylase, which decreases both serum cortisol and aldosterone levels. This side effect has been more common with continuous infusions of etomidate in the intensive care unit setting rather than with a single-dose injection used for emergency RSI. The risks and benefits of the use of etomidate in patients with sepsis are discussed in detail in the *Evidence* section at the end of the chapter.

Ketamine (Ketalar)

Usual Emergency Induction dose (mg/kg)	Onset (sec)	$t_{1/2}\alpha$ (min)	Duration (min)	$t_{1/2}\beta$ (hr)
1.5	45–60	11–17	10–20	2–3

1. **Clinical Pharmacology**

   Ketamine is a phencyclidine derivative that provides significant analgesia, anesthesia, and amnesia with minimal effect on respiratory drive. The amnestic effect is not as pronounced as that seen with the benzodiazepines. Ketamine is believed to interact with the N-methyl-D-aspartate (NMDA) receptors at the GABA-receptor complex, promoting neuroinhibition and subsequent anesthesia. Action on opioid receptors accounts for its profound analgesic effect. Ketamine releases catecholamines, stimulates the sympathetic nervous system, and therefore augments heart rate and blood pressure in those patients who are not catecholamine depleted secondary to the demands of their underlying disease. Furthermore, increases in mean arterial pressure may offset any rise in ICP, resulting in a relatively stable cerebral perfusion pressure. This is discussed in detail in the *Evidence* section. In addition to its catecholamine-releasing effect, ketamine directly relaxes bronchial smooth muscle, producing bronchodilatation. Ketamine is primarily metabolized in the liver, producing one active metabolite, norketamine, which is metabolized and excreted in the urine.

2. **Indications and Contraindications**

   Ketamine is the induction agent of choice for patients with reactive airways disease who require tracheal intubation. Because of its pharmacological profile, ketamine should also be considered the induction agent of choice for patients who are hypovolemic or hypotensive and for patients with hemodynamic instability due to sepsis. In normotensive or hypertensive patients with ischemic heart disease, catecholamine release may adversely increase myocardial oxygen demand, but it is unlikely that this effect is important in patients with significant hypotension, who are probably maximally catecholamine stimulated before the ketamine is given. Ketamine's preservation of upper airway reflexes makes it appealing for awake laryngoscopy and intubation in the difficult airway patient where the dose is titrated to effect. The pregnancy category of ketamine has not been established by the FDA.

3. **Dosage and Clinical Use**

   The induction dose of ketamine for RSI is 1.5 mg/kg IV. In patients who are catecholamine depleted, doses greater than 1.5 mg/kg IV may cause myocardial depression, exacerbating hypotension. For sedation, ketamine is titrated to effect beginning with doses that approximate 10% of the calculated induction dose of the drug. Because of its generalized stimulating effects, ketamine enhances laryngeal reflexes and increases pharyngeal and bronchial secretions. These secretions may uncommonly precipitate laryngospasm and may be bothersome during upper airway examination during awake intubation, but are not an issue during RSI. Atropine 0.01 mg/kg IV or glycopyrrolate (Robinul) 0.01 mg/kg IV may be administered in conjunction with ketamine to promote a drying effect for awake intubation, although this is usually not necessary.

4. **Adverse Effects**
The hallucinations that occasionally occur on emergence from ketamine are more common in the adult than in the child and can be eliminated by the concomitant or subsequent administration of a benzodiazepine, if desired. This is rarely an issue in emergency airway management, in which the patient is usually sedated for prolonged periods, often with benzodiazepines.

Propofol (Diprivan)

Usual Emergency Induction dose (mg/kg)	Onset (sec)	$t_{1/2}\alpha$ (min)	Duration (min)	$t_{1/2}\beta$ (hr)
1.5	15–45	1–3	5–10	1–3

1. **Clinical Pharmacology**
Propofol is an alkylphenol derivative (i.e., an alcohol) with hypnotic properties. It is highly lipid soluble. Propofol enhances GABA activity at the GABA-receptor complex. It decreases $CMRO_2$ and ICP. Propofol does not cause histamine release. Propofol causes a direct reduction in blood pressure through vasodilatation and direct myocardial depression, resulting in a decrease in cerebral perfusion pressure, which may be detrimental to a compromised patient. The manufacturer recommends that rapid bolus dosing (either single or repeated) be avoided in patients who are elderly, debilitated, or ASA III/IV in order to minimize undesirable cardiovascular depression, including hypotension. It must be used cautiously for emergency RSI in hemodynamically unstable patients. It causes greater myocardial depression and venodilation than thiopental, when used in equivalent doses.

2. **Indications and Contraindications**
Propofol is an excellent induction agent in a stable patient. Its adverse potential for hypotension and reduction in cerebral perfusion pressure limits its role as an induction agent in emergent RSI. Propofol has been used as an induction agent during tracheal intubation for reactive airways disease. There are no absolute contraindications to the use of propofol. Propofol is delivered as an emulsion in soybean oil and lecithin. Patients who are allergic to eggs generally react to the ovalbumin and not to lecithin, and propofol is not contraindicated in patients with egg allergy. Propofol is a pregnancy category B drug.

3. **Dosage and Clinical Use**
The induction dose of propofol is 1.5 mg/kg IV in a euvolemic, normotensive patient. Because of its predictable tendency to reduce mean arterial blood pressure, smaller doses are generally used when propofol is given as an induction agent for emergency RSI in compromised patients.

4. **Adverse Effects**
Propofol causes pain on injection comparable to that of methohexital, less than etomidate, and more than thiopental. This effect can be attenuated by injecting the medication through a rapidly running IV in a large vein (e.g., antecubital). Premedication with lidocaine (2–3 mL of 1% lidocaine) will also minimize the pain of injection. Propofol and

lidocaine are compatible in the same syringe and can be mixed in a 10:1 ratio (10 mL of propofol to 1 mL of 1% lidocaine). Propofol can cause mild clonus to a greater degree than thiopental, but less than etomidate or methohexital. Venous thrombophlebitis at the injection site can sometimes occur.

EVIDENCE

1. **What is the correct dosing of midazolam for RSI?** The dose of midazolam for induction of anesthesia is 0.2 to 0.3 mg/kg IV. The data to support this dose are from dosing studies conducted in the 1980s after the introduction of midazolam into clinical practice (1–9). Interestingly, Sagarin et al. (10), as a substudy of the National Emergency Airway Registry (NEAR) project, recently demonstrated that most emergency intubations performed with midazolam generally use doses in the 0.03 to 0.04 mg/kg range, dramatically less than the minimum recommended induction dose. Their analysis showed that this is likely due to inexperience with the larger doses of midazolam used for induction (10). In any case, midazolam is a poor choice as an induction agent for emergency RSI because of its relatively slow onset.

2. **Which induction agents are most hemodynamically stable?** Etomidate results in the least variation in blood pressure and heart rate when compared to the other agents used for rapid induction of anesthesia (11–15). Etomidate also appears to have less effect on cardiac function as determined by echocardiographic findings (15). This effect is seen in children and adults, including the elderly (11,14).

3. **Should etomidate be used in sepsis syndrome?** Etomidate has been widely adopted as the agent of choice for the induction phase of RSI because of its superior hemodynamic stability, reliable and predictable effects, rapidity of onset, brief duration of action, and lack of serious side effects (16).

   A single dose of etomidate will produce transient adrenal suppression through blockade of 11 β-hydroxylase, with suppression lasting up to 24 hours and perhaps beyond (17,18). Within the past 5 years, increased attention has focused on adrenal insufficiency in sepsis, the role of corticosteroids to treat these patients, and whether the use of etomidate as an induction agent constitutes an unnecessary risk (19,20). Although no studies to date have measured outcomes when sepsis patients were randomized to etomidate versus other agents, this has not deterred some authors from recommending proscription of the use of etomidate in sepsis. The most assertive of these has been published as a letter (21) and personal communication (22) in response to a report of a clinical trial involving low-dose corticosteroids in patients with septic shock (23). Annane et al. (23) reported 72 patients with septic shock received etomidate, of whom 68 subsequently failed to respond to corticotropin stimulation. A post hoc subgroup analysis of these 68 *nonresponders* revealed higher mortality rates in patients who had been randomized to receive placebo versus corticosteroids (76% vs. 55%) (22). The meaning of this finding is not clear. More recently, Lipiner-Friedman et al. (24), in a retrospective multicenter study on the use of corticosteroids in sepsis, concluded that etomidate influenced ACTH test results and was associated with a worse outcome. This study excluded etomidate use *within* 24 hours prior to the start of the study. Two hundred and thirty-seven (50%) patients received at least one dose of etomidate more than 24 hours before the study started. By their analysis, etomidate use was associated with a *moderately* increased risk of dying (odds ratio [OR] 1.53; 95% confidence interval [CI] 1.06–2.26). However, the use of vasopressors was associated with a *markedly* increased risk of dying (OR 38.52; 95% CI 20.69–71.73) (24). These findings underscore the limitations of retrospective study designs and the weakness of post-hoc analysis, in which patients were not randomized with respect to the agent being studied (in this case, etomidate). It is difficult to determine, after the fact, whether the etomidate had some real adverse effect, or whether the observed outcomes were the result of other factors. For example, it is difficult to accept that the use of vasopressors *caused* a 38-fold increase in mortality, and no one is calling for a moratorium on their use. Opposing the move against eto-midate, a study by Riché et al. (25), also retrospective, compared septic shock patients who underwent general anesthesia with or without etomidate and found no adverse effect on survival. In this study, response to a corticotrophin stimulation test did not predict survival (25). Another recent study compared the use of etomidate and other induction agents in 159 patients with septic shock and found that vasopressor therapy was required less frequently and in smaller doses when etomidate was used to induce anesthesia (18). However, this study is also subject to the same inability to control for confounders.

Etomidate has superior hemodynamic characteristics and offers, along with ket-amine, the best opportunity to avoid postintubation hypotension. For this reason, eto-midate has emerged as the induction agent of choice for emergency intubation of patients with hemodynamic instability or shock (26). Until more specific data are available, it would be premature to subject critically ill septic shock patients to worsened hypotension on the basis of a loosely inferred association drawn from retrospectively reanalyzed data.

Three approaches might be considered for the use of etomidate in patients with septic shock:

a. *Eliminate etomidate use altogether in these patients.* Although a few passionate advocates of this approach have emerged, principally in the critical care community, there is no evidence to support it. As summarized previously, there are no well-designed studies demonstrating that etomidate is detrimental to patients in septic shock. Although ketamine is also a reasonable agent for these hemodynamically compromised patients (27–31), etomidate is widely used and familiar with a wide margin of safety.

b. *Routinely administer corticosteroids to septic shock patients who have received etomidate (32).* Advocates of this approach argue that the administration of corticosteroids might correct adrenal suppression, if any, caused by etomidate (16,32). Again, although there are theoretical reasons why this might make sense, there is no evidence to support this approach; therefore, it cannot be recommended.

c. *Inform subsequent care providers that etomidate was used during intubation, so that they can consider this in their care of the patient.* In the presence of existing evidence, this would seem the appropriate approach.

4. **Is ketamine use acceptable in patients with elevated ICP?** Ketamine has not been recommended for patients with elevated ICP for more than three decades after early, small studies apparently showed increased cerebral oxygen consumption, CBF, and ICP after ketamine administration in these patients. Recently, evidence has emerged that has cast doubt on these longheld beliefs (33–39). Of most interest to those performing emergency intubation, the cerebral hemodynamic effects of ketamine are not as detrimental as previously believed. In spontaneously breathing volunteers, ketamine increases CBF and cerebral metabolism. In patients undergoing controlled ventilation and sedation, however, ketamine does not appear to increase ICP. When ketamine is used for sedation and analgesia in intubated head injured patients, the cerebral perfusion pressure is stable when compared with opioid/benzodiazepine combinations, mean arterial pressure is maintained, and vasopressor use is decreased (36–39).

It has been repeatedly shown that systemic hypotension is harmful in brain injury. Systolic blood pressure of 90 mm Hg or less in the emergency department is the single risk factor most highly associated with mortality in severe blunt head injury (35). Any mechanism by which hypotension can be avoided in traumatic brain injury should be encouraged. Ketamine maintains mean arterial pressure and has been shown not to increase ICP in ventilated patients. Ketamine should be considered for use in the multiply injured patient with head injury who is hypotensive on induction (39). A similar argument could be extended to medical causes of elevated ICP (tumor, hemorrhage.) In these patients, too, it would seem prudent to use an alternative agent when the blood pressure is normal or high, but ketamine is reasonable to consider when hypotension is present.

5. **What is the best induction agent in patients with seizures?** Etomidate has been shown to increase activity in certain electroencephalogram (EEG) leads in comparison to other sedatives when given to patients induced for general anesthesia. Thiopental, propofol, and midazolam all suppress EEG activity more quickly and completely than etomidate (40). Propofol, midazolam, or thiopental is a logical choice for RSI in the status seizure patient, followed by an infusion in the postintubation phase and ongoing EEG monitoring. Use of etomidate in the patient with status seizure is not contraindicated, but there are clearly superior agents for this indication (see Chapter 33).

6. **What is the best induction agent for patients with severe bronchospasm?** Ketamine and propofol both cause bronchodilation when used for induction (41–45). Eames et al. (43) prospectively demonstrated that 2.5 mg/kg of propofol was superior to either 0.4 mg/kg etomidate or 5 mg/kg thiopental in decreasing mean airway pressure during bronchoscopy in 75 patients. Simon, et al. (44) demonstrated immediate improvement after propofol in 6 of 18 intubated patients with severe asthma on ventilators, compared to 8 of 13 who were placed on halothane anesthesia. Hemmingsen, et al. (45) demonstrated a clinically and statistically significant improvement in respiratory dynamics after prospectively infusing ketamine or placebo to 14 asthmatics on ventilators. Etomidate causes a mild increase in airway resistance, but thiopental causes a significant rise in bronchospasm and resistance (43,46). Midazolam data are lacking. Ketamine is the recommended drug for patients without known coronary artery disease because it is readily available, can be given IV push, and results in an increase in hemodynamic parameters such as heart rate and blood pressure, in contrast to propofol.

7. **What is the role of the induction agent in intubation success?** The choice of sedative used for intubation may influence intubation success rates, especially if lower doses of a paralytic agent are used. A retrospective analysis of the NEAR data suggests that thiopental, methohexital, and propofol have higher first attempt intubation success rates compared to etomidate, benzodiazepines, ketamine, or no induction agent (47). Skinner, et al. (48) found that propofol was better than etomidate; however, Fuchs-Buder, et al. (49) found no difference between thiopental and etomidate with rocuronium paralysis. Hans et al. found ketamine superior to Pentothal, when rocuronium 0.6 mg/kg was the paralytic (50). El-Orbany et al. (51,52) found no difference between thiopental, propofol, and etomidate when rapacuronium was used as the paralytic agent. Although there is no clear winner, these variations underscore the importance of the induction agent to RSI success. Even though neuromuscular blockade is used, the dose and selection of the induction agent influence success, probably because of additive relaxation at the early phase of neuromuscular paralysis at which intubation is first attempted. Correct dosing of both the neuromuscular blocking agent and the sedative agent are required to achieve optimal intubating conditions during RSI.

8. **In the obese patient, how should I dose the induction agent?** This is discussed in Chapter 35.

REFERENCES

1. Berggren L, Eriksson I. Midazolam for induction of anaesthesia in outpatients: a comparison with thiopentone. *Acta Anaesthesiol Scand* 1981;25(6):492–496.

2. Crawford ME, Carl P, Bach V, et al. A randomized comparison between midazolam and thiopental for elective cesarean section anesthesia. I. Mothers. *Anesth Analg* 1989;68(3):229–233.

3. Driessen JJ, Booij LH, Crul JF, et al. [Comparative study of thiopental and midazolam for induction of anesthesia.] *Anaesthesist* 1983;32(10):478–482.

4. Izuora KL, Foulkes-Crabbe DJ, Kushimo OT, et al. Open comparative study of the efficacy, safety and tolerability of midazolam versus thiopental in induction and maintenance of anaesthesia. *West Afr J Med* 1994;13(2):73–80.

5. Jensen S, Schou-Olesen A, Huttel MS. Use of midazolam as an induction agent: comparison with thiopentone. *Br J Anaesth* 1982;54(6):605–607.

6. Lebowitz PW, Cote ME, Daniels AL, et al. Cardiovascular effects of midazolam and thiopentone for induction of anaesthesia in ill surgical patients. *Can Anaesth Soc J* 1983;30(1):19–23.

7. Lebowitz PW, Cote ME, Daniels AL, et al. Comparative cardiovascular effects of midazolam and thiopental in healthy patients. *Anesth Analg* 1982;61(9):771–775.

8. Pakkanen A, Kanto J. Midazolam compared with thiopentone as an induction agent. *Acta Anaesthesiol Scand* 1982;26(2):143–146.

9. Salonen M, Kanto J, Iisalo E. Induction of general anesthesia in children with midazolam—is there an induction dose? *Int J Clin Pharmacol Ther Toxicol* 1987;25(11):613–615.

10. Sagarin MJ, Barton ED, Sakles JC, et al. Underdosing of midazolam in emergency endotracheal intubation. *Acad Emerg Med* 2003;10(4):329–338.

11. Guldner G, Schultz J, Sexton P, et al. Etomidate for rapid-sequence intubation in young children: hemodynamic effects and adverse events. *Acad Emerg Med* 2003;10(2):134–139.

12. Benson M, Junger A, Fuchs C, et al. Use of an anesthesia information management system (AIMS) to evaluate the physiologic effects of hypnotic agents used to induce anesthesia. *J Clin Monit Comput* 2000;16(3):183–190.

13. Jellish WS, Riche H, Salord F, et al. Etomidate and thiopental-based anesthetic induction: comparisons between different titrated levels of electrophysiologic cortical depression and response to laryngoscopy. *J Clin Anesth* 1997;9(1):36–41.

14. Sokolove PE, Price DD, Okada P. The safety of etomidate for emergency rapid sequence intubation of pediatric patients. *Pediatr Emerg Care* 2000;16(1):18–21.

15. Gauss A, Heinrich H, Wilder-Smith OH. Echocardiographic assessment of the haemodynamic effects of propofol: a comparison with etomidate and thiopentone. *Anaesthesia* 1991;46(2):99–105.

16. Murray H, Marik PE. Etomidate for endotracheal intubation in sepsis: acknowledging the good while accepting the bad. *Chest* 2005;127(3):707–709.

17. Lundy JB, Slane ML, Frizzi JD. Acute adrenal insufficiency after a single dose of etomidate. *J Intensive Care Med* 2007;22(2):111–117.

18. Ray DC, McKeown DW. Effect of induction agent on vasopressor and steroid use, and outcome in patients with septic shock. *Crit Care* 2007;11(3):R56.

19. den Brinker M, Joosten KF, Liem O, et al. Adrenal insufficiency in meningococcal sepsis: bioavailable cortisol levels and impact of interleukin-6 levels and intubation with etomidate on adrenal function and mortality. *J Clin Endocrinol Metab* 2005;90(9):5110–5117.

20. Mohammad Z, Afessa B, Finkielman JD. The incidence of relative adrenal insufficiency in patients with septic shock after the administration of etomidate. *Crit Care* 2006;10(4):R105.

21. Annane D, Sebille V, Bellissant E. Corticosteroids for patients with septic shock. *JAMA* 2003;289(1):43–44.

22. Jackson WL Jr. Should we use etomidate as an induction agent for endotracheal intubation in patients with septic shock?: a critical appraisal. *Chest* 2005;127(3):1031–1038.

23. Annane D, Sebille V, Charpentier C, et al. Effect of treatment with low doses of hydrocortisone and fludrocortisone on mortality in patients with septic shock. *JAMA* 2002;288(7): 862–871.

24. Lipiner-Friedman D, Sprung CL, Laterre PF, et al. Adrenal function in sepsis: the retrospective Corticus cohort study. *Crit Care Med* 2007;35(4):1012–1018.

25. Riché FC, Boutron CM, Valleur P, et al. Adrenal response in patients with septic shock of abdominal origin: relationship to survival. *Intensive Care Med* 2007;33(10):1761–1766.

26. Green R. Etomidate and RSI: how important is post-intubation hypotension? *CJEM* 2007;9(1):3; author reply 4.

27. Hemmingsen C, Nielsen JE. Intravenous ketamine for prevention of severe hypotension during spinal anaesthesia. *Acta Anaesthesiol Scand* 1991;35(8):755–757.

28. Katz RI, Lagasse RS, Levy A, et al. Hemodynamic stability and patient satisfaction after anesthetic induction with thiopental sodium, ketamine, thiopental-fentanyl, and ketamine-fentanyl. *J Clin Anesth* 1993;5(2):134–140.

29. Furuya A, Matsukawa T, Ozaki M, et al. Intravenous ketamine attenuates arterial pressure changes during the induction of anaesthesia with propofol. *Eur J Anaesthesiol* 2001;18(2): 88–92.

30. Oklu E, Bulutcu FS, Yalcin Y, et al. Which anesthetic agent alters the hemodynamic status during pediatric catheterization? Comparison of propofol versus ketamine. *J Cardiothorac Vasc Anesth* 2003;17(6):686–690.

31. Goh PK, Chiu CL, Wang CY, et al. Randomized double-blind comparison of ketamine-propofol, fentanyl-propofol and propofol-saline on haemodynamics and laryngeal mask airway insertion conditions. *Anaesth Intensive Care* 2005;33(2):223–228.

32. Zed PJ, Mabasa VH, Slavik RS, et al. Etomidate for rapid sequence intubation in the emergency department: is adrenal suppression a concern? *CJEM* 2006;8(5):347–350.

33. Kolenda H, Gremmelt A, Rading S, et al. Ketamine for analgosedative therapy in intensive care treatment of head-injured patients. *Acta Neurochir (Wien)* 1996;138(10):1193–1199.

34. Albanese J, Arnaud S, Rey M, et al. Ketamine decreases intracranial pressure and electroencephalographic activity in traumatic brain injury patients during propofol sedation. *Anesthesiology* 1997;87(6):1328–1334.

35. Schreiber MA, Aoki N, Scott BG, et al. Determinants of mortality in patients with severe blunt head injury. *Arch Surg* 2002;137(3):285–290.

36. Bourgoin A, Albanese J, Wereszczynski N, et al. Safety of sedation with ketamine in severe head injury patients: comparison with sufentanil. *Crit Care Med* 2003;31(3):711–717.

37. Langsjo JW, Kaisti KK, Aalto S, et al. Effects of subanesthetic doses of ketamine on regional cerebral blood flow, oxygen consumption, and blood volume in humans. *Anesthesiology* 2003;99(3):614–623.

38. Bourgoin A, Albanese J, Leone M, et al. Effects of sufentanil or ketamine administered in target-controlled infusion on the cerebral hemodynamics of severely brain-injured patients. *Crit Care Med* 2005;33(5):1109–1113.

39. Himmelseher S, Durieux ME. Revising a dogma: ketamine for patients with neurological injury? *Anesth Analg* 2005;101(2):524–534.

40. Choi YF, Wong TW, Lau CC. Midazolam is more likely to cause hypotension than etomidate in emergency department rapid sequence intubation. *Emerg Med J* 2004;21(6):700–702.

41. Conti G, Dell'Utri D, Vilardi V, et al. Propofol induces bronchodilation in mechanically ventilated chronic obstructive pulmonary disease (COPD) patients. *Acta Anaesthesiol Scand* 1993;37(1):105–109.

42. Conti G, Ferretti A, Tellan G, et al. Propofol induces bronchodilation in a patient mechanically ventilated for status asthmaticus. *Intensive Care Med* 1993;19(5):305.

43. Eames WO, Rooke GA, Wu RS, et al. Comparison of the effects of etomidate, propofol, and thiopental on respiratory resistance after tracheal intubation. *Anesthesiology* 1996;84(6):1307–1311.

44. Simon A, Nebel B, Metz G. [Emergency intubation and ventilation therapy in severe bronchial asthma.] *Pneumologie* 1990;44(Suppl 1):657–658.

45. Hemmingsen C, Nielsen PK, Odorico J. Ketamine in the treatment of bronchospasm during mechanical ventilation. *Am J Emerg Med* 1994;12(4):417–420.

46. Wu RS, Wu KC, Sum DC, et al. Comparative effects of thiopentone and propofol on respiratory resistance after tracheal intubation. *Br J Anaesth* 1996;77(6):735–738.

47. Sivilotti ML, Filbin MR, Murray HE, et al. Does the sedative agent facilitate emergency rapid sequence intubation? *Acad Emerg Med* 2003;10(6):612–620.

48. Skinner HJ, Biswas A, Mahajan RP. Evaluation of intubating conditions with rocuronium and either propofol or etomidate for rapid sequence induction. *Anaesthesia* 1998;53(7): 702–706.

49. Fuchs-Buder T, Sparr HJ, Ziegenfuss T. Thiopental or etomidate for rapid sequence induction with rocuronium. *Br J Anaesth* 1998;80(4):504–506.

50. Hans P, Brichant JF, Hubert B, et al. Influence of induction of anaesthesia on intubating conditions one minute after rocuronium administration: comparison of ketamine and thiopentone. *Anaesthesia* 1999;54(3):276–279.

51. El-Orbany MI, Joseph NJ, Salem MR. Tracheal intubating conditions and apnoea time after small-dose succinylcholine are not modified by the choice of induction agent. *Br J Anaesth* 2005;95(5):710–714.

52. El-Orbany MI, Wafai Y, Joseph NJ, et al. Does the choice of intravenous induction drug affect intubation conditions after a fast-onset neuromuscular blocker? *J Clin Anesth* 2003;15(1):9–14.

19

Neuromuscular Blocking Agents

David A. Caro and Erik G. Laurin

INTRODUCTION

Neuromuscular blocking agents (NMBAs) are the cornerstone of rapid sequence intubation (RSI) and are used to facilitate rapid endotracheal intubation while minimizing the risks of aspiration or other adverse physiological events. NMBAs are used in conjunction with a sedative-induction agent for RSI because the NMBAs do not provide analgesia, sedation, or amnesia. Similarly, appropriate sedation is essential when neuromuscular blockade is maintained postintubation.

The pharmacology of NMBAs is based on their effects at the postjunctional cholinergic nicotinic receptors in the neuromuscular junction. Under normal circumstances, the nerve synthesizes acetylcholine (ACH) and stores it in small packages (vesicles). Nerve stimulation results in these vesicles migrating to the nerve surface, rupturing and discharging ACH into the junctional clefts between the nerve and the muscle as well as into those clefts that invaginate into the muscle fiber. The ACH attaches to ACH receptors, promoting muscle fiber depolarization that culminates in a muscle cell action potential and muscle cell contraction. Once the ACH diffuses away from the cleft, some undergoes reuptake into the prejunctional neuron, although most is hydrolyzed by acetylcholinesterase (ACHE). NMBAs are either agonists (depolarizers of the motor end plate) or antagonists ("nondepolarizers"). The antagonists attach to the receptors and competitively block ACH from accessing ACH receptors. Because they are in competition with ACH for the motor end plate, they can be displaced from the end plate by increasing concentrations of ACH, the end result of reversal agents (cholinesterase inhibitors such as neostigmine, edrophonium, and pyridostigmine) that inhibit ACHE and allow acetylcholine to accumulate and reverse the block.

In clinical practice, there are two classes of NMBAs: the noncompetitive or depolarizing NMBAs, of which succinylcholine (Anectine) is the prototype and the only one in common clinical use. The competitive or nondepolarizing agents are divided into two main classes: the benzylisoquinolinium compounds and the aminosteroid compounds. The benzylisoquinolines, d-tubocurarine (Tubarine), dimethyltubocurarine (Metocurine), atracurium (Tracrium), cisatracurium (Nimbex), and mivacurium (Mivacron) share common properties. The aminosteroids, vecuronium (Norcuron), pancuronium (Pavulon), and rocuronium (Zemuron) also share common attributes, which are distinct from those of the benzylisoquinolines.

Depolarizing (Competitive) NMBA: Succinylcholine

Intubating dose (mg/kg)	Onset (sec)	$t_{1/2}\alpha$ (min)	Duration (min)	$t_{1/2}\beta$ (hr)	Pregnancy Category
1.5	45 seconds	<1 minute	6–10	5	C

The ideal muscle relaxant to facilitate tracheal intubation would have a rapid onset of action, rendering the patient paralyzed within seconds; a short duration of action, returning the patient's normal protective reflexes within 3 to 4 minutes; no significant adverse side effects; and metabolism and excretion independent of liver and kidney function. Unfortunately, such an agent does not exist. Succinylcholine (SCh) comes closest to meeting these desirable goals. Despite the historic and well-known adverse effects of SCh and the continuous advent of new competitive NMBAs, SCh remains the drug of choice for emergency RSI in both adults and children.

A. *Clinical pharmacology*

SCh is actually two molecules of ACH linked back to back by an ester bridge, and as such, is chemically similar to ACH. It stimulates all nicotinic and muscarinic cholinergic receptors of the sympathetic and parasympathetic nervous system, not just those at the neuromuscular junction. Stimulation of cardiac muscarinic receptors can cause bradycardia, especially when repeated doses are given to small children. Although SCh can be a negative inotrope, this effect is so minimal as to have no clinical relevance. SCh also releases trace amounts of histamine, but this effect is also not clinically significant. Once SCh reaches the neuromuscular junction, it binds tightly to the ACH receptors, resulting in depolarization that manifests initially as fasciculations, then subsequent paralysis. The onset, activity, and duration of action of SCh are resistant to ACHE and dependent on rapid hydrolysis by pseudocholinesterase, an enzyme of the liver and plasma not present at the neuromuscular junction. Therefore, diffusion away from the neuromuscular junction motor end plate and back into the vascular compartment is ultimately responsible for SCh metabolism. This extremely important pharmacological concept explains why only a fraction of the initial intravenous (IV) dose of SCh ever reaches the motor end plate to promote paralysis. More important, it is for this reason that larger, rather than smaller, doses of SCh should always be given in emergency RSI. Incomplete paralysis may jeopardize the patient by compromising respiration and may not provide adequate relaxation to facilitate otherwise easy endotracheal intubation. Succinylmonocholine, the initial metabolite of SCh, sensitizes the cardiac muscarinic receptors in the sinus node to repeat does of SCh, which may then cause bradycardia that will respond to atropine. At room temperature, SCh retains 90% of its activity for up to 3 months. Refrigeration mitigates this degradation. Therefore, if SCh is stored at room temperature, it should be dated and regularly exchanged to the operating room, where it will be rapidly used.

B. *Indications and contraindications*

SCh remains the NMBA of choice for emergency RSI because of its rapid onset and relatively brief duration of action. A personal or family history of malignant hyperthermia is an absolute contraindication to the use of SCh. Inherited disorders that lead to abnormal or insufficient cholinesterases contraindicate SCh use in elective anesthesia, but are not an issue in emergency airway management. Certain conditions place patients at risk for SCh-related hyperkalemia and represent absolute contraindications to SCh. These patients should be intubated using a competitive, nondepolarizing NMBA. Relative contraindications to the use of SCh are dependent on the skill and proficiency of the intubator and the individual patient's clinical circumstance. The role of difficult airway assessment in the decision regarding whether a patient should undergo RSI is discussed in Chapters 2 and 7.

C. *Dosage and clinical use*

In the normal-size adult patient, the recommended dose of SCh for emergency RSI is 1.5 mg/kg IV. In a rare, life-threatening circumstance when SCh must be given intramuscularly (IM) because of inability to secure venous access, a dose of 4 mg/kg IM may be used. Absorption and delivery of drug will be dependent on the patient's circulatory status. Intramuscular administration may result in a prolonged period of vulnerability for the patient, during which respirations will be compromised, but relaxation is not sufficient to permit intubation. Active bag-mask ventilation will usually be required before laryngoscopy in this circumstance.

Although length-based drug dosing will lead to the correct dose of SCh for children, adults, including obese adults, are dosed on a total body weight basis (see Chapter 35). In the emergency department, it may be impossible to know the exact weight of a patient, and weight estimates, especially of supine patients, have been shown to be notoriously inaccurate. In those uncertain circumstances, it is better to err on the side of a higher dose of SCh to ensure adequate patient paralysis. The serum half-life of SCh is less than 1 minute, so doubling the dose theoretically increases the duration of block by only 60 seconds. The margin of safety in dosing SCh is up to a cumulative dose of 6 mg/kg. At doses greater than 6 mg/kg, the typical phase 1 depolarization block of SCh becomes a phase 2 block, which changes the pharmacokinetic displacement of SCh from the motor end plate; that is, it becomes competitive rather than noncompetitive. This may prolong the duration of paralysis but is otherwise clinically irrelevant. The risk of an inadequately paralyzed patient who is difficult to intubate because of an inadequate dose of SCh greatly outweighs the minimal potential for adverse effects from excessive dosing.

In children younger than 10 years of age, length-based dosing is recommended, but if weight is used as the determinant, the recommended dose of SCh for emergency RSI is 2 mg/kg IV, and in the newborn (younger than 12 months of age), the appropriate dose is 3 mg/kg IV. Some practitioners routinely administer atropine to children younger than 12 months old who are receiving SCh, but there is no high-quality evidence to support this practice. There is similarly no evidence that it is harmful, so it is considered optional. When adults or children of any age receive a second dose of SCh, bradycardia may occur, and atropine should be readily available.

D. *Adverse effects*

The recognized side effects of SCh include fasciculations, hyperkalemia, bradycardia, prolonged neuromuscular blockade, malignant hyperthermia, and trismus/masseter muscle spasm. Each is discussed separately.

1. Fasciculations

Fasciculations are believed to be produced by stimulation of the nicotinic ACH receptors. Fasciculations occur simultaneously with increases in intracranial pressure (ICP), intraocular pressure, and intragastric pressure, but these are not the result of concerted muscle activity. Of these, only the increase in ICP is potentially clinically important.

The exact mechanisms by which these effects occur are not well elucidated. The use of nondepolarizing agents to pretreat fasciculations in an attempt to prevent increases in ICP has been emphasized in the past. A systematic review failed to show sufficient evidence for this practice in acute brain injury, but did show level II evidence of a modest effect in patients undergoing neurosurgery with brain tumors.

The relationship between muscle fasciculation and subsequent postoperative muscle pain is controversial. Studies have been variable with respect to prevention of fasciculations and subsequent muscle pain. The theoretical concern in open globe injury is extrusion of vitreous, but there has not been a single published report of this. In fact, many anesthesiologists continue to use SCh as a muscle relaxant in cases of open globe injury, with or without an accompanying defasciculating agent. Similarly, the increase in intragastric pressure that has been measured has never been shown to be of any clinical significance, perhaps because it is offset by a corresponding increase in the lower esophageal sphincter pressure.

2. Hyperkalemia

Under normal circumstances, serum potassium increases minimally (0–0.5 mEq/L) when SCh is administered. In certain pathological conditions, however, a rapid and dramatic increase in serum potassium can occur in response to SCh. These pathological hyperkalemic responses occur by two distinct mechanisms: receptor upregulation and rhabdomyolysis. In either situation, potassium increase may approach 5 to 10 mEq/L within a few minutes and result in hyperkalemic dysrhythmias or cardiac arrest.

Two forms of postjunctional receptors exist: mature (junctional) and immature (extrajunctional). Each receptor is composed of five proteins arranged in a circular fashion around a common channel. Both types of receptors contain two alpha subunits. ACH must attach to both alpha subunits to open the channel and effect depolarization and muscle contraction. When receptor upregulation occurs, the mature receptors at and around the motor end plate are gradually converted over a 4- to 5-day period to immature receptors that propagate throughout the entire muscle membrane. Immature receptors are characterized by low conductance and prolonged channel opening times (four times longer than mature receptors), resulting in increasing release of potassium. Most of the entities associated with hyperkalemia during emergency RSI are the result of receptor upregulation. Interestingly, these same extrajunctional nicotinic receptors are relatively refractory to nondepolarizing agents, so larger doses of vecuronium, pancuronium, or rocuronium may be required to produce paralysis. This is not an issue in emergency RSI, where full intubating doses several times greater than the ED_{95} for paralysis are used.

Rhabdomyolysis is the other mechanism by which hyperkalemia may occur. It is most often associated with myopathies, especially inherited forms of muscular dystrophy. When severe hyperkalemia occurs related to rhabdomyolysis, the mortality approaches 30%, almost three times higher than that in cases of receptor upregulation. This mortality increase may be related to coexisting cardiomyopathy. SCh is a toxin to unstable membranes in any patient with a myopathy and should be avoided.

Patients with the following conditions are at risk of SCh-induced hyperkalemia:

a. **Burns**

In burn victims, the extrajunctional receptor sensitization becomes clinically significant 5 days postburn. It lasts an indefinite period of time, at least until there is complete healing of the burned area. If the burn becomes infected or healing is delayed, the patient remains at risk for hyperkalemia. It is prudent not to administer SCh to burned patients beyond day 5 post-burn if any question exists regarding the status of their burn. The percent of body surface area burned does not correlate well with the magnitude of hyperkalemia. Significant hyperkalemia has been reported in patients with as little as 8% total body surface area burn (less than the surface of one arm), but this is rare. Most emergency intubations for burns are performed well within the safe 5-day window after the burn occurs, but if later intubation is required, rocuronium or vecuronium provide excellent alternatives for emergency RSI in these situations (see Chapter 26).

b. **Denervation**

The patient who suffers a denervation event, such as spinal cord injury or stroke, is at risk for hyperkalemia from approximately the fifth day post event until there is healing or total muscle fiber atrophy (generally 6 months post event). Patients with progressive neuromuscular disorders such as multiple sclerosis or amyotrophic lateral sclerosis are perpetually at risk for hyperkalemia. Likewise, patients with transient neuromuscular disorders such as Guillain-Barré syndrome or wound botulism can develop hyperkalemia after day 5, depending on the severity of their disease. As long as the neuromuscular disease is dynamic, there will be augmentation of the extrajunctional receptors and the risk for hyperkalemia. The hyperkalemic response cannot be attenuated by administering defasciculating doses of nondepolarizing NMBAs, and therefore, these specific clinical situations should be considered absolute contraindications to SCh during the designated time periods.

c. **Crush injuries**

The data regarding crush injuries are scant. The hyperkalemic response begins about 5 days postinjury, similar to denervation, and persists for several months after healing seems complete. The mechanism appears to be receptor upregulation.

d. **Severe infections**

This entity seems to relate to established, serious infections, usually in the intensive care unit environment. The mechanism is receptor upregulation, but the initiating event is not established. Total body disuse atrophy and chemical denervation of the ACH receptors, particularly if muscle relaxants are chronically infused, appear to drive the pathological receptor changes. Again, the at-risk time period is 5 days after initiation of the infection and continues indefinitely as long as the disease process is dynamic. Intra-abdominal sepsis has most prominently been identified as the culprit, but any serious, prolonged, debilitating infection should prompt concern.

e. **Prolonged Immobility**

Hospitalized patients who are bedbound and relatively immobile for long periods can develop severe SCh-related hyperkalemia from disuse atrophy, as described previously. Another common setting is the elderly patient who has been ill and immobile (e.g. "found down") for several days at home, then enters the emergency care system and RSI is performed as part of the stabilization efforts.

f. **Myopathies**

SCh is absolutely contraindicated in patients with inherited myopathies, such as muscular dystrophy. Myopathic hyperkalemia can be devastating because of the combined effects of receptor upregulation and rhabdomyolysis. This is a particularly difficult problem in pediatrics, when a child with occult muscular dystrophy receives SCh. SCh has a black box warning advising against its use in elective pediatric anesthesia, but it continues to be the muscle relaxant of choice for emergency intubation. Any patient suspected of a myopathy should be intubated with nondepolarizing muscle relaxants rather than SCh.

g. **Pre-existing hyperkalemia**

The risk of SCh-induced cardiac dysrhythmias in patients who are hyperkalemic prior to SCh administration is not clearly determined. Although there is widespread belief that patients with acute hyperkalemia, such as from acute renal failure or diabetic ketoacidosis, are more likely to exhibit cardiac disturbances from SCh than patients with chronic or recurrent hyperkalemia, such as chronic renal failure, there is no evidence to support this. Most likely, the severity of pre-existing hyperkalemia dictates the response because these patients are subject to the same potential rise of 0 to 0.5 mEq/L of potassium. The only study evaluating the use of SCh in large numbers of patients with chronic renal failure, including those with hyperkalemia prior to intubation, failed to identify any adverse effects. A reasonable approach is to assume that SCh is safe to use in patients with renal failure unless the ECG (either monitor tracing or 12-lead ECG) shows evidence of acute hyperkalemia (high T waves or prolongation of QRS).

3. **Bradycardia**

The controversy regarding bradycardia following the administration of SCh in young children is discussed in Chapter 20. In both adults and children, repeated doses of SCh may produce bradycardia, and administration of atropine may become necessary.

4. **Prolonged neuromuscular blockade**

Prolonged neuromuscular blockade may result from an acquired pseudocholinesterase (PCHE) deficiency, a congenital absence of PCHE, or the presence of an atypical form of PCHE, any of the three of which will delay the degradation of SCh and prolong paralysis. Acquired PCHE deficiency may be a result of liver disease, pregnancy, burns, oral contraceptives, metoclopramide, bambuterol, or esmolol. Atypical or abnormal genetic variants of PCHE can be disclosed by testing the patient's PCHE against dibucaine. A 20% reduction in normal levels will increase apnea time about 3 to 9 minutes. The most severe variant (0.04% of population) will prolong paralysis for 4 to 8 hours.

5. **Malignant hyperthermia**

A personal or family history of malignant hyperthermia (MH) is an absolute contraindication to the use of SCh. MH is a myopathy characterized by a genetic skeletal muscle membrane abnormality of the Ry[1] ryanodine receptor. It can be triggered by halogenated anesthetics, SCh, vigorous exercise, and even emotional stress. Following the initiating event, its onset can be acute and progressive or delayed for hours. Generalized awareness of MH, earlier diagnosis, and the availability of dantrolene (Dantrium) have decreased the mortality from as high as 70% to less than 5%. Acute loss of intracellular calcium control results in a cascade of rapidly progressive events manifested primarily by increased metabolism, muscular rigidity, autonomic instability, hypoxia, hypotension, severe lactic acidosis, hyperkalemia, myoglobinemia, and disseminated intravascular coagulation. Temperature elevation is a late manifestation. The presence of more than one of these clinical signs is suggestive of MH. Masseter spasm has been claimed to be the hallmark of MH. However, SCh can promote isolated masseter spasm as an exaggerated response at the neuromuscular junction, especially in children. Therefore, masseter spasm alone is not pathognomonic of MH.

The treatment for MH consists of discontinuing the known or suspected precipitant and the immediate administration of dantrolene sodium (Dantrium). Dantrolene is essential to successful resuscitation and should be given as soon as the diagnosis is seriously entertained. Dantrolene is a hydantoin derivative that acts directly on skeletal muscle to prevent calcium release from the sarcoplasmic reticulum without affecting calcium reuptake. The initial dose is 2.5 mg/kg IV and is repeated every 5 minutes until muscle relaxation occurs or the maximum dose of 10 mg/kg is administered. Dantrolene is free of any serious side effects. In addition, measures to control body temperature, acid–base balance, and renal function must be used. All cases of MH require constant monitoring of pH, arterial blood gases, and serum potassium. Immediate and aggressive management of hyperkalemia with the administration of calcium gluconate, glucose, insulin, and sodium bicarbonate may be necessary. Interestingly, full paralysis with nondepolarizing NMBAs will prevent SCh-triggered MH. MH has never been reported related to use of SCh in the emergency department. The MH emergency hotline number is 1–800-MH-HYPER 1-800-644-9737 (U.S. and Canada) or 315-464-7079, 24 hours a day, 7 days a week. Ask for "index zero." The e-mail address for the Malignant Hyperthermia Association of the United States (MHAUS) is mhaus@norwich.net, and the Web site is www.mhaus.org.

6. **Trismus/masseter muscle spasm**
SCh can transiently raise mandibular muscle tone. This is not true spasm, and laryngoscopy is usually unaffected. On occasion, SCh may cause transient trismus/masseter muscle spasm, especially in children. This is manifested as jaw muscle rigidity associated with limb muscle flaccidity. Pretreatment with defasciculating doses of nondepolarizing NMBAs will not prevent masseter spasm. If masseter spasm interferes with intubation, an intubating dose of a competitive nondepolarizing agent (e.g., rocuronium 1 mg/kg) should be administered and will relax the involved muscles. The patient may require bag-mask ventilation until relaxation is complete and intubation is possible. In such circumstances, serious consideration should be given to the diagnosis of MH (see previous discussion).

Nondepolarizing (Competitive) NMBA

A. *Clinical pharmacology*
The nondepolarizing NMBAs actually compete with and block the action of ACH at the postjunctional cholinergic nicotinic receptors in the neuromuscular junction. The blockade is accomplished by competitively binding to one or both of the alpha subunits in the receptor, preventing ACH access to both alpha subunits, which is required for muscle depolarization. This competitive blockade is characterized by the absence of fasciculations and the reversal of paralysis by ACHE inhibitors that prevent metabolism of ACH and allow its reaccumulation and retransmission at the motor end plate, promoting a

muscle contraction. These drugs are metabolized and eliminated by Hoffman degradation, liver metabolism, and renal excretion.

The nondepolarizing NMBAs are divided into two groups: the benzylisoquinolinium compounds (e.g., d-tubocurarine, atracurium, mivacurium) and the aminosteroid compounds (e.g., vecuronium, pancuronium, rocuronium). Of the two groups, the aminosteroid compounds are the only agents used commonly for emergency RSI and postintubation paralysis.

In general, the aminosteroid compounds do not release histamine and do not cause ganglionic blockade. They vary inversely regarding their potency and time to onset (more potent agents require longer time to onset), and they exhibit differences in their vagolytic effects (i.e., moderate in pancuronium, slight in rocuronium, absent in vecuronium).

These compounds are further subdivided based on their duration of action, which is determined by their metabolism and excretion. None has the brief duration of action of SCh. Pancuronium is longer lasting than vecuronium or rocuronium. Although pancuronium is excreted primarily by the kidney, 10% to 20% is metabolized in the liver. Vecuronium is more lipophilic, hence more easily absorbed. It is eliminated primarily in the bile and is very stable cardiovascularly. Rocuronium is lipophilic and excreted in the bile. We recommend only rocuronium or vecuronium for emergency RSI (see Chapter 26).

The nondepolarizing NMBAs can be reversed by administering ACHE inhibitors such as neostigmine (Prostigmine) 0.06 to 0.08 mg/kg IV after significant (40%) spontaneous recovery has occurred. Atropine 0.02 mg/kg IV or glycopyrrolate (Robinul) 0.2 mg IV should be given to block excessive muscarinic stimulation. Reversal of blockade with neostigmine is rarely, if ever, indicated following emergency airway management. A new selective rocuronium reversal agent, called sugammadex (Org 25969), is in phase III studies at the time of this writing. Its hollow, cone-shaped molecular structure encapsulates rocuronium and promotes dissociation of the rocuronium from the ACH receptor, thereby reversing the neuromuscular block without the muscarinic side effects of the ACHE inhibitors. Spontaneous breathing is restored in approximately 1 minute, compared to more than 5 minutes with the ACHE inhibitors. In addition, sugammadex is rapidly effective, regardless of the extent of the neuromuscular block, and it is not necessary for any spontaneous recovery to occur before reversal is initiated. A rapid reversal agent such as this may be clinically useful in emergency RSI, especially if rapid reversal is desired for a failed airway. See *Evidence* section for details.

B. *Indications and contraindications*

The nondepolarizing NMBAs serve a multipurpose role in emergency airway management. They have been widely used as pretreatment agents to attenuate increases in ICP that occurs in response to succinylcholine administration, but we no longer recommend them for this purpose. Rocuronium or vecuronium can be used for emergency RSI when SCh is contraindicated (see Chapter 26), and any of the competitive agents is appropriate for maintenance of postintubation paralysis, when this is desired (see Chapter 3). There are no known contraindications to nondepolarizing NMBAs. Patients with myasthenia gravis are sensitive to NMBAs and may experience greater, or more prolonged, paralysis at any given dose.

	Intubating dose (mg/kg)	Time to intubation level paralysis (sec)	Duration (min)
Vecuronium	0.01 to prime, then 0.15	75–90	60–75
Rocuronium	1	60–75	40–60

C. *Dosage and clinical use*

1. For RSI when SCh is contraindicated, the drug of choice is rocuronium 1.0 mg/kg IV, which produces intubation-level paralysis consistently within 60 seconds, especially when an adequate dose of induction (sedative) agent is used. If rocuronium is not available, vecuronium can be given using a modified priming regimen. A priming dose of 0.01 mg/kg is given, followed 3 minutes later by an intubating dose of 0.15 mg/kg. Pancuronium is not recommended for emergency RSI (see Chapter 26).

2. For postintubation management when continued neuromuscular blockade is desired, vecuronium 0.1 mg/kg IV or pancuronium 0.1 mg/kg IV is appropriate, in concert with adequate sedation (see Chapter 3).

   Table 19-1 lists the onset and duration of action for routine paralyzing doses of all commonly used NMBAs. The onset times and durations are for the specific doses listed, which are lower than the doses used for intubation, and vary with dose for each agent.

D. *Adverse effects*

Of the three aminosteroid compounds, pancuronium is the least expensive but may be less desirable because it has a tendency to produce tachycardia. Vecuronium and rocuronium are more expensive but do not cause tachycardia. All competitive NMBAs are generally less desirable for intubation than SCh because of either delayed time to paralysis, prolonged duration of action, or both. Their onset can be shortened by administering the rather larger intubating dose (as opposed to the ED95 dose (Table 19-1) used for surgical paralysis), but this further prolongs the duration of action. Availability of rapidly effective reversal agents, such as sugammadex, may greatly expand the role of competitive NMBAs in emergency RSI.

TABLE 19-1

Onset and Duration of Action of Neuromuscular Blocking Drugs

Drug	Dose (mg/kg)	Time to maximal blockade (min)	Time to recovery (min) 25%	Time to recovery (min) 75%
Quarternary amine				
Succinylcholine	1.0	1.1	8	11 (90%)
Benzylisoquinolinium compounds				
Tubocurarine	0.5	3.4	—	130
Metocurine	0.4	4.1	107	—
Atracurium	0.4	2.4	38	52
Doxacurium	0.05	5.9	83	116
Mivacurium	0.15	1.8	16	25
Cisatracurium	0.1	7.7	46	63
Aminosteroid compounds				
Pancuronium	0.08	2.9	86	—
Vecuronium	0.1	2.4	44	56
Rocuronium	0.6	1.0	43	66

From Hunter JM. Drug therapy: new neuromuscular blocking drugs. *N Engl J Med* 1995;332:1691–1699, with permission.

EVIDENCE

1. **What is the advantage to RSI with an NMBA versus intubation with deep sedation alone?** RSI with a paralytic agent is the current standard of care for routine emergency intubation. NMBAs have been safely and successfully used in the emergency setting since the late 1970s to provide paralysis for intubation (1–3). Cicala and Westbrook (4) demonstrated an improved intubation success rate with neuromuscular blockade over deep anesthesia without neuromuscular blockade. This finding has been replicated many times, most recently by Naguib and his colleagues in two separate studies. In one study, patients received doses of SCh ranging from 0 to 2 mg/kg, after induction with propofol and fentanyl. Seventy percent of the group receiving no SCh had poor intubating conditions or failed intubation, despite full induction of general anesthesia (5). By comparison, more than 80% of the patients receiving 1.5 mg/kg or more of SCh had excellent intubating conditions. In an earlier study, the same investigators found acceptable intubating conditions in more than 95% of patients receiving SCh versus only 30% of those undergoing general anesthesia without neuromuscular blockade (6). The same results have been observed when rocuronium is used for intubation. In one study, 65% of patients who received general anesthesia without rocuronium had unacceptable intubating conditions, compared to zero patients who received rocuronium (7). In a study by Bozeman et al. (8), comparing etomidate-alone intubation to RSI using etomidate and SCh in an air medical setting, good or acceptable intubating conditions occurred in 79% of the RSI group versus 13% of the etomidate group. Success rates were 92% for RSI, 25% for etomidate alone (8). Multiple prospective studies confirm the high success rate of RSI with NMBAs when performed by experienced operators (9–11), with a lower rate of complications compared to sedatives alone (12,13).

2. **Are any of the nondepolarizing NMBAs as good as SCh for emergency RSI?** Multiple studies have compared SCh to rocuronium and vecuronium for intubation, but only a few have approximated the conditions and circumstances of an emergency RSI (9,14,15). Three review articles compared intubation success rates and intubating conditions for SCh versus rocuronium, and all three concluded that the two drugs are similar but not identical (16–18). SCh produces slightly better intubating conditions and has a statistically significant reduced number of intubation attempts when compared to intubating doses of rocuronium (19). A recent Cochrane review of rocuronium versus SCh for RSI concluded that, in adults, SCh produced "excellent" intubating conditions more often than rocuronium, but "adequate" ("excellent or good") intubating conditions were produced equally with either NMBA (20). In a subgroup analysis, the intubating conditions were equivalent only if propofol was used as the sedative agent. In children, the conclusion was that SCh and rocuronium produced equivalent intubating conditions, but the studies were few and varied in design. The Cochrane review included 26 papers, of which only two used true RSI (intubation in <60 seconds), and none were done by emergency physicians in the emergency department. There are little data comparing SCh and rocuronium for emergency department RSI by emergency physicians, but one study of 520 intubations found SCh produced slightly better intubating conditions than rocuronium (16). The mean onset time of paralysis for SCh was 39 ± 13 seconds, and for rocuronium was 44 ± 15 seconds, which was neither statistically nor clinically significant. Importantly, the dose of rocuronium is critical to the success of rapid intubation. This has been elegantly studied, and the correct dose of rocuronium for RSI is 1.0 mg/kg, not 0.6 mg/kg as is commonly recommended. The duration for the 1.0 mg/kg dose is 46 minutes (18,21,22). SCh has been repeatedly shown to produce better intubating conditions at 45 to 60 seconds compared to

pancuronium, vecuronium, and atracurium in well-designed prospective studies (23–25).

3. **Can I give an NMBA intramuscularly?** IV administration of NMBAs is vastly preferred to other routes, but infrequently a situation arises in which IV or intraosseous access cannot be obtained. IM administration of NMBAs has been described, with multiple agents (SCh, rocuronium, and mivacurium) studied. Invariably, the onset to paralysis is delayed. Schuh (26) performed a prospective comparison of SCh via IM and IV routes and found that the IM dose required is 3.0 to 4.0 mg/kg and time to onset is 5 to 6 minutes. Sutherland, Bevan, and Bevan (27) performed a prospective study that demonstrated obliteration of muscle twitch at 4.0 ± 0.6 minutes with an IM dose of 4 mg/kg. Each of the studies assessing IM rocuronium combines it with prior halothane use, which is not applicable to the emergency airway management situation. Reynolds et al. (28,29) prospectively demonstrated that deltoid injection of 1.0 mg/kg in infants and 1.8 mg/kg in children created adequate or good intubating conditions in 2.5 and 3.0 minutes, respectively. Kaplan et al. (30), however, found that equivalent doses gave inadequate intubating conditions at 2.5 and 3.0 minutes, and only half of the children receiving these doses had adequate intubating conditions at 3.5 and 4 minutes. The majority of patients had adequate conditions only after 7 to 8 minutes. Although IM administration of NMBAs has been described, its use in the emergent situation should be limited to the rare situation when absolutely no IV or intraosseous access can be obtained.

4. **What is the correct dose of SCh for RSI?** Although recent studies have demonstrated acceptable intubating conditions with doses of SCh as low as 0.3 mg/kg, these studies have not replicated the conditions extant for emergency RSI (6,31). Intubating conditions appear directly related to the dose of SCh used, with excellent intubating conditions in more than 80% of patients receiving 1.5 mg/kg or more of SCh (5). Increasing the dose of SCh from 0.5 mg/kg to 2 mg/kg increased the duration of action only from 5.2 to 7.5 minutes, reinforcing the notion that the half-life of SCh in vivo is about 1 minute, as shown by Kato et al. (5,32). Earlier studies have also shown that 1.0 mg/kg of SCh provides better intubating conditions than does placebo, 0.3 mg/kg or 0.5 mg/kg (6,33). In addition, use of 1.5 mg/kg of SCh is associated with less muscle fasciculation and myalgia than the 1.0 mg/kg dose (31). There is sufficient evidence that decreasing doses of succinylcholine produce inferior intubating conditions; hence, our firm recommendation that 1.5 mg/kg be considered the dose for emergency RSI.

5. **What is the correct dose of rocuronium for RSI?** Rocuronium has been studied in the context of intubation, although not precisely in the setting of RSI. Most studies induce general anesthesia, then compare escalating doses of rocuronium and, occasionally, succinylcholine. Early studies suggested that rocuronium doses of 0.6 mg/kg are inferior to doses of 0.9 to 1.2 mg/kg (15). The most valuable information, however, is provided by Kirkegaard-Nielsen et al. (7), who randomized patients to various doses of rocuronium for intubation at 60 seconds and showed that 1.0 mg/kg is the optimal dose.

6. **SCh use in patients with open eye injuries.** SCh has been linked to increases in intraocular pressure. Concern has been raised about its use in penetrating eye injuries (34). However, there has never been a case report of vitreous extrusion following the use of SCh in a patient with an open globe injury (35). The more pressing concern for the protection of the injured eye is the prevention of stimuli associated with laryngoscopy (36). Pretreatment with a nondepolarizing NMBA is recommended in patients with open globe injuries, but without supporting evidence.

7. **Timing of hyperkalemia after significant (>5% body surface area) burns.** Schaner et al. (37) and Gronert et al. (38) found the greatest risk 18 to 66 days postburn in two studies in 1969 and 1975, and Viby-Mogensen et al. (39) found dangerous rises in serum potassium as early as 9 days postburn. SCh can be safely used within the

first week of a burn, but should be withheld after the first week through clinical healing of the burn wound. We recommend a 5 day post-burn cut-off.

8. **SCh use in denervation injuries (stroke, Guillain-Barré syndrome, polio, spinal cord trauma, myasthenia gravis, etc.).** Denervation injuries cause a change in the number and function of junctional and extrajunctional ACH receptors at 4 to 5 days postinjury (40,41). This can result in massive serum potassium increases that can cause cardiac arrest. SCh can be safely used up to 5 days postdenervation and not again until complete muscle atrophy has occurred or the event is no longer dynamic.

9. **SCh use in myopathic patients (muscular dystrophy, rhabdomyolysis, crush injuries, prolonged immobility, etc.).** Myopathies cause hyperkalemia by a similar mechanism as denervation, that is, changes in ACH receptor function and density (42). Congenital myopathies are considered an absolute contraindication to SCh; its use with the myopathies can result in rhabdomyolysis and resuscitation-resistant hyperkalemic arrest (43,44). Hyperkalemia and occult, undiagnosed myopathy must be considered in children who experience cardiac arrest after SCh (45,46). When a patient with known rhabdomyolysis is encountered, SCh should be avoided.

10. **SCh use in patients with pre-existing hyperkalemia.** There are few studies of the risk of SCh administration in hyperkalemic patients (47,48). Unfortunately, no studies examine the outcome of large numbers of patients with pre-existing hyperkalemia. In fact, even the prevalence of pre-existing hyperkalemia in emergency department patients undergoing RSI is rarely described (16). In a meta-analysis, Thapa and Brull (49) identified only four controlled studies of patients with and without renal failure, and there were no cases in which serum potassium rose by more than 0.5 mEq/L. In two cases series, 22 of 23 patients with chronic renal failure had maximum serum potassium increases of 0.7 mEq/L. The other patient had an increase of 1.2 mEq/L, which resolved without treatment in a few minutes (49). The largest series, involving more than 40,000 patients undergoing general anesthesia, identified 38 adults and children with hyperkalemia (5.6–7.6 mEq/L) at the time they received SCh. None of the 38 had an adverse event, and the authors calculated that the maximum likelihood of an adverse event related to SCh in hyperkalemic patients is 7.9% (50). The long-held dogma to avoid SCh in any patient with renal failure is not valid, and SCh's independence of renal excretion makes it an excellent agent to consider when renal function is impaired (51,52). Some small studies have shown no instances of cardiac arrest when using SCh in the setting of renal failure (49,53), as long as the pre-SCh potassium was not elevated. We recommend that when hyperkalemia is present, or believed to be present (e.g., patient with end-stage renal disease), and the ECG shows stigmata of hyperkalemia (peaked T waves or increased QRS duration), an alternative agent, usually rocuronium, should be used for RSI. Otherwise, renal failure, or nominal hyperkalemia (i.e., without ECG changes), is not a contraindication to SCh.

10. **SCh use in patients with severe (especially intraabdominal) infections.** Intraabdominal infections lasting longer than 1 week are susceptible to SCh-induced hyperkalemia (54). SCh-induced hyperkalemia risk increases with increasing severity of infection (55).

11. **Treatment for SCh-induced MH.** Discontinue any anesthetic use. Dantrolene, 2 mg/kg IV, is the recommended therapy, and it can be repeated every 5 minutes to a total dose of 10 mg/kg (56). In a review of 21 patients with presumed MH, 11 patients immediately treated with dantrolene survived, and 3 of 4 patients who did not receive treatment until 24 hours later died (6 patients were excluded because of insufficient evidence that MH was the cause of decompensation) (57).

12. **Sugammadex evidence.** The molecular shape of sugammadex allows it to encapsulate rocuronium and reverse neuromuscular blockade (58,59). Early studies demonstrate safe and effective reversal of rocuronium neuromuscular blockade in less than 2 minutes (60–63). (See also Chapter 26.)

ACKNOWLEDGMENT

The authors wish to recognize the significant contributions made by Robert Schneider, MD, to versions of this chapter in previous editions of this manual.

REFERENCES

1. Roberts DJ, Clinton JE, Ruiz E. Neuromuscular blockade for critical patients in the emergency department. *Ann Emerg Med* 1986;15:152–156.
2. Thompson JD, Fish S, Ruiz E. Succinylcholine for endotracheal intubation. *Ann Emerg Med* 1982;11:526–529.
3. Brown EM, Krishnaprasad D, Smiler BG. Pancuronium for rapid induction technique for tracheal intubation. *Can Anaesth Soc J* 1979;26:489–491.
4. Cicala R, Westbrook L. An alternative method of paralysis for rapid-sequence induction. *Anesthesiology* 1988;69:983–986.
5. Naguib M, Samarkandi AH, El-Din ME, et al. The dose of succinylcholine required for excellent endotracheal intubating conditions. *Anesth Analg* 2006;102:151–155.
6. Naguib M, Samarkandi A, Riad W, et al. Optimal dose of succinylcholine revisited. *Anesthesiology* 2003;99:1045–1049.
7. Kirkegaard-Nielsen H, Caldwell JE, Berry PD, et al. Rapid tracheal intubation with rocuronium: a probability approach to determining dose. *Anesthesiology* 1999;91(1):131–136.
8. Bozeman WP, Kleiner DM, Huggett V, et al. A comparison of rapid-sequence intubation and etomidate-only intubation in the prehospital air medical setting. *Prehosp Emerg Care* 2006;10(1):8–13.
9. Sagarin MJ, Chiang V, Sakles JC, et al. National Emergency Airway Registry (NEAR) investigators. Rapid sequence intubation for pediatric emergency airway management. *Pediatr Emerg Care* 2002;18:417–423.
10. Tayal VS, Riggs RW, Marx JA, et al. Rapid-sequence intubation at an emergency medicine residency: success rate and adverse events during a two-year period. *Acad Emerg Med* 1999;6:31–37.
11. Sakles JC, Laurin EG, Rantapaa AA, et al. Airway management in the emergency department: a one-year study of 610 tracheal intubations. *Ann Emerg Med* 1998;31:325–332.
12. Li J, Murphy-Lavoie H, Bugas C, et al. Complications of emergency intubation with and without paralysis. *Am J Emerg Med* 1999;17:141–143.
13. Gnauck K, Lungo JB, Scalzo A, et al. Emergency intubation of the pediatric medical patient: use of anesthetic agents in the emergency department. *Ann Emerg Med* 1994;23:1242–1247.
14. Vijayakumar E, Bosscher H, Renzi FP, et al. The use of neuromuscular blocking agents in the emergency department to facilitate tracheal intubation in the trauma patient: help or hindrance? *J Crit Care* 1998;13:1–6.
15. Magorian T, Flannery KB, Miller RD. Comparison of rocuronium, succinylcholine, and vecuronium for rapid-sequence induction of anesthesia in adult patients. *Anesthesiology* 1993; 79:913–918.
16. Laurin EG, Sakles JC, Panacek EA, et al. A comparison of succinylcholine and rocuronium for rapid-sequence intubation of emergency department patients. *Acad Emerg Med* 2000;7: 1362–1369.
17. Mazurek AJ, Rae B, Hann S, et al. Rocuronium versus succinylcholine: are they equally effective during rapid-sequence induction of anesthesia? *Anesth Analg* 1998;87:1259–1262.
18. Andrews JI, Kumar N, van den Brom RH, et al. A large simple randomized trial of rocuronium versus succinylcholine in rapid-sequence induction of anaesthesia along with propofol. *Acta Anaesthesiol Scand* 1999;43:4–8.

19. Perry JJ, Lee J, Wells G. Are intubating conditions using rocuronium equivalent to those using succinylcholine? *Acad Emerg Med* 2002;9:813–823.

20. Perry JJ, Lee J, Wells G. Rocuronium versus succinylcholine for rapid sequence induction intubation. *Cochrane Database Syst Rev* 2003;1:CD002788.

21. Cheng CA, Aun CS, Gin T. Comparison of rocuronium and suxamethonium for rapid tracheal intubation in children. *Paediatr Anaesth* 2002;12:140–145.

22. McCourt KC, Salmela L, Mirakhur RK, et al. Comparison of rocuronium and suxamethonium for use during rapid sequence induction of anaesthesia. *Anaesthesia* 1998;53:867–871.

23. Barr AM, Thornley BA. Thiopentone and pancuronium crash induction: a comparison with thiopentone and suxamethonium. *Anaesthesia* 1978;33:25–31.

24. Mehta MP, Sokoll MD, Gergis SD. Accelerated onset of non-depolarizing neuromuscular blocking drugs: pancuronium, atracurium and vecuronium: a comparison with succinylcholine. *Eur J Anaesthesiol* 1988;5:15–21.

25. Martin C, Bonneru JJ, Brun JP, et al. Vecuronium or suxamethonium for rapid sequence intubation: which is better? *Br J Anaesth* 1987;59:1240–1244.

26. Schuh FT. The neuromuscular blocking action of suxamethonium following intravenous and intramuscular administration. *Int J Clin Pharmacol Ther Toxicol* 1982;20:399–403.

27. Sutherland GA, Bevan JC, Bevan DR. Neuromuscular blockade in infants following intramuscular succinylcholine in two or five percent concentration. *Can Anaesth Soc J* 1983;30:342–346.

28. Reynolds LM, Lau M, Brown R, et al. Bioavailability of intramuscular rocuronium in infants and children. *Anesthesiology* 1997;87:1096–1105.

29. Reynolds LM, Lau M, Brown R, et al. Intramuscular rocuronium in infants and children: dose-ranging and tracheal intubating conditions. *Anesthesiology* 1996;85:231–239.

30. Kaplan RF, Uejima T, Lobel G, et al. Intramuscular rocuronium in infants and children: a multicenter study to evaluate tracheal intubating conditions, onset, and duration of action. *Anesthesiology* 1999;91:633–638.

31. Schreiber JU, Lysakowski C, Fuchs-Buder T, et al. Prevention of succinylcholine-induced fasciculation and myalgia: a meta-analysis of randomized trials. *Anesthesiology* 2005;103(4):877–884.

32. Kato M, Shiratori T, Yamamuro M, et al. Comparison between in vivo and in vitro pharmakokinetics of succinylcholine in humans. *J Anesth* 1999;13:189–192.

33. Donati F. The right dose of succinylcholine. *Anesthesiology* 2003;99:1037–1038.

34. Cunningham AJ, Barry P. Intraocular pressure—physiology and implications for anesthetic management. *Can Anaesth Soc J* 1986;33:195–208.

35. Vachon CA, Warner DO, Bacon DR. Succinylcholine and the open globe: tracing the teaching. *Anesthesiology* 2003;99:220–224.

36. Miller RD. *Anesthesia*, 5th ed. Philadelphia: Churchill Livingstone; 2000:423, 2178.

37. Schaner PJ, Brown RL, Kirksey TD, et al. Succinylcholine-induced hyperkalemia in burned patients—part I. *Anesth Analg* 1969;48:764–770.

38. Gronert GA, Dotin LN, Ritchey CR, et al. Succinylcholine-induced hyperkalemia in burned patients—part II. *Anesth Analg* 1969;48:958–962.

39. Viby-Mogensen J, Hanel HK, Hansen E, et al. Serum cholinesterase activity in burned patients. II: anaesthesia, suxamethonium and hyperkalaemia. *Acta Anaesthesiol Scand* 1975;19:169–179.

40. Martyn JA, White DA, Gronert GA, et al. Up-and-down regulation of skeletal muscle acetylcholine receptors: effects on neuromuscular blockers. *Anesthesiology* 1992;76:822–843.

41. Gronert GA, Lambert EH, Theye RA. The response of denervated skeletal muscle to succinylcholine. *Anesthesiology* 1973;39:13–22.

42. Gronert GA, Theye RA. Pathophysiology of hyperkalemia induced by succinylcholine. *Anesthesiology* 1975;43:89–99.

43. Gronert GA. Cardiac arrest after succinylcholine: mortality greater with rhabdomyolysis than receptor upregulation. *Anesthesiology* 2001;94:523–529.

44. Smith CL, Bush GH. Anaesthesia and progressive muscular dystrophy. *Br J Anaesth* 1985;57:1113–1118.

45. Larach MG, Rosenberg H, Gronert GA, et al. Hyperkalemic cardiac arrest during anesthesia in infants and children with occult myopathies. *Clin Pediatr (Phila)* 1997;36:9–16.

46. Pedrozzi NE, Ramelli GP, Tomasetti R, et al. Rhabdomyolysis and anesthesia: a report of two cases and review of the literature. *Pediatr Neurol* 1996;15:254–257.

47. Roth F, Wuthrich H. The clinical importance of hyperkalaemia following suxamethonium administration. *Br J Anaesth* 1969;41:311–316.

48. Schow AJ, Lubarsky DA, Olson RP, Gan TJ. Can succinylcholine be used safely in hyperkalemic patients? *Anesth Analg* 2002;95(1):119–122.

49. Thapa S, Brull SJ. Succinylcholine-induced hyperkalemia in patients with renal failure: an old question revisited. *Anesth Analg* 2000;91:237–241.

50. Schow AJ, Lubarsky DA, Olson RP, et al. Can succinylcholine be used safely in hyperkalemic patients? *Anesth Analg* 2002;95:119–122.

51. Powell DR, Miller R. The effect of repeated doses of succinylcholine on serum potassium in patients with renal failure. *Anesth Analg* 1975;54:746–748.

52. Koide M, Waud BE. Serum potassium concentrations after succinylcholine in patients with renal failure. *Anesthesiology* 1972;36:142–145.

53. Kotani T, Nishio I, Kou H, et al. Effect of succinylcholine on serum potassium concentration in children with chronic renal failure. *Masui* 1993;42:20–24.

54. Kohlschutter B, Baur H, Roth F. Suxamethonium-induced hyperkalaemia in patients with severe intra-abdominal infections. *Br J Anaesth* 1976;48:557–562.

55. Khan TZ, Khan RM. Changes in serum potassium following succinylcholine in patients with infections. *Anesth Analg* 1983;62:327–331.

56. Gronert GA, Antognini JF, Pessah IN. Malignant hyperthermia. In: Miller RD, ed. *Anesthesia*, 5th ed. Philadelphia: Churchill Livingstone; 2000:1033–1050.

57. Kolb ME, Horne ML, Martz R: Dantrolene in human malignant hyperthermia: a multicenter study. *Anesthesiology* 1982;56:254.

58. Welliver M. New drug sugammadex: a selective relaxant binding agent. *AANA J* 2006;74: 357–363.

59. Sacan O, White PF, Tufanogullari B, et al. Sugammadex reversal of rocuronium-induced neuromuscular blockade: a comparison with neostigmine-glycopyrrolate and edrophonium-atropine. *Anesth Analg* 2007;104(3):569–574.

60. Suy K, Morias K, Cammu G, et al. Effective reversal of moderate rocuronium- or vecuronium-induced neuromuscular block with sugammadex, a selective relaxant binding agent. *Anesthesiology* 2007;106(2):283–288.

61. Gijsenbergh F, Ramael S, Houwing N, et al. First human exposure of Org 25969, a novel agent to reverse the action of rocuronium bromide. *Anesthesiology* 2005;103(4):695–703.

62. Groudine SB, Soto R, Lien C, et al. A randomized, dose-finding, phase II study of the selective relaxant binding drug, sugammadex, capable of safely reversing profound rocuronium-induced neuromuscular block. *Anesth Analg* 2007;104(3):555–562.

63. Sparr HJ, Vermeyen KM, Beaufort AM, et al. Early reversal of profound rocuronium-induced neuromuscular blockade by sugammadex in a randomized multicenter study: efficacy, safety, and pharmacokinetics. *Anesthesiology* 2007;106(5):935–943.

20

Approach to the Pediatric Airway

Robert C. Luten and John D. McAllister

THE CLINICAL CHALLENGE

Airway management in the pediatric patient presents many potential challenges, including age-related drug dosing and equipment sizing, anatomical variation that continuously evolves as development proceeds from infancy to adolescence, and the performance anxiety that invariably accompanies the resuscitation of a critically ill child. Clinical competence in managing the airway of a critically ill or injured child requires an appreciation of age- and size-related factors, and a degree of familiarity and comfort with the fundamental approach to pediatric airway emergencies.

The principles of airway management in children and adults are the same. Medications used to facilitate intubation, the need for alternative airway management techniques, and many other aspects of airway management are generally the same in the child and adult. There are, however, a few important differences that must be considered in emergency airway management situations. These differences are most exaggerated in the first 2 years of life, after which the pediatric airway gradually evolves into the adult airway.

This discussion focuses on the main differences between adults and children and their significance in airway management.

APPROACH TO THE PEDIATRIC PATIENT

General Issues

A recent review of the pediatric resuscitation process attempted to define elements of the mental (cognitive) burden of providers when dealing with the unique aspects of critically ill children compared with adults. Age- and size-related variables unique to children introduce the need for more complex, nonautomatic, or knowledge-based mental activities, such as calculating drug doses and selecting equipment. The concentration required to undertake these activities may subtract from other important mental activity such as assessment, evaluation, prioritization, and synthesis of information, referred to in the resuscitative process as critical thinking activity. The cumulative effect of these factors leads to inevitable time delays and a corresponding increase in the potential for decision-making errors in the pediatric resuscitative process. This is in sharp contrast to adult resuscitation, where drug doses, equipment sizing, and physiological parameters are usually familiar to the provider, leading to more automatic-type decisions that free the adult provider's attention for critical thinking. In children, the decision-making process is prolonged due to the cognitive burden of age-related anatomical and physiological variation, and the calculation of drug doses. Drug dosing determinations are subject to error, particularly as doses are weight related, and the ultimate dose selected tends to vary significantly by age. The use of resuscitation aids in pediatric resuscitation significantly reduces the cognitive load (and error) related to drug dosing calculations and equipment selection by relegating these activities to a lower order of mental function (referred to as "automatic" or "rule based"). The result is reduced error, attenuation of psychological stress, and an increase in critical thinking time. Table 20-1 is a length-based, color-coded equipment reference chart (Broselow-Luten–based "resuscitation guide") for pediatric airway management that eliminates error-prone strategies based on age and weight. Both equipment and drug dosing information are included in the Broselow-Luten system and can be accessed by a single length measurement or patient weight.

Specific Issues

Anatomical and Functional Issues

The approach to the child with airway obstruction (the most common form of a difficult pediatric airway) incorporates several unique features of the pediatric anatomy.

TABLE 20-1
Equipment Selection

Length (cm)-based pediatric equipment chart

	Pink[a]	Red	Purple	Yellow	White	Blue	Orange	Green
Weight (kg)	6–7	8–9	10–11	12–14	15–18	19–23	23–31	31–41
Length (cm)	60.75–67.75	67.75–75.25	75.25–85	85–98.25	98.25–110.75	110.75–122.5	122.5–137.5	137.5–155
Endotracheal tube size (mm)	3.5	3.5	4.0	4.5	5.0	5.5	6.0 cuff	6.5 cuff
Lip-tip length (mm)	10–10.5	10.5–11	11–12	12.5–13.5	14–15	15.5–16.5	17–18	18.5–19.5
Laryngoscope Size+blade	1 Straight	1 Straight	1 Straight	2 Straight	2 Straight	2 Straight or curved	2 Straight or curved	3 Straight or curved
Suction catheter	8F	8F	8F	8–10F	10F	10F	10F	12F
Stylet	6F	6F	6F	6F	6F	14F	14F	14F
Oral airway	50 mm	50 mm	60 mm	60 mm	60 mm	70 mm	80 mm	80 mm
Nasopharyngeal airway	14F	14F	18F	20F	22F	24F	26F	30F
Bag/valve device	Infant	Infant	Child	Child	Child	Child	Child/adult	Adult
Oxygen mask	Newborn	Newborn	Pediatric	Pediatric	Pediatric	Pediatric	Adult	Adult
Vascular access	22–24/23–25	22–24/23–25	20–22/23–25	18–22/21–23	18–22/21–23	18–20/21–23	18–20/21–22	16–20/18–21
Catheter/butterfly	Intraosseous	Intraosseous	Intraosseous	Intraosseous	Intraosseous	Intraosseous	Intraosseous	
Nasogastric tube	5–8F	5–8F	8–10F	10F	10–12F	12–14F	14–18F	18F
Urinary catheter	5–8F	5–8F	8–10F	10F	10–12F	10–12F	12F	12F

(continued)

TABLE 20-1
Equipment Selection (Continued)

	Pink[a]	Red	Purple	Yellow	White	Blue	Orange	Green
Chest tube	10–12F	10–12F	16–20F	20–24F	20–24F	24–32F	24–32F	32–40F
Blood pressure cuff	Newborn/ infant	Newborn/ infant	Infant/ child	Child	Child	Child	Child/ adult	Adult
Laryngeal mask airway (LMA)[b]	1.5	1.5	2	2	2	2–2.5	2.5	3

Directions for use: (a) measure patient length with centimeter tape or with a Broselow tape; (b) using measured length in centimeters or Broselow tape measurement, access appropriate equipment column; (c) column for endotracheal tubes, oral and nasopharyngeal airways, and LMAs, always select one size smaller and one size larger than recommended size.

[a]For infants smaller than the pink zone, but not preterm, use the same equipment as the pink zone.
[b]Based on manufacturer's weight-based guidelines:

Mask size	Patient size
1	≤5 kg
1.5	5–10 kg
2	10–20 kg
2.5	20–30 kg
3	>30 kg

Permission to reproduce with modification from Luten RC, Wears RL, Broselow J, et al. Managing the unique size related issues of pediatric resuscitation: reducing cognitive load with resuscitation aids. *Ann Emerg Med* 1992;21:900–904.

a. Children obstruct more readily than adults. The pediatric airway, as opposed to the adult airway, is especially susceptible to airway obstruction due to swelling. See Table 22-2 in Chapter 22, which outlines the effect of 1-mm edema on airway resistance in the infant (4-mm airway diameter) versus the adult (8-mm airway diameter). Nebulized racemic epinephrine causes local vasoconstriction and can reduce mucosal swelling and edema to some extent. For diseases such as croup, where the anatomical site of swelling occurs at the level of the cricoid ring, the narrowest part of the pediatric airway, racemic epinephrine can have dramatic results. Disorders located in areas with greater airway calibre, such as the supraglottic swelling of epiglottitis or the retropharyngeal swelling of an abscess, rarely see results as dramatic. In these latter examples, especially in epiglottitis, efforts to force a nebulized medication on a child may agitate the child, leading to increased airflow velocity and dynamic upper airway obstruction.

b. Noxious interventions can lead to dynamic airway obstruction and precipitate respiratory arrest. The work of breathing in the crying child increases 32-fold, elevating the threat of dynamic airway obstruction and hence the principle of maintaining children in a quiet, comfortable environment during evaluation and management for potential airway obstruction; another reason to "leave them alone" (Fig. 20-1A–C).

c. Bag-mask ventilation (BMV) may be of particular value in the child who has arrested from upper airway obstruction. Note in Figure 20-1C that efforts by the patient to alleviate the obstruction may actually exacerbate it because increased inspiratory effort creates a more negative extrathoracic pressure, leading to collapsing of the malleable extrathoracic trachea. The application of positive pressure via BMV causes the opposite effect by stenting the airway open and relieving the dynamic component of obstruction (Fig. 20-1C and D). This mechanism explains the recommendation to try BMV as a temporizing measure, even if the patient arrests from obstruction. Case reports of successful resuscitation in patients that arrest from epiglottitis by BMV have borne this out.

d. Apart from differences related to size, there are certain anatomical peculiarities of the pediatric airway. The glottic opening is situated at the level of the first cervical vertebra (C-1) in infancy. This level transitions to the level of C-3 to C-4 by age 7 and to the level of C-5 to C-6 in the adult. Thus, the glottic opening tends to be higher and more anterior in children as opposed to adults. The size of the tongue with respect to the oral cavity is larger in children, particularly infants. These two factors lead to the recommendation that a straight laryngoscope blade be used in children younger than 3 years to elevate this distensible anatomy and enhance visualization of the glottic aperture (Table 20-2).

Blind nasotracheal intubation is difficult and relatively contraindicated in children younger than 10 years for at least two reasons: children have large tonsils and adenoids that may bleed significantly when traumatized, and the angle between the epiglottis and the laryngeal opening is also more acute than that in the adult.

Children possess a small cricothyroid membrane. In children younger than 3 to 4 years of age, it is virtually nonexistent. For this reason, needle cricothyrotomy may be difficult, and surgical cricothyrotomy is virtually impossible and contraindicated in infants and small children as old as 10 years.

Although younger children possess a relatively high, anterior airway with the attendant difficulties in visualization of the glottic aperture, this anatomical pattern is fortunately rather consistent from one child to another, so this difficulty can be anticipated. Adults may have difficult airways related to body habitus, arthritis, or chronic disease, modified by variations in individual underlying anatomy, and so are less consistent from one individual to another.

In summary, children younger than 2 years have higher anterior airways. In children older than 8 years, the airway tends to be similar to the adult, whereas years 2

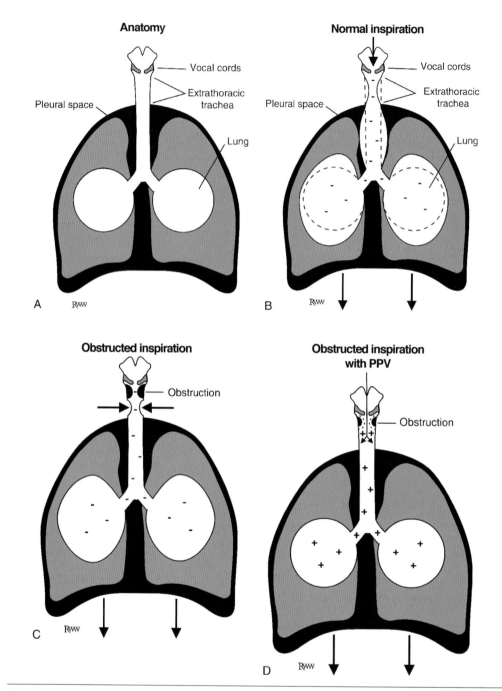

Figure 20-1 ● **Intra- and Extrathoracic Trachea and the Dynamic Changes that Occur in the Presence of Upper Airway Obstruction.** **A:** Normal anatomy. **B:** The changes that occur with normal inspiration; that is, dynamic collapsing of the upper airway associated with the negative pressure of inspiration on the extrathoracic trachea. **C:** Exaggeration of the collapse secondary to superimposed obstruction at the subglottic area. **D:** Positive pressure ventilation (PPV) stents the collapse/obstruction versus the patient's own inspiratory efforts, which increase the obstruction. *Source:* Adapted from Cote CJ, Ryan JF, Todres ID, et al., eds. *A practice of anesthesia for infants and children*, 2nd ed. Philadelphia: WB Saunders; 1993, with permission.

TABLE 20-2
Anatomical Differences Between Adults and Children

Anatomy	Clinical significance
Large intraoral tongue occupying relatively large portion of the oral cavity	Straight blade preferred over curved to push distensible anatomy out of the way to visualize the larynx
High tracheal opening: C-1 in infancy vs. C-3 to C-4 at age 7, C-4 to C-5 in the adult	High anterior airway position of the glottic opening compared with that in adults
Large occiput that may cause flexion of the airway, large tongue that easily collapses against the posterior pharynx	Sniffing position is preferred. The larger occiput actually elevates the head into the sniffing position in most infants and children. A towel may be required under shoulders to elevate torso relative to head in small infants
Cricoid ring is the narrowest portion of the trachea as compared with the vocal cords in the adult	Uncuffed tubes provide adequate seal because they fit snugly at the level of the cricoid ring Correct tube size essential because variable expansion cuffed tubes not used
Consistent anatomical variations with age with fewer abnormal variations related to body habitus, arthritis, chronic disease	Younger than 2 years, high anterior; 2 to 8 years, transition; older than 8 years, small adult
Large tonsils and adenoids may bleed; more acute angle between epiglottis and laryngeal opening results in nasotracheal intubation attempt failures.	Blind nasotracheal intubation not indicated in children; nasotracheal intubation failure
Small cricothyroid membrane	Needle cricothyrotomy difficult, trachea is the landmark, surgical cricothyrotomy impossible in infants and small children

to 8 represent a transition period. Figure 20-2 demonstrates anatomical differences particular to children.

Physiological Issues

Although there are many physiological differences between children and adults, the one of most importance with respect to emergency airway management (Box 20-1) is that children have a basal oxygen consumption that is approximately twice that of adults. Coupling that factor with the decrease in functional residual capacity (FRC) to body weight ratio seen in children compared to adults means that children desaturate much more rapidly than adults given an equivalent duration of preoxygenation. The clinician must anticipate and communicate this possibility to the staff and be prepared to provide supplemental oxygen by BMV if the patient's oxygen saturation drops below 90%.

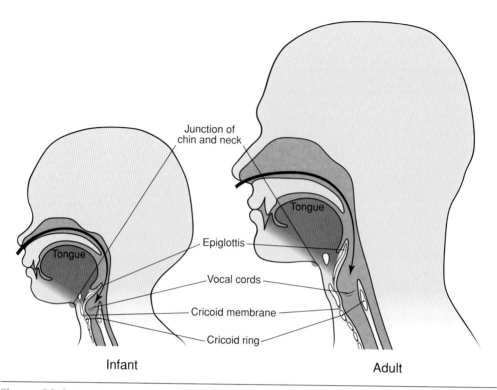

Figure 20-2 ● The anatomical differences particular to children are (a) higher, more anterior position of the glottic opening (note the relationship of the vocal cords to the chin/neck junction); (b) relatively larger tongue in the infant, which lies between the mouth and glottic opening; (c) relatively larger and more floppy epiglottis in the child; (d) the cricoid ring is the narrowest portion of the pediatric airway versus the vocal cords in the adult; (e) position and size of the cricothyroid membrane in the infant; (f) sharper, more difficult angle for blind nasotracheal intubation; and (g) larger relative size of the occiput in the infant.

Drug Dosage and Selection

Drug dosage determinations are most appropriately and safely done using resuscitation aids such as the Broselow-Luten system previously described.

The dose of succinylcholine (SCh) in children is different from that in adults. SCh is rapidly metabolized by plasma esterases and distributed to extracellular water. Children

---

BOX 20-1 Physiological Differences

Physiological difference	Significance
Basal O_2 consumption is twice adult values (>6 mL/kg/minute). Proportionally smaller functional residual capacity as compared with adults.	Shortened period of protection from hypoxia for equivalent preoxygenation time as compared with adults. Infants and small children often require bag-mask ventilation while maintaining cricoid pressure to avoid hypoxia.

have a larger volume of extracellular fluid water relative to adults: at birth 45%; at age 2 months, approximately 30%; at age 6 years, 20%; and at adulthood, 16% to 18%. The recommended dose of SCh, therefore, is higher on a per kilo basis in children than adults (2 mg/kg vs. 1–1.5 mg/kg).

In 1993, the U.S. Food and Drug Administration (FDA), in conjunction with pharmaceutical companies, revised the package labeling for SCh in the wake of reports of hyperkalemic cardiac arrest following the administration of SCh in patients with previously undiagnosed neuromuscular disease. Initially, it stated that SCh was contraindicated for elective anesthesia in pediatric patients because of this concern, although the wording was subsequently altered to embrace a risk–benefit analysis when deciding to use SCh in children. However, both the initial advisory warning and the revised warning continue to recommend SCh for emergency or full-stomach intubation in children. Pediatric drug doses are provided in Table 20-3.

Equipment Selection

Table 20-1 references length-based recommendations for emergency equipment in pediatric patients. Appropriately sized equipment can be chosen with a centimeter length measurement or with a Broselow tape.

A word of caution with respect to the storage of airway management equipment for children: Despite best efforts (e.g., equipment lists or periodic checks), it is not uncommon for newborn equipment to be mixed in with or placed in proximity to the smallest pediatric equipment—"the pink zone." This practice may lead to newborn equipment being used in older children for whom it may not function properly or may, in fact, be dangerous. Examples include the #0 laryngoscope blade, which is too short to allow visualization of the airway; the 250-cc newborn BMV, which provides inadequate ventilation volumes; and various other equipment, such as oral airways that can cause airway obstruction if

TABLE 20-3
Drugs—Pediatric Considerations

Drug	Dosage	Pediatric-specific comments
Premedications		
Lidocaine	1.5 mg/kg IV	Head injury, asthma, older than 10 years
Fentanyl	1–3 μg/kg IV	In head injury, older than 10 years
Induction agents		
Midazolam	0.3 mg/kg IV	Use 0.1 mg/kg if hypotensive
Thiopental	3–5 mg/kg IV	Lower dose to 1 mg/kg or delete if perfusion poor
Etomidate	0.3 mg/kg IV	
Ketamine	1–2 mg/kg IV, 4 mg/kg IM	
Propofol	2–3 mg/kg IV	
Paralytics		
Succinylcholine	2 mg/kg IV	Have atropine drawn up and ready
Pan/vecuronium	0.2 mg/kg IV	May increase to 0.3 mg/kg of vecuronium for RSI. (0.1 mg/kg for maintenance of paralysis)
Rocuronium	1.0 mg/kg IV	(for rapid sequence intubation (RSI))

TABLE 20-4
Dangerous Equipment

Equipment	Problem
#0 or #00 laryngoscope endotracheal tube (ET) blades	Valuable time can be lost trying to visualize the glottic opening if mistaken for a #1 blade.
Curved #1 laryngoscope ET blades	Straight blades are preferred because • The epiglottis is picked up directly, not indirectly, by compressing the hyoepiglottic ligament in the vallecula. • The tongue and mandibular anatomy are more easily elevated from the field of vision.
250-cc bag-mask ventilation	Cannot generate adequate tidal volumes.
Cuffed ET tubes <5.0 mm	If leak pressures are not monitored, ischemia of the tracheal mucosa may develop with the potential for scarring and stenosis.
Oral airways <50 mm	Unless appropriate size oral airways are used, they may act to increase, rather than relieve, obstruction.
Any *other* equipment too small	Sizing is critical to function!

Note. Only appropriate size is functional. It is a frequent occurrence for very small sizes to be placed in the pediatric area without attention to appropriateness of size. The results can be devastating.

too small, or a curved laryngoscope blade that may not reach and pick up the relatively large epiglottis, or effectively remove the large tongue from the laryngoscopic view of the airway. See Table 20-4.

a. **Endotracheal tubes**

The correct ETT size for the patient can be determined by a length measurement and by referring to the equipment selection chart. The formula

$$(16 + \text{age in years})/4$$

is also a reasonably accurate method of determining the correct tube size. However, the formula cannot be used in children younger than 1 year and is only useful if an accurate age is known, which cannot always be determined in an emergency. Uncuffed endotracheal tubes (ETTs) are recommended in the younger pediatric age groups, and cuffed tubes are used for size 5.5 mm and up (Fig. 20-3).

When intubating a young child, there is a tendency to insert the ETT too far, usually into the right mainstem bronchus. Insertion of the ETT to a predetermined, appropriate distance will avoid this. Various formulas have been proffered as aids to determine the correct insertion distance (e.g., internal diameter [ID] of the tube times 3). For example, a 3.5-mm ID tube ought to be inserted 3.5 × 3 = 10.5 cm at the lip. Alternatively, a length-based chart can be used.

b. **Tube securing devices**

An all too frequent complication following intubation is inadvertent extubation. ETTs must be secured at the mouth, and since head and neck movement translates

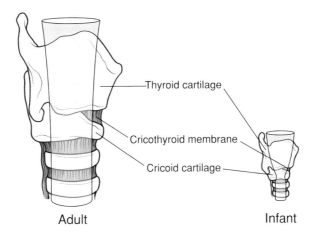

Adult   Infant

Figure 20-3 ● Airway Shape. Note the position of the narrowest portion of the pediatric airway, which is at the cricoid ring, creating a funnel shape, versus a straight pipe as seen in the adult, where the vocal cords form the narrowest portion. This is the rationale for using the uncuffed tube in the child; it fits snugly, unlike the cuffed tube used in the adult, which is inflated once the tube passes the cords to produce a snug fit. *Source:* Modified with permission from Cote CJ, Todres ID. The pediatric airway. In: Cote CJ, Ryan JF, Todres ID, et al., eds. *A practice of anesthesia for infants and children*, 2nd ed. Philadelphia: WB Saunders; 1993.

in ETT movement, a cervical collar is employed (Fig. 20-4). In the infant, small movements are capable of dislocating the ETT into the esophagus, emphasizing the importance of head and neck immobilization. The ETT at the mouth is traditionally secured by taping the tube to the cheek. Alternatively, various commercial devices are available.

c. Oxygen masks

The simple rebreather mask used for most patients provides a maximum of 35% to 60% oxygen and requires a flow rate of 6 to 10 L/minute. A nonrebreather mask can provide approximately 70% oxygen in children if a flow rate of 10 to 12 L/minute is used. For emergency airway management, and particularly for preoxygenation for rapid sequence intubation (RSI), the pediatric nonrebreather mask is preferable. Adult nonrebreather masks can be used for older children but are too large to be used for infants and small children. Properly configured bag-mask systems (i.e., those that have a one-way exhalation valve [e.g., "duck bill"] and small dead space) are capable of delivering oxygen concentrations >90%, if correctly used. The spontaneously breathing patient opens the duck-billed valve on inspiration, and on expiration, the expired CO_2 is vented into the atmosphere. Adult type units tend not to be used in infants and small children where the capacity to generate sufficient negative inspiratory pressure to open the duck bill valve may be lacking, leading some to prefer pediatric nonrebreather masks.

d. Oral airways

Oral airways should only be used in children who are unconscious. In the conscious or semiconscious child, these airways can incite vomiting. Oral airways can be selected based on the Broselow tape measurement or can be approximated by selecting an oral airway that fits the distance from the angle of the mouth to the tragus of the ear.

e. Nasopharyngeal airways

Nasopharyngeal airways are helpful in the obtunded but responsive child. The correctly sized nasopharyngeal airway is the largest one that comfortably fits in the naris

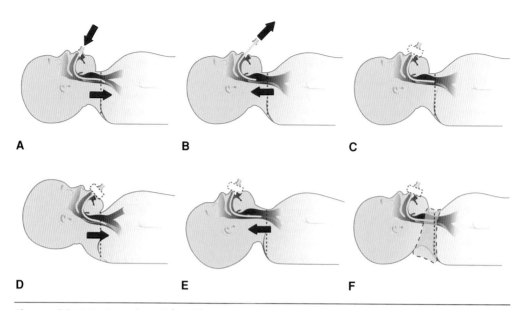

Figure 20-4 ● Securing Tube Placement. Unsecured tube sliding in/down **(A)**. Unsecured tube sliding out/up **(B)**. Tube secured to prevent in/out, up/down movement **(C)**. Secured tube moving down and in as head flexes **(D)**. Secured tube moving up/out as head extends **(E)**. Neck movement prevented by cervical collar, thus preventing tube movement in the trachea **(F)**.

but does not produce blanching of the nasal skin. The correct length is from the tip of the nose to the tragus of the ear, and usually corresponds to the nasopharyngeal airway with the correct diameter. Care must be taken to suction these airways regularly to avoid blockage.

f. Nasogastric tubes

BMV may lead to insufflation of the stomach, hindering full diaphragmatic excursion and preventing effective ventilation. A nasogastric (NG) tube should be placed soon after intubation to decompress the stomach in any patient who has undergone BMV and requires ongoing mechanical ventilation post intubation. Often in such patients, the abdomen is distended or tense, making the problem obvious, but other times it is difficult to identify the difference between this and the normally protuberant abdomen of the young child. If there is any difficulty in ventilation, particularly related to apparently high resistance, an NG tube should be placed. Length-based systems identify the appropriate NG tube size.

g. Bag-mask ventilation equipment

For emergency airway management, the self-inflating bag is preferred over the anesthesia ventilation bag. The BMV should have an oxygen reservoir so that at 10 to 15 L of oxygen flow, one can provide a F_iO_2 of 90% to 95%. The smallest bag that should be used is 450 mL. Neonatal bags that are smaller (250 mL) do not provide effective tidal volume even for small infants. Many of the BMV devices have a pop-off valve. The pop-off valve is usually set at approximately 35 to 45 cm of water pressure (CWP) and is used to prevent barotrauma. Emergency airway management often requires higher peak airway pressures, so the bag should be configured without a pop-off valve or with a pop-off valve that can be defeated. Practically, it is a good practice to store the BMV device with the pop-off valve defeated so that initial attempts to ventilate the patient can achieve sufficient peak airway pressure to achieve ventilation. Chapter 21 discusses this issue in more detail and offers suggestions to prevent its occurrence.

h. End-tidal CO₂ detectors

Colorimetric end-tidal carbon dioxide ($ETCO_2$) detectors are as useful in children as in adults. A pediatric size exists for children weighing <15 kg. The adult model should be used for children weighing >15 kg. The resistance to airflow created by the pediatric-size device may make ventilation of the older child, where the larger size is more appropriate, more difficult.

i. Airway alternatives (Table 20-5)

Orotracheal intubation is the procedure of choice for emergency airway management of the pediatric patient, including those patients with potential cervical spine injury where RSI with inline manual stabilization is preferred. Nasotracheal intubation is relatively contraindicated in children for the reasons previously discussed.

Cricothyrotomy is the preferred emergency surgical airway in adults. The cricothyroid space emerges as one ages and is really only accessible after the age of 10 years. "Needle cricothyrotomy" in children younger than 8 to 10 years is the term used when one accesses the airway in a percutaneous manner in young children even though it is recognized that the point of entry into the airway is often the trachea as opposed to the cricothyroid space.

The only other device that has been demonstrated to be of use in failed airway management in young children is the laryngeal mask airway, which is supplied in sizes small enough for young infants and newborns, and, as a temporizing measure, might be useful when intubation cannot be done or fails. The Combitube is easy to insert, but currently there are no models for pediatric patients less than 48 inches tall. These and other adjuncts are discussed in Chapter 21.

INITIATION OF MECHANICAL VENTILATION

In pediatrics, two modes of ventilation are used for emergency ventilation. For newborns and small infants, pressure-limited ventilators are traditionally used. For larger infants and older children, volume-limited ventilators are used, as in adults. One can arbitrarily set 10 kg as the weight below which pressure-limited ventilators should be used, although volume-limited ventilators have been used effectively in smaller children. Generally speaking, the younger the child, the more rapid is the ventilatory rate. The initial ventilatory rate in infants is typically set between 20 and 25 per minute. Inspiratory/expiratory ratios are set at 1:2. The typical peak inspiratory pressure at initiation of ventilation is between 15 and 20

TABLE 20-5
Alternatives for Airway Support

Bag-mask ventilation	May be the most reliable temporizing measure in children. Equipment selection, adjuncts, and good technique are essential.
Orotracheal intubation (usually with rapid sequence intubation)	Still the procedure of choice for emergent airway in potential cervical spine injury and most other circumstances.
Needle cricothyrotomy	Recommended as last resort in infants and children, but data lacking.
Laryngeal mask	Possible alternative but requires further evaluation.
Blind nasotracheal intubation	Not indicated for children younger than 10 years.

CWP. These initial settings in a pressure-controlled ventilation mode will usually give a tidal volume of 8 to 12 mL/kg. These initial settings are adjusted according to subsequent clinical evaluation and chest rise. Positive end-expiratory pressure should also be set at 3 to 5 cm of water and F_iO_2 at 1.0. Once initial settings have been established, it is critical that the patient be quickly re-evaluated and adjustments made, particularly as pulmonary compliance, airways resistance, and leak volumes change with time, precluding adequate ventilation with the initial settings of pressure-controlled ventilation. Clinical evaluation of ventilatory adequacy is more important than formulae or guidelines for ensuring adequate ventilation. Once adjustments are made and the patient appears clinically to be ventilated and oxygenating, blood gas determinations, or continuous pulse oximetry and $ETCO_2$ monitoring, should be used for confirmation and to guide additional adjustments (Table 20-6 and Box 20-2).

RSI TECHNIQUES FOR CHILDREN

The procedure of RSI in children is essentially the same procedure as in adults with a few important differences outlined as follows:

TABLE 20-6
Initiation of Mechanical Ventilation

I. Initial settings		
Ventilator type	Pressure limited	Volume limited
Respiratory rate	20–25/minute	12–20/min, by age
Positive end-expiratory pressure	3–5 cm H_2O	3–5 cm H_2O
F_iO_2	1.0 (100%)	1.0 (100%)
Inspiratory time	≥0.6 seconds	≥0.6 seconds
Inspiratory/expiratory ratio	1:2	1:2
Pressure/volume settings	For pressure ventilation, start with peak inspiratory pressure (PIP) of 15–20 cm H_2O. Assess chest rise and adjust to higher pressures as needed. For volume ventilation, start with tidal volumes of 8–12 mL/kg. Start at lower volumes and increase to a PIP of 20–30 cm H_2O. *These are initial setting guidelines only. Assess chest rise and adjust accordingly.*	
II. Evaluate clinically and make adjustments	Most patients will be ventilated with volume-cycled ventilators. Poor chest rise, poor color, and decreased breath sounds require *higher* tidal volume. Check for pneumo, blocked tube. Ensure that tube size and position are optimal and leaks are not present. For patients ventilated with pressure-cycled ventilators, these findings may indicate the need to increase the peak inspiratory pressure.	
III. Laboratory information	Arterial blood gas should be performed approximately 10–15 minutes after settings are stabilized. Additional samples may be necessary after each ventilator adjustment, unless ventilatory status is monitored by $ETCO_2$ and S_pO_2.	

BOX 20-2 Emergency Pediatric Airway Management—Practical Considerations

---

Anatomical
- Anticipate high anterior glottic opening.
- Do not hyperextend the neck.
- Uncuffed tubes are used in children younger than 8 years.
- Use straight blades in young children.

Physiological
- Anticipate possible desaturation.

Drug dosage and equipment selection
- Use length-based system. Do *not* use memory or do calculations.
- Nasogastric tube is an important airway adjunct in infants.
- Stock pediatric nonrebreather masks.

Airway alternatives for failed or difficult airway
- Surgical cricothyrotomy—contraindicated until age 10 years.
- Blind nasotracheal intubation—contraindicated until age 10 years.
- Combitube—only if >4 feet tall.
- Needle cricothyrotomy—acceptable.

A. Preparation
  - Use resuscitation aids that address age- and size-related issues in drug dosing and equipment selection (e.g., Broselow-Luten tape).
B. Preoxygenation
  - Be meticulous. Children desaturate more rapidly than adults.
C. Pretreatment
  - None. Atropine is optional but may be drawn up and kept at bedside used principally in infants less than one year of age.
D. Paralysis with induction
  - Induction agent selection as for adult: dose by length or weight.
  - SCh 2 mg/kg IV or rocuronium 1 mg/kg.
E. Protection and positioning
  - Apply Sellick's maneuver.
F. Placement with proof
  - Anticipate desaturation; bag ventilate if oxygen saturation (S_pO_2) is less than 90%.
  - Confirm tube placement with $ETCO_2$ as for adult.
G. Postintubation management
  Mechanical ventilation in the child can be accomplished using either pressure-controlled or volume-controlled techniques. Regardless of the technique used, one should ensure that the chest rise is adequate. The Broselow-Luten length-based system gives guidelines for approximate starting tidal volumes and ventilator rates. In almost all cases, children who are intubated and mechanically ventilated should be paralyzed and sedated in the emergency department to prevent deleterious rises in intracranial or intrathoracic pressures.

EVIDENCE

   1. **When is "a kid a kid" from the standpoint of airway management?** The term "kids are different" is a long-used term to bring attention to the unique differences

between children and adults. From an airway management perspective, those differences are most pronounced in the first year of life, after which there is a gradual transition, both anatomically and physiologically, to adulthood. Although arbitrary, for simplicity's sake, and because many children requiring airway management cannot be weighed, we define "children" as patients who fit on the Broselow tape. Those that do not are considered adults for dosing, equipment selection, and other recommendations. Children who are larger than the last zone on the tape are usually at least 80 lb (36 kg), at least 5 feet tall (>150 cm or ~60 inch), and at least 10 years old.

2. **What are the particular barriers to successful airway management in children?** Pediatric emergency airway management is often fraught with a lack of familiarity and complicated by a degree of complexity that for the average emergency airway manager may translate into errors and time delay. This mental burden (or "cognitive load") can be reduced by the use of resuscitation aids. Time is saved and error reduced.

    Time delay and error are associated with the management of children in emergency situations (1). Pediatric emergencies are complicated by the fact that children vary in size, creating logistical difficulties, especially with respect to drug dosing and equipment selection. A recent review analyzed the effect of these variables on the mental burden in the resuscitative process and demonstrated how resuscitation aids can help mitigate their effect (2). Simulated emergency patient encounters have confirmed that the Broselow-Luten color-coded emergency system reduces time delay and errors by eliminating the cognitive burden associated with these situations (3).

    Other factors also contribute to an increased cognitive load in managing children. To the extent that the process can be simplified (e.g., limiting the number of recommended medications, reducing the complexity and number of decisions required), time is freed up for critical thinking that can then be dedicated to the priorities of airway management. RSI in children is a good example. The management of children in extremis can be stressful. RSI should be kept simple and uncomplicated to reduce stress.

3. **Should I use a nondepolarizing relaxant to defasciculate prior to using SCh in children?** Defasciculation has been recommended in past editions of this text to attenuate the rise in intracranial pressure (ICP) seen in patients with intracranial pathology. As discussed in Chapter 17, this recommendation has been dropped for this edition of the text. Rapid and atraumatic tracheal intubation is the primary goal for all head-injured trauma patients. Minimizing the complexity of RSI by eliminating the defasciculation step contributes positively to this intent. Our view is that the SCh-induced increase in ICP in this setting is not relevant, and that even if there is a modest increase in ICP with SCh, the consequences of poor airway and ventilatory management outweigh any potential benefit. The deleterious effects of hypoxia, hypercarbia, noxious stimulation associated with laryngoscopy, delay in securing airway, and aspiration are much more significant. Defasciculation therapy is therefore not recommended in the emergency setting, and the ICP concerns are not a significant contraindication to SCh.

4. **Should atropine be used as a premedication for RSI in children?** The evidence does not support this. However, it is an issue that is difficult to definitively resolve based on current literature. Traditionally, atropine has been used to prevent the bradycardia associated with a single dose of SCh in children, a rare, but serious event. A few recent studies failed to show a difference in response to SCh with or without atropine in children (4,5), with similar numbers in the atropine- and non–atropine-treated groups developing transient, self-limited decreases in heart rate. The absence of evidence of benefit, however, should not be construed as "proof" when dealing with uncommon events, although this evidence is of note. Atropine also has significant, but rare side effects (6). Thus, we are currently not recommending its routine use in this situation.

There is a theoretical benefit for giving atropine when manipulating the airway of infants younger than 1 year due to their disproportionate predominance in vagal tone, coupled with a relatively greater dependency on heart rate for cardiac output (7). However, most bradycardic episodes are due to hypoxia or are a transient, vagally mediated reflex response that resolves spontaneously. It is better to treat the hypoxia or the reflex if it occurs.

In summary, in an effort to keep the process of RSI in children as simple as possible, we are not recommending the routine use of atropine. In special circumstances, such as with infants younger than 1 year (3, 4, and 5 kg, and pink or red zones on the Braselow-Luten tape and airway card), atropine should be considered an option.

5. **Should opioids be used as pretreatment medications in children?** There is excellent evidence that premedication with synthetic opioids prior to direct laryngoscopy and tracheal intubation attenuates the increase in ICP, intraocular pressure (IOP), mean arterial pressure, myocardial oxygen consumption, and pulmonary artery pressure caused by this noxious stimulus. The attenuation of the reflex sympathetic response to laryngoscopy and intubation conferred by pretreatment with an opioid is dose dependent and generally requires 3 to 5 minutes for peak effect (fentanyl). During this time, the side effects of a narcotic can be significant (respiratory depression, cough, decreased locus of control, hypotension, stiff chest). RSI in an emergency is usually a life-threatening cardiorespiratory event that already has created a stress-induced increase in catechols. For this reason, and because the dosing and administration of small doses of opioids in children is fraught with the potential for overdose, we do not routinely recommend use of opioids *in children* and place more emphasis on induction of general anesthesia and rapid onset of muscle relaxation to create ideal intubating conditions.

6. **Should lidocaine be used as a pretreatment medication in children?** Lidocaine has been recommended for children with presumed elevation of ICP (usually due to head trauma) to prevent further rises in ICP related to laryngoscopy and intubation (8). Most of the data for this recommendation, however, is extrapolated from adult studies and nontraumatic elevated ICP situations.

There are no data to support or refute the use of lidocaine in children to prevent or mitigate the reflex bronchospasm related to airway manipulation. Studies related to the use of lidocaine in children to blunt the sympathetic response to intubation are inconsistent (9,10).

We therefore do not recommend the use of lidocaine pretreatment for children younger than 10 years undergoing RSI.

7. **Succinylcholine versus rocuronium as a paralytic in children—which is the preferred agent?** In the 1990s, the FDA warned against the use of SCh in children following case reports of hyperkalemic cardiac arrest following the administration of SCh to patients with undiagnosed neuromuscular disease. The pediatric anesthesia community at that time challenged the FDA decision on the basis of the risk versus benefit in patients requiring emergency intubation, leading to a modification of their position to a "caution." There is no body of evidence that specifically addresses the relative risks and benefits of SCh versus rocuronium in children to guide recommendations. Both are used, and preferences are personal.

Currently, SCh remains the agent of choice for emergency full-stomach intubations (11,12). Although rocuronium is preferred in pediatrics by some practitioners, for simplicity's sake, we recommend SCh as first-line treatment for adults and children.

8. **Are uncuffed ETTs now recommended in pediatric emergency airway management?** The issue of whether cuffed ETTs are safe or required in children younger than 8 to 10 years has been debated for some time because of the anatomical and functional seal afforded by the subglottic area. Two studies have addressed this issue (13,14). Deakers et al. (13) studied 282 patients intubated either in the operating room, emergency department, or intensive care unit. In their observational prospective, nonrandomized

study, they found no difference in postextubation stridor, the need for reintubation, or long-term upper airway symptomatology. Khine et al. (14) compared the incidence of postextubation croup, inadequate ventilation, anaesthetic gases in the environment, and the requirement for a second laryngoscopy due to the tube being too large. In this study, which looked at children younger than 8 years only, the authors found no difference in croup, more attempts at intubation with uncuffed tubes, less gas flow required with cuffed tubes, or less gas leakage into the environment.

Even though it may seem that the use of cuffed tubes in younger children does not result in any postextubation sequelae, it must be made clear that these studies monitored cuff inflation pressures, a practice that is uncommonly performed in emergency intubations. For this reason, it seems reasonable to recommend the use of uncuffed ETTs to avoid excessive tracheal mucosal pressure with the potential sequelae of scarring and stenosis. However, for some patients in whom high mean airway pressures are expected, such as those with acute respiratory diseases and asthma, the placement of a cuffed tube with the cuff initially deflated, and inflated if necessary, may be appropriate. The most recent Pediatric Advanced Life Support standards (15) recommend cuffed tubes, but with the qualifier *only if leak pressures are monitored.*

9. **Why do children desaturate more quickly than adults with comparable degrees of preoxygenation?** The infant uses 6 mL of oxygen per kilogram per minute as compared with the adult who uses 3 mL per kilogram per minute. The FRC reduction in an apneic child is far greater than in the apneic adult. This is due to the differences in the elastic forces of the chest wall and the lung. In children, the chest wall is more compliant, and the lung elastic recoil is less than in adults. An analysis of these forces reveals that if they are brought into equilibrium as in the apneic patient, a value of FRC around 10% of TLC is predicted instead of the observed value of slightly less than 40%. These same factors also reduce the FRC in the spontaneously breathing patient, albeit to a lesser degree. FRC is further reduced with the induction of anesthesia and by the supine position. The clinical implication of the decreased effective FRC combined with increased oxygen consumption is that the preoxygenated, paralyzed infant has a disproportionately smaller store of intrapulmonary oxygen to draw on as compared to the adult. Pulmonary pathology in critically ill patients may further reduce the ability to preoxygenate. It is therefore critical that these factors be considered when preoxygenating and intervening in pediatric patients. BMV with cricoid pressure may be required to maintain oxygen saturation above 90% during RSI, especially if multiple attempts are required or the child has a disorder that compromises the ability to preoxygenate (16,17).

REFERENCES

1. Oakley P. Inaccuracy and delay in decision making in pediatric resuscitation, and a proposed reference chart to reduce error. *Br Med J* 1988;297:817–819.

2. Luten R, Wears R, Broselow J, et al. Managing the unique size related issues of pediatric resuscitation: reducing cognitive load with resuscitation aids. *Acad Emerg Med* 2002;9: 840–847.

3. Shah AN, Frush KS. *Reduction in error severity associated with use of a pediatric medication dosing system: a crossover trial.* Presented at the AAP 2001 National Conference and Exhibition, Section on Critical Care, October, 2001.

4. McAuliffe G, Bisonnette B, Boutin C. Should the routine use of atropine before succinylcholine in children be reconsidered? *Can J Anaesth* 1995;42:724–729.

5. Fleming B, McCollough M, Henderson SO. Myth: atropine should be administered before succinylcholine for neonatal and pediatric intubation. *Can J Emerg Med* 2005;7(2):114–117.

6. Tsou CH, Chiang CE, Kao T, et al. Atropine-triggered idiopathic ventricular tachycardia in an asymptomatic pediatric patient. *Can J Anaesth* 2004;51(8):856–857.

7. Rothrock SG, Pagane J. Pediatric rapid sequence intubation incidence of reflex bradycardia and effects of pretreatment with atropine. *Pediatr Emerg Care* 2005;21(9):637–638.

8. Zaritsky AL, Nadkarni VM, Hickey RW, et al. *PALS Provider Manual.* Dallas, TX: American Heart Association; 2002.

9. Splinter WM. Intravenous lidocaine does not attenuate the haemodynamic response of children to laryngoscopy and tracheal intubation. *Can J Anaesth* 1990;37(Pt 1):440–443.

10. Tanaka K. Effects of intravenous injections of lidocaine on hemodynamics and catecholamine levels during endotracheal intubation in infants and children. *Aichi Gakuin Daigaku Shigakkai Shi* 1989;27:345–358.

11. Robinson AL, Jerwood DC, Stokes MA. Routine suxamethonium in children: a regional survey of current usage. *Anaesthesia* 1996;51:874–878.

12. Weir PS. Anaesthesia for appendicectomy in childhood: a survey of practice in Northern Ireland. *Ulster Med J* 1997;66:34–37.

13. Deakers TW, Reynolds G, Stretton M, et al. Cuffed endotracheal tubes in pediatric intensive care. *J Pediatr* 1994;125:57–62.

14. Khine HH, Corddry DH, Kettrick RG, et al. Comparison of cuffed and uncuffed endotracheal tubes in young children during general anesthesia. *Anesthesiology* 1997;86:627–631.

15. American Heart Association. Pediatric Advanced Life Support. *Circulation* 2005;112:IV-167–IV-187.

16. Angostoni E, Mead J. Statics of the respiratory system. In: Fenn WO, Rahn H, eds. *Handbook of Physiology.* Washington, DC: American Physiologic Society; 1964.

17. Lumb A. Elastic forces and lung volumes. In: *Nunn's Applied Respiratory Physiology*, 5th ed. Oxford, England: Butterworth-Heineman; 2000:51–53.

21

Pediatric Airway Techniques

Robert C. Luten and Steven A. Godwin

TECHNIQUE

For the most part, the airway devices and techniques used in older children and adolescents are no different than those used in adults. The same cannot be said of small children (younger than 3 years) and infants (younger than 1 year), mostly related to two factors: the airway anatomy in these age groups is substantially different from the adult form, and some of the commonly used rescue devices are not available in pediatric sizes (e.g., Combitube). We limit our discussion to those rescue devices that are available for the pediatric population *and* that have evidence of successful use in children.

Mastering these techniques is straightforward and necessary if one is to manage the emergent pediatric airway. The following discussion describes the appropriate use of the various airway modalities in pediatrics, with emphasis on age appropriateness.

Techniques Used in All Children

Bag-mask Ventilation and Endotracheal Intubation

Refer to Chapter 5 for a detailed description of bag-mask ventilation (BMV) and endotracheal intubation. As in adults, oral and nasopharyngeal airways are important adjuncts to BMV, especially in small children where the tongue is relatively large in relation to the volume of the oral cavity. Recommendations and the rationale for the use of specific equipment (curved or straight blades, cuffed vs. uncuffed tubes) are described in Chapter 20. Use of size-appropriate equipment for pediatric airway management is critical to success, even in the most experienced hands. Proper BMV technique is particularly important in pediatric patients because the indication for intervention is most often primarily related to a respiratory disorder, and the child is likely to be hypoxic. In addition, pediatric patients are subject to more rapid oxyhemoglobin desaturation (see Chapter 20), meaning that BMV with cricoid pressure (Sellick's maneuver) applied is frequently required during the preoxygenation and paralysis phases of rapid sequence intubation (RSI). Pediatric BMV requires smaller tidal volumes, higher rates, and size-specific equipment. The pediatric airway is particularly amenable to positive pressure ventilation, even in the presence of upper airway obstruction (see Chapter 20).

1. **Tips for successful BMV and endotracheal intubation in infants and children**
   Although BMV in the pediatric population fails infrequently, it must be done correctly: the mask seal must be adequate, the airway open, and the rate and volume of ventilation appropriate to the patient's age. Two errors of technique tend to occur. First, there is a tendency in the excitement of the situation to press the mask portion of the unit downward in an attempt to obtain a tight seal, resulting in neck flexion and upper airway obstruction. Second, there is a tendency to bag at an excessive rate.
   a. **Positioning**
      Children have a relatively large occiput compared with adults. In the supine position, the occiput of the unsupported, relaxed patient may produce flexion of the head and neck and resultant airway obstruction. Proper positioning of the patient therefore is key to prevent obstruction and provide optimal alignment of the axes of the airway (see Chapter 20). Optimal alignment of the laryngeal, pharyngeal, and oral axes in adults usually requires elevation of the occiput to flex the neck on the torso and extend the head at the atlanto-occipital joint. Because of the larger relative size of the occiput in small children, elevation of the occiput is usually unnecessary, and extension of the head may actually cause obstruction. Slight anterior displacement of the atlanto-occipital junction is all that is needed (i.e., pulling up on the chin to create the sniffing position). In small infants, elevation of the shoulders with a towel may be needed to counteract the effect of the large occiput that causes the head to flex forward on the chest. As a general rule, once correctly positioned, the external auditory canal should lie just anterior to the shoulders. Whether this position requires support beneath the occiput

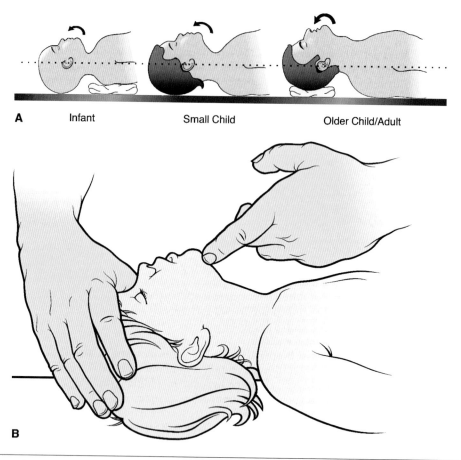

Figure 21-1 ● **A:** Clinical determination of optimal airway alignment, using a line passing through the external auditory canal and anterior to the shoulder (see text for details). **B:** Application of the line to determine optimal position. In this small child, the occiput obviates the need for head support, yet the occiput is not so large as to require support of the shoulders. Note that the line traversing the external auditory canal passes anterior to the shoulders. With only slight extension of the head on the atlanto-occipital joint, the sniffing position is achieved.

(older child/adult), the shoulders (small infant), or no support (small child) (Fig. 21-1A) can be determined using this rule of thumb. These are guidelines only, and each individual patient is different. A quick trial to find the optimal position may be of use. Figure 21-1B demonstrates the most common position for intubating the small child, the so-called sniffing position, and how this is achieved in this size child.

b. **BMV**

Always place an oral airway in the unconscious child before ventilating with a bag and mask because the pediatric tongue is large relative to the size of the oropharynx and is more prone to obstruct the upper airway. The positioning described in the previous paragraph is usually obtained while applying the one-handed, C-grip technique. The thumb and forefinger place and support the mask from the bridge of the nose to the cleft of the chin, avoiding the eyes. The bony prominences of the chin are lifted up by the rest of the fingers, placing the head in mild extension to form the sniffing position. Care is taken to avoid pressure on the airway anteriorly to prevent collapsing and obstructing the pliable trachea.

Further elevation of the jaw with one or two hands in a jaw thrust–like maneuver can only enhance airway patency. The cadence for bagging can be facilitated by the mnemonic "squeeze, release, release," which will allow adequate time for exhalation during the cycle. If ventilation is not immediately obtained with these maneuvers, positioning should be reassessed and a nasopharyngeal airway be placed to supplement the oropharyngeal airway.

c. **Endotracheal intubation**

Even with optimal positioning, external manipulation of the airway (e.g., BURP maneuver, see Chapter 5) may increase visualization of the glottis. This may be especially helpful in small children who have anterior airways, and trauma patients who cannot be optimally aligned.

d. **BMV and cricoid pressure**

Studies in children have shown that cricoid pressure not only prevents passive regurgitation, but also prevents gastric insufflation, even with ventilation pressures greater than 40 cm H_2O. This is especially important in infants, in whom gastric distention may compromise ventilation and increase the risk of aspiration.

e. **Pop-off (also know as positive pressure relief) valves: the good and the bad**

A pop-off valve is designed to prevent the delivery of excessive pressure to the lower airway in an attempt to limit the risk of barotrauma. These valves are incorporated in the infant and pediatric resuscitation bags of most manufacturers. At a preset level, an escape valve opens, limiting the peak pressure that can be delivered, usually 35 to 45 cm of water pressure (CWP), depending on the manufacturer. The bag-mask units tend to be packaged by the manufacturer with the valve ready to function, thereby limiting the risk of barotrauma with initial ventilation attempts. However, in the face of upper airway obstruction, increased airway resistance, or decreased pulmonary compliance, higher pressures may be required. In situations such as these, the operator should disable the valve. With some devices, this must be done manually, although some manufacturers provide a built-in feature that disables the positive pressure relief valve.

In addition to the pop-off valve, many manufacturers incorporate manometer ports into the bag so that one can monitor peak airway pressures as they perform BMV. A leak at the site of the manometer port may interfere with one's ability to achieve airway pressures sufficient to effect adequate gas exchange.

Even though trouble shooting inadequate BMV starts with evaluating the adequacy of mask seal and assessing airway patency, the performance of a "leak test" immediately before beginning BMV will detect the status of the pop-off valve, and also tests for a leak at the manometer site. The leak test is performed by removing the mask from the BVM, occluding the mask port with the palm of one hand, and squeezing the bag with the other hand. If the bag remains tight, no escape of gas, or "leak," has occurred. If the bag does not remain tight, gas is escaping from the system, most commonly from the pop-off valve or the manometer port, although other causes for the leak may be present. The pressure leakage from an open manometer port occurs immediately on compressing the bag as opposed to the open pop-off valve, which vents once a pressure of 35 to 40 CWP is exceeded. The amount of volume lost will vary, depending on the size of the leak. This test is also useful for screening adult bags for malfunctions and leaks. After a negative test (i.e., the bag remains tight with squeezing), the port occluding palm hand should be released, and the bag squeezed to confirm that gas escapes properly from the outlet valve.

Laryngeal Mask Airway

The laryngeal mask airway (LMA) is a safe and effective airway management device for children undergoing general anesthesia and is considered a rescue option in the event of a failed airway in children and infants. Placement of the LMA in children requires some training but is a relatively easily learned skill, particularly if the correct size of mask is chosen. The LMA has also been used successfully in difficult pediatric airways and should be considered as an alternative device for emergency airway management in these patients. As in the adult, difficult pediatric intubations have also been facilitated by the use of the LMA in combination with such devices as the bronchoscope.

The LMA has a few important associated complications, which are especially prevalent in smaller infants, including partial airway obstruction by the epiglottis, loss of adequate seal with patient movement, and air leakage with positive pressure ventilation. To avoid obstruction by the epiglottis in these younger children and infants, some authors have suggested a rotational placement technique where the mask is inserted through the oral cavity "upside-down" and then rotated 180 degrees as it is advanced into the hypopharynx. The LMA is contraindicated in the pediatric patient or adult with intact protective airway reflexes, and therefore, is not suitable for awake airway management unless the patient is adequately sedated and the airway is topically anesthetized. It is also contraindicated if foreign body aspiration is present or suspected because it may aggravate an already desperate situation and is likely to fail to provide adequate ventilation and oxygenation because the obstruction is distal to the device. The LMA comes in multiple sizes to accommodate children from neonate to adolescent. (See also Chapter 10.)

Needle Cricothyrotomy

Although virtually every textbook chapter, article, or lecture on pediatric airway management refers to the technique of needle cricothyrotomy as the recommended last-resort rescue procedure, there is little literature to support its use and safety. Few of the "experts" who write about needle cricothyrotomy have significant experience performing the procedure on live humans. Newer devices, such as the LMA and others, may further reduce the infrequent need for needle cricothyrotomy, but nevertheless, any clinician who manages pediatric emergencies as part of his or her practice must be familiar with the procedure and its indications, and have the appropriate equipment readily accessible in the emergency department.

Needle cricothyrotomy is indicated as a life-saving, last-resort procedure in children younger than 8 to 10 years who present or progress to the "can't intubate, can't ventilate" scenario and whose obstruction is proximal to glottic opening. The classic indication is epiglottitis where BMV and intubation are judged to have failed (although true failure of BMV is rare in epiglottitis, and failure is more often caused by a failure of technique than by a truly insurmountable obstruction). Other indications include facial trauma, angioedema, and other conditions that preclude access to the glottic opening from above. Needle cricothyrotomy is rarely helpful in patients who have aspirated a foreign body that cannot be visualized by direct laryngoscopy because these foreign bodies are usually in the lower airway. It would also be of questionable value in the patient with croup because the obstruction is subglottic. In these patients, the obstruction is more likely to be bypassed by an endotracheal tube (ETT) introduced orally into the trachea with a stylet, than blindly by needle cricothyrotomy.

Various commercially available needles are also available for percutaneous needle cricothyrotomy as well (Table 21-1). The simplest equipment, appropriate for use in infants, consists of the following:
• 14-gauge over-the-needle catheter
• 3.0-mm ETT adapter
• 3-mL or 5-mL syringe

It is a good practice to preassemble the kit, place it in a clear bag, seal the bag, and tape it in an accessible place in the resuscitation area.

TABLE 21-1
Recommended Commmercial Catheters

These catheters are available commercially and can be used as an option:

Jet ventilation catheter (Ravussin). Sizes 13 and 14 gauge, not the16-gauge catheter. Although listed as jet ventilation catheters, we recommend them only for use with bag-mask ventilation.
http://www.hospitecnica.com.mx/productos/VBMventilator%20jet.pdf

6F Cook Emergency Transtracheal Airway Catheters. They are available in two sizes, 5 and 7.5 cm. We only recommend the 5-cm catheter.
http://www.cookmedical.com/cc/dataSheet.do?id=1307

1. **Procedure**

Place the child in the supine position with the head extended over a towel under the shoulder. This forces the trachea anteriorly such that it is easily palpable and can be stabilized with two fingers of one hand. The key to success is strict immobilization of the trachea throughout the procedure. The following statement appears in many textbooks describing this procedure: "Carefully palpate the cricothyroid membrane." In reality, it is difficult to do this in an infant and is not essential. Indeed, in smaller children, it may be impossible to precisely locate the cricothyroid membrane, so the proximal trachea is often accessed. The priority is an airway and provision of oxygen. Complications from inserting the catheter elsewhere into the trachea besides the cricothyroid membrane are addressed later. Consider the trachea as one would a large vein, and cannulate it with the catheter-over-needle device directed caudad at a 30-degree angle. Aspirate air to ensure tracheal entry, and then slide the catheter gently off the needle, removing the needle. Attach the 3.0-mm ETT adapter to the catheter and commence bag ventilation. The provider will note exaggerated resistance to bagging. This is normal and is related to the small diameter of the catheter and the turbulence created by ventilating through it. It is not generally the result of a misplaced catheter or poor lung compliance secondary to pneumothorax. It is helpful to practice BMV through a catheter to experience the feel of the significantly increased resistance. The required pressures are well above the limits of the pop-off valve; therefore, it must be disabled in order to permit gas flow through the catheter. Jet ventilation has also been advocated, although extreme caution must be exercised to prevent barotrauma. Jet ventilation should be considered only by those familiar with its use and in children older than 5 to 6 years. However, even in this age group, if adequate oxygen saturation can be maintained with the bag technique described previously, this is preferable to jet ventilation. If jet ventilation is used, the ventilator must have a pressure control valve system. Start with low pressure (20 PSI), and titrate to adequate chest rise and fall and oxygen saturation, using exceedingly brief bursts of ventilation while observing chest rise, followed by sufficient exhalation time again judged by watching the chest fall. Percutaneous needle ventilation techniques are contraindicated in patients with complete upper airway obstruction.

Techniques Used in Adolescents and Adults

Blind Nasotracheal Intubation

Nasotracheal intubation in children is uniformly discouraged and is frequently considered contraindicated. This recommendation is based on the fact that the sharp angle of the nasopharynx and pharyngotracheal axis in children precludes a reasonable likelihood of success with this technique when performed blindly. A second reason is that children are at

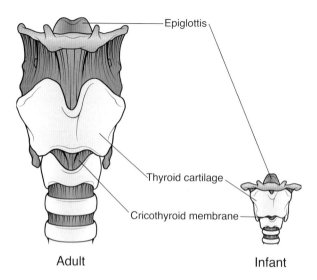

Figure 21-2 ● Cricothyroid Membrane. Comparative size of the adult *(left)* versus pediatric *(right)* cricothyroid membrane. Note that not only is the larynx smaller, but also the actual membrane is smaller proportionately in comparison, involving one-fourth to one-third the anterior tracheal circumference versus two-thirds to three-fourths in the adult. This pediatric drawing is that of a toddler, which accommodates a 4.5-mm endotracheal tube.

increased risk for hemorrhage because of the preponderance of highly vascular and delicate adenoidal tissue. The direct visualization technique is, however, commonly used in small infants and children for chronic ventilator management in the intensive care unit setting. Using direct visualization with a laryngoscope once the ETT has passed into the oro- and hypopharynx, tracheal placement is aided with Magill forceps. However, this technique is not helpful in emergency airway management. In general, the technique of blind nasotracheal intubation, which is essentially the same as that described for adults in Chapter 9, has few, if any, primary indications in pediatric emergency airway management, and in any case, is not recommended for patients younger than 10 years.

Combitube

The Combitube represents an excellent, easily learned rescue airway device that is available only for patients of height greater than 48 inches, so is of limited application in pediatric emergency airway management. The use of the Combitube is identical to that described in Chapter 10.

Surgical Cricothyrotomy

The cricothyroid membrane in small infants and children is minimally developed (Fig. 21-2). Identification of the key landmarks is at best extremely difficult, even in the noncrisis situation. The low likelihood of success, combined with the high anticipated complication rate from attempts to perform this procedure in an emergency, make it contraindicated in small children and infants. Surgical or cricothyrotome-based cricothyrotomy should not be attempted in children younger than 10 years, except in extraordinary circumstances. In children younger than 10 years, needle cricothyrotomy with BMV is recommended. As with adults, adolescents may have easily identifiable and accessible anatomy, and therefore, cricothyrotomy may be a reasonable rescue technique

---

BOX 21-1 Summary Recommendations for Invasive Airway Procedures in Children

---

5 years old
Needle cricothyrotomy and bag ventilation

5–10 years old
Consider needle cricothyrotomy and bag ventilation[a]
Percutaneous Seldinger technique and bag ventilation
(Transtracheal jet ventilation [TTJV] regulated to low PSI is discouraged unless done
   by experienced operator)

>10 years
Operator preference
Needle cricothyrotomy with TTJV *or* Surgical cricothyrotomy

[a]There is less evidence to support this recommendation in this age group; however, it may be the only available option and should be converted to a more definitive airway.

---

in this age group. Cricothyrotomy using a commercially available kit (Pedi-trake) has not been shown to be successful or even safe. Box 21-1 summarizes recommendations for invasive airway procedures in children.

EVIDENCE

1. **Does a needle cricothyrotomy with BMV in children provide sufficient oxygenation and ventilation to avoid hypoxia and hypercarbia?** The evidence surrounding pediatric needle cricothyrotomies is based on an animal study by Cote et al. (1) using a 30-kg dog model. Cote was able to demonstrate that dogs representative in size of a 9- to 10-year-old child could be oxygenated through a 12-gauge catheter and 3.0 ETT adapter with a bag for at least 1 hour (the study duration). Rises in $PaCO_2$ levels were noted, but were not believed to be significant because children normally tolerate mild degrees of hypercarbia well (1).

   One adult retrospective study reported that 48 patients were successfully oxygenated and ventilated using transtracheal ventilation through a 13-gauge intratracheal catheter for up to 360 minutes. Transtracheal jet ventilation (TTJV) was used primarily in 47 of these patients, although 6 patients did receive conventional bagging measures until TTJV circuits could be initiated. During manual transtracheal ventilation, each patient demonstrated increases in $PaCO_2$ on blood gases but maintained PaO_2 values greater than 100 mm Hg (2).

2. **The LMA should be considered as both a rescue device and an alternative airway in the management of difficult emergency pediatric airways.** Most of the literature regarding the use of LMAs in children has been compiled from the anesthesia experience in the operating room. Therefore, little information is available for the use of the LMA in the acute emergency setting. However, an observational study by Lopez-Gil et al. has demonstrated that the skill for placement of the LMA could be rapidly learned by anesthesia residents with a low complication rate (3,4). Published case reports have demonstrated success of the LMA in the pediatric patient with difficult airways, including isolated severe retrognathia, Dandy-Walker syndrome, and Pierre Robin syndrome (5,6).

At least one prospective study reports a higher incidence of airway obstruction, higher ventilatory pressures, larger inspiratory leaks, and more complications in smaller children (those weighing <10 kg) with LMA use than in the older child. These authors recommend that the risk–benefit should be carefully weighed in younger children before using the LMA with paralysis and positive pressure ventilation. Importantly, the success rate for placement of the LMA in this study that was performed in elective cases undergoing prolonged ventilation was high at 98% (7). Although airway managers should be aware of these potential complications, this study is not generalizable to the emergency setting and should not deter providers from implementing this as a *rescue device* in infants or young children with failed airways, or as a planned approach to an infant or young child with an identified difficult airway. In the failed airway situation, the LMA may be a lifesaving bridge, providing effective oxygenation and ventilation until a definitive airway can be secured.

REFERENCES

1. Cote CJ, Eavey RD, Todres ID, et al. Cricothyroid membrane puncture: oxygenation and ventilation in a dog model using an intravenous catheter. *Crit Care Med* 1988;16:615–619.
2. Ravussin P, Freeman J. A new transtracheal catheter for ventilation and resuscitation. *Can Aneaesth Soc J* 1985;32:60–64.
3. Lopez-Gil, Brimacombe J, Alvarez M. Safety and efficacy of the laryngeal mask airway: a prospective survey of 1,400 children. *Anaesthesia* 1996;51:969–972.
4. Lopez-Gil, Brimacombe J, Cebrian J, et al. Laryneal mask airway in pediatric practice: a prospective study of skill acquisition by anesthesia residents. *Anesthesiology* 1996;84:807–811.
5. Selim M, Mowafi H, Al-Ghamdi A, et al. Intubation via LMA in pediatric patients with difficult airways. *Can J Anaesth* 1999;46:891–893.
6. Stocks RM, Egerman R, Thompson JW, et al. Airway management of the severely retrognathic child: use of the laryngeal mask airway. *Ear Nose Throat J* 2002;81:223–226.
7. Park C, Bahk JH, Ahn WS, et al. The laryngeal mask airway in infants and children. *Can J Anaesth* 2001;48:413–417.

22

The Difficult Pediatric Airway

Robert C. Luten and Niranjan Kissoon

TECHNIQUE

Securing an airway in a patient, adult or child, is made more challenging or difficult for two principal reasons:

1. The patient's normal airway anatomy is modified because of an acute insult
2. The patient with an abnormal airway (e.g., a congenital anomaly) requires airway management for an unrelated cause, such as respiratory failure due to an asthma exacerbation

The approach to the emergent difficult airway is described in Chapter 7, which should be read before this chapter. Pediatric difficult airways, especially those encountered in emergency situations, are far less common than in adults, not well studied, and not extensively covered in any textbook. For purposes of this discussion, difficult pediatric airways are divided functionally into difficult airways secondary to:

1. Acute infectious disease
2. Acute noninfectious disease
3. Congenital anomalies, most commonly with a superimposed indication for emergency airway management unrelated to the airway abnormality (e.g., respiratory failure secondary to asthma or pneumonia)

Difficult Airways Secondary to Acute Infectious Disease

Examples of entities in which an otherwise normal anatomy is altered by an infectious process include
1. Epiglottitis
2. Croup (usually not a difficult intubation; Table 22-1)
3. Retropharyngeal abscess
4. Bacterial tracheitis
5. Ludwig's angina
   Most often, children with the disorders described in this and in the next section present because the normal anatomy is altered, usually by swelling, which leads to varying degrees of airway obstruction. The pediatric patient is especially susceptible to airway obstruction from swelling, often from conditions that are less threatening to the adult. This is illustrated in Table 22-2, which outlines the effect of 1-mm of edema on airway resistance in the infant (4-mm airway diameter) versus adult (8-mm airway diameter). These figures reflect the quietly breathing infant or adult. If the child cries, the work of breathing is increased 32-fold, hence the principle of maintaining children in a quiet, nonthreatening, and comfortable environment during evaluation and in preparation for management.
   Table 22-1 outlines the two most notorious infectious diseases involving the upper airway with potential for obstruction in children, epiglottitis and croup. Epiglottitis is rarely seen in the Western world since the introduction of the *Haemophilus* influenza vaccine, and croup, commonly referred to in the differential diagnosis of epiglottitis, is usually a clinically distinct entity that is rarely a difficult intubation because the obstruction is subglottic. It is of value still to discuss epiglottitis because it represents the prototype indication for needle cricothyrotomy (see Chapter 21) as an obstruction proximal to the glottic opening when bag-mask ventilation (BMV) and intubation fail. Other, noninfectious problems causing obstruction proximal to the glottic opening include facial trauma, angioedema, and caustic ingestions and burns involving the hypopharynx. To put these "most-feared" diseases in perspective, the following points should be kept in mind:
A. These problems have in common the fact that airway intervention in the emergency department (ED) should never be attempted unless deterioration occurs or is imminent. If one adheres to this principle and then follows a stepwise approach as outlined in Table 22-1, results will be optimal and complications, especially iatrogenic complications, will be avoided.

TABLE 22-1

Management of The "Most-Feared" Pediatric Airway Problems

Disease	Pathology and deterioration	Approach	FB removal maneuvers	BMV two-person techniques	Intubation	Needle cricothyrotomy
Epiglottitis	Rapidly progressing disease process affecting the supraglottic structures (epiglottis, aryepiglottic folds). Patients usually present in minimal distress. Decompensation rarely occurs unless the patient is overstimulated or manipulated, leading to dynamic airway obstruction. Otherwise, decompensation is the result of progressive deterioration over time secondary to fatigue, although the respiratory arrest may occur precipitously.	Stable → observe → transfer to OR for definitive airway Decompensation BMV → Intubation → Needle cric	Not indicated	Effective *in most* patients who deteriorate. Technique: two-handed seal, with another rescuer providing sufficient pressure to overcome the obstruction.	Usually successful. Use tube size 1 mm smaller. Use stylet. Suction, visualize, press on chest, and look for bubble.	Probably one of the few indications for needle cric *if* BMV and intubation are unsuccessful.

(continued)

TABLE 22-1
Management of The "Most-Feared" Pediatric Airway Problems (Continued)

Disease	Pathology and deterioration	Approach	FB removal maneuvers	BMV two-person techniques	Intubation	Needle cricothyrotomy
Croup	Slowly progressive (hours to days) disease process affecting the subglottic trachea, causing dynamic inspiratory augmented obstruction. Deterioration is usually progressive rather than sudden and related to respiratory muscle fatigue, and as in the case of epiglottis, the arrest may also occur precipitously.	Racemic epi Steroids stable → ICU Decompensation → BMV → Intubation	Not indicated	Effective. Positive pressure overcomes obstruction by acting as a stent. Will probably require high pressures.	Proximal airway normal; therefore, should not be problematic. Consider ETT one size smaller and use stylet.	Not indicated because obstruction is distal.

FB aspiration	Patients with aspirated FBs have the potential for decompensation secondary to acute airway obstruction. The level of obstruction may vary from the hypopharynx, above or below the glottis, to the mainstem bronchus.	Stable → observe → transfer for removal Decompensation ↑ FB removal maneuvers ↑ Direct visualization and removal with Magill forceps ↑ Intubation to force FB distally into mainstem bronchus	Indicated if *appropriate* (i.e., patient totally obstructs)	Should not be used before attempts to remove FB. May be obviated by intubation.	Last resort in an effort to push FB distally.	Usually not indicated because FB will be distal to the obstruction if other efforts have failed.

FB, foreign body; BMV, bag-mask ventilation; OR, operating room; epi, epinephrine; ICU, intensive care unit; ETT, endotracheal tube.

TABLE 22-2
Effect of 1-mm Edema on Airway Resistance

	Change in cross-sectional area	Change in resistance
Infant	44% decrease	200% increase
Adult	25% decrease	40% increase

B. Epiglottitis and croup are distinct clinical entities, that rarely, if ever, require radiologic studies to distinguish the two. The fact that textbooks group them together in the differential diagnosis of acute life-threatening upper airway obstruction is misleading because the differentiation is usually clinically obvious.

C. Croup, as opposed to epiglottitis or foreign body aspiration, will respond to medical intervention (inhaled epinephrine), which usually obviates the need for intubation.

D. Retropharyngeal abscess in children usually presents without airway compromise, although it is virtually always found in textbooks in the differential diagnosis of acute life-threatening airway obstruction. The same is true of Ludwig's angina, an even less common disease. The term *para-airway diagnoses* is used to describe conditions involving the airway above the level of the glottis. These conditions rarely require emergency airway intervention of the pediatric patient in the ED. A retropharyngeal abscess most commonly presents with odynophagia and neck stiffness. Lateral neck films reveal thickening of the retropharyngeal space. Most of these patients have retropharyngeal cellulitis and respond to antibiotics. If an abscess is present, incision and drainage is required, but rarely, if ever, is it necessary to actively manage the airway in the ED.

Difficult Airways Secondary to Noninfectious Causes

1. Foreign body
2. Burns
3. Anaphylaxis
4. Caustic ingestion
5. Trauma
6. Other swellings (angioedema, Quinke disease, etc.)

Foreign body aspiration is probably the most feared pediatric airway problem. They should be managed "expectantly," meaning that no intervention should be attempted in the ED and that resources should be summoned to provide definitive care (removal) in the operating room setting. If the patient converts to complete obstruction, immediate intervention is required. With complete obstruction of the airway, oxygen desaturation, rendering the patient unconscious, ordinarily occurs within 1 minute or so. A stepwise approach should be followed.

A. *The conscious child*

Although controversy exists regarding the ideal emergency procedure for relief of choking, the Heimlich maneuver is suggested by the American Heart Association for children older than 1 year. For children younger than 1 year, a series of five back blows followed by five chest thrusts is recommended.

If the patient is conscious, the correct initial treatment is the application of these maneuvers, which should be repeated until the foreign body is expelled or the patient loses consciousness. To summarize

- Children younger than 1 year: five back blows followed by five chest thrusts.
- Children older than 1 year: repetitive abdominal thrusts.
- Attempt ventilation.
- Continue this sequence as long as the child is conscious.

Attempting instrumentation to remove the foreign body of a completely obstructed upper airway while the patient is still conscious is not wise. If the maneuvers are successful in removing the foreign body, and the patient can phonate and breathe normally, an observation period of 12 to 24 hours is advised.

The disposition of a child with a stable partial obstruction to the operating room as described previously may not be possible if expert resources are unavailable or unwilling, and an alternative plan, preferably crafted in advance as time is of the essence, must be activated. Removal of the foreign body in the ED should only be done if other options are unavailable. The approach to the partially obstructed airway is described elsewhere (see Chapter 36).

Recognizing that conscious children are unlikely to cooperate with efforts to remove the foreign body sedation is important. As described in the *Tips and Pearls* section of Chapter 30, the intravenous titration of ketamine beginning at the induction dose (1–2 mg/kg), or 4 mg/kg intramuscularly, produces dependable deep sedation/anesthesia while maintaining respiratory drive and reflexes.

B. *The unconscious child*

If the maneuvers are unsuccessful in removing the foreign body and the patient loses consciousness, or if the patient with an upper airway foreign body presents unconscious, direct laryngoscopy should be attempted. This is a "crash airway" (see Chapter 2), and the administration of a neuromuscular blocking agent is not indicated for the initial attempt. However, if the child presents with clenched teeth or other signs of substantial muscle activity, use of succinylcholine to achieve relaxation in order to identify and remove the foreign body may be necessary. If the foreign body can be identified under direct laryngoscopy, it should be removed.

Occasionally, BMV using high pressure (usually a two-person, two-handed technique is required to achieve an adequate seal) may be successful. If ventilation is successful in these cases, it is usually because the foreign body has been forced beyond the glottis and subglottic region into one of the mainstem bronchi.

If BMV is unsuccessful, the child should be intubated and an attempt made to advance the foreign body into either mainstem bronchus. The tube should then be withdrawn above the carina and ventilation of the unobstructed lung attempted. Resuscitation guides such as the Broselow-Luten tape provide a "lip-to-tip" distance number as an objective guide for positioning the endotracheal tube (ETT) in the trachea of a child. With the ETT positioned at the stipulated distance at the lip, the distal opening of the ETT is halfway between the vocal cords and the carina, although clinical verification is always recommended. Occasionally, soft foreign bodies such as foodstuff or adenoidal tissue, if a nasal intubation was performed, may lodge within the ETT, necessitating withdrawal of the ETT. In the event that the patient breathes spontaneously following this maneuver, BMV or intubation may not be required.

Percutaneous approaches (e.g., needle cricothyrotomy) are rarely indicated in foreign body aspirations, and will only be successful if the foreign body is lodged in the airway above the entrance of the needle into the airway (e.g., a ball bearing seen to be lodged below the vocal cords at the cricoid ring on laryngoscopy that cannot be extracted with instruments). In the event that the foreign body cannot be visualized on direct laryngoscopy, it is unlikely that a percutaneous approach will be distal to the object, rendering the procedure ineffective. An overview of the sequence is presented in Table 22-1, and detail is provided in Figure 22-1.

In both adults and children, if the foreign body becomes lodged causing complete obstruction and cannot be retrieved or expelled by blind maneuvers, attempts at BMV followed by advancement of the foreign body into a mainstem bronchus as described previously should be immediately performed.

C. *Timing the intervention*

As is the case for adults, the anticipated clinical course of the presenting condition becomes a key determinant in the decision whether to actively intervene in the airway

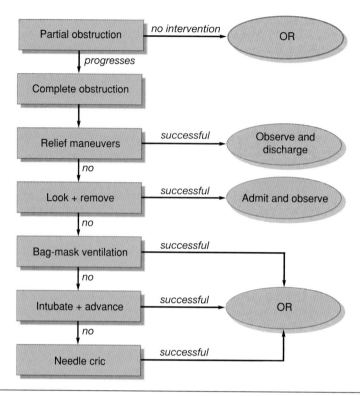

Figure 22-1 ● Stepwise approach for the management of an aspirated foreign body.

(e.g., intubate) or to observe the patient for possible deterioration. Table 22-3 groups disorders from both infectious and noninfectious causes according to timing of intervention based on anticipated clinical course.

The *expectant intervention group* represents patients in whom the intervention itself may be more hazardous than a period of close observation, during which preparation is

TABLE 22-3
Timing of Intervention According to Anticipated Clinical Course

Expectant intervention group: Intervene *only* if deterioration occurs:
1. Assemble subspecialty multidisciplinary team for definitive management:
   Foreign body
   Epiglottitis
2. Obtain subspecialty assistance if deterioration appears likely:
   Para-airway *diagnoses* (diseases such as retropharyngeal or peritonsillar abscess or Ludwig's angina that are usually stable on presentation and deterioration is uncommon)

Early intervention group: Intervene *early* (preventively):
Burns
Anaphylaxis: usually responds to medical treatment; anaphylactoid-like reactions such as angioedema respond less reliably to medical treatment, particularly if angiotensin-converting enzyme inhibitor is the culprit
Caustic ingestions
Trauma

rapidly undertaken for definitive management. In these children, the airway should be actively managed in the ED only if deterioration occurs. The rationale in these cases is that intervention is best done in a controlled environment by a multidisciplinary team with expertise in the management of difficult airways. Treatment in less than ideal conditions may lead to untoward outcomes.

The signs and symptoms of impending airway obstruction in children are important indicators that guide the approach to the *early intervention group*. These disorders, if left to expectant treatment, have a greater potential for deterioration. An example is the burn or caustic ingestion patient who is beginning to develop a raspy voice. This symptom heralds the potential for deterioration, although the degree and pace of progression cannot be predicted. However, it must be assumed that progression to the point of obstruction is possible, in which case should intubation become necessary, it will be extremely difficult if not impossible. For this reason, intervention earlier rather than later is recommended. Patients with compromised airways secondary to anaphylactic or anaphylactoid reactions (e.g., angioedema) who do not respond to immediate medical treatment similarly require early intervention to prevent a more difficult, unmanageable problem later.

As discussed previously, children are anatomically less able to accommodate airway swelling than adults and can deteriorate precipitously.

Difficult Airways Secondary to Congenital Anomalies

Patients with difficult airways secondary to congenital anomalies receive the most attention in discussions of difficult airways in pediatrics. However, they are encountered only rarely in the ED, much less frequently than groups 1 and 2. Also, the literature concerning these patients usually describes elective situations, managed by experienced pediatric anesthesiology subspecialists in well-equipped operating rooms with the intubation done under controlled conditions. This kind of discussion is not relevant to the management of the airway if these children present emergently.

Most patients with congenital anomalies presenting to the ED require intubation for reasons unrelated to their difficult airway (e.g., a child with Pierre Robin syndrome with respiratory failure secondary to asthma). The best approach for these patients is to obtain expert subspecialty assistance as early as possible and, as with all patients, to aggressively manage the medical condition to try to obviate the need for intubation. Unlike the conditions discussed previously in this chapter, there is some luxury of time here because those factors that progressively increase the likelihood of being confronted with a difficult airway are not operative. Delay in managing the airway may result in some deterioration of the patient, but will not make the airway itself any more difficult, except possibly by limiting the time available to successfully intubate a severely hypoxemic child.

The micrognathic mandible is the most common anatomical feature in the child rendering intubation difficult, although there are others. The small mandible reduces the space ("mandibular space") into which the tongue and submandibular tissue must be compressed with the laryngoscope blade to visualize the glottic opening. A significantly recessed (micrognathic) mandible can be recognized by drawing a line that touches the forehead and maxilla and continues inferiorly (Fig. 22-2). In a patient with grossly normal anatomy, the line also touches the tip of the chin. In the micrognathic patient, a gap between the line and the tip of the chin is observed. In such patients, as described in the Difficult Airway Algorithm, an awake look (sedated) to assess the degree to which the tongue can be displaced into the mandibular space may be attempted before opting for rapid sequence intubation (RSI).

For patients in extremis or in crash situations, the clinician is left with no other options than those used in other patients. Often, such simple procedures as BMV or endotracheal intubation are successful in these patients and should remain as the mainstay of therapy.

Therapeutic options for the pediatric difficult airway are outlined in Table 22-4.

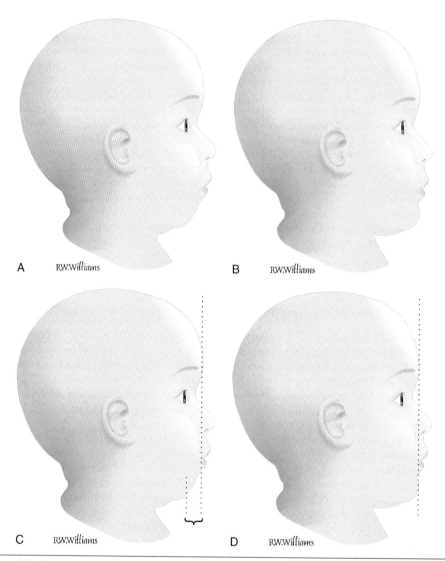

Figure 22-2 ● It may not always be obvious that a given patient possesses a difficult airway (**A**). When compared with a normal child, the differences may be more striking (**A** vs. **B**). In the individual patient, however, a line drawn inferiorly from the forehead, touching the maxilla, will also touch the mandible (**D**). The failure to do so demonstrates a degree of micrognathia (**C**), which must be correlated with the clinical picture. Source: Extrapolated from Frankville D. ASA refresher course. Parkridge, IL: American Society of Anesthesiologists; 2001:126.

EVIDENCE

Unfortunately, little evidence is published on the recognition and management of the difficult pediatric airway in an emergency. Most of the descriptions of difficult pediatric airways deal with children with congenital anomalies. The literature on predicting the difficulty airway employing a systematic clinical evaluation is confined to adults and may not necessarily be applicable to children (1; Table 22-5). It is anticipated that the National Emergency

TABLE 22-4
Therapeutic Options for The Difficult Airway

The difficult airway algorithm applies to both children and adults with few exceptions; most notably, blind nasotracheal intubation is contraindicated in children younger than 10 years, as is surgical cricothyrotomy. Combitube, a useful adjunct in adults, is not manufactured for patients less than 48 inches tall. Otherwise, the same approach and options are recommended for both children and adults, the only difference being that they are required less often.

There are a variety of airway devices for use in the pediatric patient. However, because of lack of frequency of use, except in elective subspecialty situations, only a few have been used in emergencies and even fewer by emergency practitioners. It is probably best to limit the number of options in an effort to gain the maximum experience with them. The following devices and procedures are listed according to appropriateness in different levels of clinical acuity.

Crash situation
   Noninvasive
      Endotracheal (ET) intubation (infancy to adulthood)
      Laryngeal mask airway (LMA; infancy to adulthood)
      Combitube (>48 inch. tall)
   Invasive
      Needle cricothyrotomy[a] (<5+ years)
      Seldinger cricothyrotomy (>5 years)[a]
      Surgical or Seldinger cricothyrotomy (>10 years)

Stable situation
   ET intubation (awake) (infancy to adulthood)
   ET intubation (rapid sequence intubation; infancy to adulthood)
   Combitube (>48 inch. in height; patient must be obtunded)
   LMA (infancy to adulthood)
   Fiberoptic intubation (infancy to adulthood)
   Blind nasotracheal intubation (>10 years)

Stable Expectant Management Patients

All emergency departments should have a plan in place for managing patients with disorders such as foreign body aspiration, epiglottitis, etc. This usually requires prior agreement of consultants willing to respond immediately to those emergencies.

---

[a]For children younger than 5 years, bag-mask ventilation (BMV) is recommended with these options. In children ages 5–10 years, transtracheal jet ventilation (TTJV) has been recommended, but requires an adjustable pressure regulator. There is little literature to support TTJV recommendation for pediatric emergency airway management, just as there is little literature to support needle cricothyrotomy and BMV. However, because the risk of complications related to TTJV is very high, it should be used with extreme caution in children and is best reserved for use only by clinicians familiar with TTJV. BMV with immediate conversion to a more definitive airway may be the only prudent option.

Airway Registry project will enable the characterization of the scope of the difficult airway in pediatrics and provide "best practice" approaches to its management.

  1. **Heimlich maneuver.** There is a controversy in the literature as to the ideal emergency procedure for relief of choking due to foreign body aspiration (2,3). However, the Heimlich maneuver is suggested by the American Heart Association as the maneuver

TABLE 22-5
A Sample Comparison of Pediatric and Adult Risk Factors

A. *Risk factors for adult difficult airway usually not present in infants and young children:*
 1. Obesity
 2. Decreased neck mobility
 3. Teeth abnormalities
 4. Temporomandibular joint problems
B. *Risk factors for pediatric difficult airway not present in adults:*
 1. Small airway caliber susceptible to obstruction from infection
 2. Discomfort secondary to dealing with age- and size-related variables
 3. Discomfort secondary to infrequency of patient encounters

to be tried initially for children older than 1 year. In children younger than 1 year, the danger of intra-abdominal injury precludes its use, and a combination of back blows and chest thrusts is recommended (4). Although little evidence exists, it is recommended that if obstruction is incomplete and the patient is phonating, then no intervention should be attempted. This approach is predicated on the fact that the force of a cough generates five to six times the airflow velocity of other maneuvers and is more likely to expel the foreign body. Moreover, there is concern that these interventions may have the potential to convert a partial obstruction to a total obstruction.

REFERENCES

 1. Kopp VJ, Bailey A, Calhoun PE, et al. Utility of the Mallampati classification for predicting difficult intubation in pediatric patients. *Anesthesiology* 1995;83:3A1147.
 2. Redding JS. The choking controversy: critique of evidence on the Heimlich maneuver. *Crit Care Med* 1979;7:475–479.
 3. Heimlich HJ. First aid for choking children: back blows and chest thrusts cause complications and death. *Pediatrics* 1982;70:120–125.
 4. Zaritsky A, Nadkarni V, Hickey R, et al., eds. *PALS Provider Manual*. Dallas, TX: American Heart Association; 2002.

23

Airway Management in the Prehospital Setting

Richard D. Zane and Michael F. Murphy

THE CLINICAL CHALLENGE

Many of the principles of prehospital airway management are similar to those in the emergency department (ED), with the obvious exception that the prehospital environment is necessarily austere. Patient management in the prehospital setting is done without many of the resources and backup assistance that are readily available in the ED. In addition, patient care must often be provided in awkward circumstances such as in private homes, in stairwells, in the seat of a damaged automobile, or on the street, where lighting and position are often not ideal. Local protocols, regional and topographic differences in transport time, the availability or unavailability of neuromuscular blocking agents, limited and varied equipment, limited backup, and mandatory transport of the patient all introduce considerations and issues that are not only different from those in the ED, but also different from one prehospital system to another.

APPROACH TO THE AIRWAY

The following factors have motivated the most striking changes in the approach to airway management in emergency medical services (EMS) since the last edition of this manual:

- The emergence of extraglottic devices (EGDs) as first-choice alternatives to bag-mask ventilation (BMV) in unresponsive patients for basic life support (BLS) providers
- The use of EGDs *instead of* endotracheal intubation (ETI) by advanced life support (ALS) urban ground ambulance services in unresponsive patients
- The emergence of "nonparalytic rapid sequence intubation (RSI)" as an alternative to "paralytic RSI" in which a full or tailored dose of an induction agent, but no neuromuscular blocking agent is administered
- Confusion in the literature as to whether ETI is of benefit in ground ambulance ALS EMS services
- A distinct pattern of improved outcomes with RSI where helicopter EMS (HEMS) (also known as air medical transport) had been used.
- The use of high-fidelity human patient simulation training to improve performance

Factors contributing to improved RSI success rates for prehospital providers have also been identified:

- High-quality initial and ongoing airway management training
- Intense medical oversight and quality management programs
- Frequent exposure to patients in need of active airway management

Improved outcomes for services embracing RSI is contingent on three factors:

1. Knowing how to correctly perform RSI
2. Being able to identify those patients where RSI should not be preformed (i.e., identifying the Difficult Airway [see Chapter 7])
3. Being able to rescue the airway in the event that intubation is unsuccessful and BMV fails

The decision to intubate the patient in the prehospital setting is based on the same principles as those applied in the ED (see Chapter 1). A prehospital algorithm for the decision to intubate is shown in Figure 23-1. The initial step is a quick evaluation of the patient, with a particular focus on assessment of the airway and ventilation. If the patient is maintaining the airway, protecting the airway, and ventilating and oxygenating adequately, then intubation is rarely indicated in the prehospital setting. However, failure to maintain or protect the airway or to exchange gases adequately mandates intubation unless the problem can be corrected by other means or transport is very short.

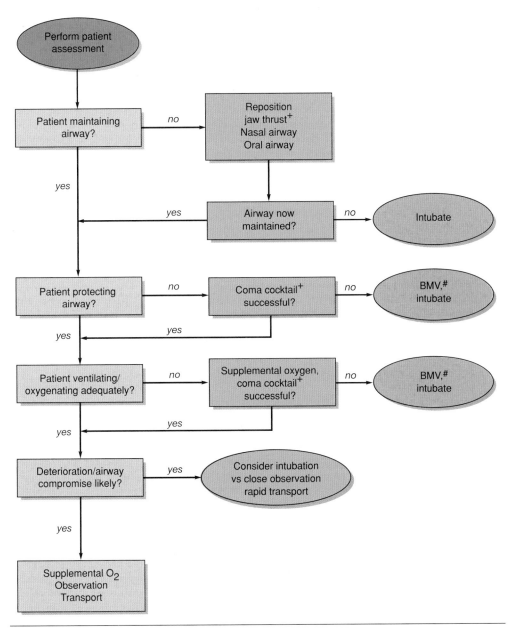

Figure 23-1 ● Decision to Intubate. *Caution in trauma; + naloxone, glucose; #BMV, bag-mask ventilation.

TECHNIQUE

If the patient is not maintaining his or her own airway, as evidenced by obstructed or noisy breathing, deep coma with unresponsiveness, or apnea, then the jaw-thrust maneuver should be immediately applied to attempt to establish a patent upper airway. Unless the patient has a contraindication to manipulation of the head and neck (e.g., blunt trauma with possible cervical spine injury), the head should be extended on the neck, and the mandible should be thrust forward by pressure applied bilaterally at the angles of the mandible. This is best done using the ring or small fingers of the rescuer's hands so that the remaining fingers can be free to apply and properly seal a mask for ventilation.

If the patient does not begin breathing spontaneously when the jaw-thrust maneuver is applied, then BMV should be initiated, with placement of nasal and oral airways (see Chapter 5). In most circumstances, BMV in this setting should be followed by ETI as soon as adequate preparations have been made, and providing the EMT is trained and credentialled to intubate. If BMV is unsuccessful, despite careful attention to proper technique, then immediate intubation or placement of an alternate airway device, such as a Combitube or laryngeal mask airway (LMA), is indicated (see Chapter 10). As mentioned previously, there is a school of thought emerging that the use of an EGD may leapfrog ahead of BMV as the first-line technique. This is based on the relative ease of use and high ventilation success rates seen with EGDs relative to the more difficult technique of BMV.

After a patent airway has been established, the next evaluation should determine whether the patient is protecting the airway from aspiration. Aspiration of gastric contents is a serious adverse event and must be prevented. Failure to maintain a patent airway usually also indicates loss of protective airway reflexes. It is appropriate to administer a "coma cocktail," which typically includes naloxone in doses of 0.4 to 2 mg as a specific reversal agent for opioid-induced respiratory depression, and glucose, 25 g intravenously, for possible hypoglycemia. In some systems, point-of-care glucose testing is performed rather than empiric glucose administration. If the coma cocktail is unsuccessful in reversing the patient's coma sufficient to permit self-protection of the airway, then BMV and intubation are indicated.

If the patient is maintaining and protecting the airway, the next assessment is of the adequacy of ventilation and oxygenation. If the patient is hypoventilating and a coma cocktail has not already been administered, this should now be done. Oxygenation failure, such as in pulmonary edema, may respond simply to supplemental oxygen via a nonrebreather mask or via bag and mask with assisted respirations. If neither supplemental oxygen nor administration of reversal agents can establish adequate oxygenation, then BMV is indicated, followed by intubation.

Finally, there is a population of patients for whom intubation may be indicated despite adequate airway maintenance and protection and acceptable levels of oxygenation and ventilation. An example is a pulmonary edema patient who is rapidly tiring but is maintaining oxygen saturations at 90%. If long transport time to the hospital is anticipated and the patient is not responding to other interventions, such that it is anticipated that the patient likely will deteriorate and require intubation before arrival at hospital, then early, anticipatory intubation may be appropriate before development of frank hypoxemia with worsening metabolic and respiratory acidosis. Other examples include a patient with drug overdose and rapidly decreasing level of consciousness, the cyclic antidepressant overdose patient who has had a generalized seizure, or certain cases of upper airway trauma in which ongoing airway bleeding or expansion of a hematoma might threaten the patient. In such cases, careful evaluation and consultation with medical control is essential. In most circumstances, expeditious transport of the patient with supplemental oxygen via a nonrebreather mask is the appropriate course of action. Nevertheless, in certain circumstances, intubation may be both prudent and indicated (Fig. 23-1).

Once a decision to intubate is made, the next step is to choose the best method for intubation, based on individual patient circumstances and the attributes of the EMS system and the intubator. The choice will depend on whether neuromuscular blockade is permitted, the availability of airway adjuncts and rescue devices, and whether prehospital cricothyrotomy is possible and permitted, along with a number of individual operator attributes.

If the patient is unresponsive and exhibits agonal cardiac or respiratory activity, the situation is analogous to the crash airway scenario depicted in Chapter 2. The choice here is between BMV, insertion of an alternate airway device (Combitube or LMA), oral tracheal intubation, and blind nasotracheal intubation. Regardless, the patient should have an airway established and oxygenation maintained using a bag and mask until intubation is attempted.

If the patient has a relatively clear upper airway (no trauma, no foreign body, and no obstruction) and is breathing spontaneously, then blind nasotracheal intubation may be reasonable (see Chapter 9). However, apnea is a relative contraindication to blind nasotracheal intubation because the patient's breath sounds are used to guide the tube into place. Similarly, abnormal anatomy or a foreign body in the upper airway also constitutes relative contraindications to this technique. In addition, blind nasotracheal intubation has a lower success rate and higher complication rate than oral intubation. Nevertheless, in some systems and in certain patients, blind nasotracheal intubation may be the preferable method. This may be especially true if the patient's jaw is clenched and the use of neuromuscular blockade is not an option. Also, blind nasotracheal intubation may be a better choice if the patient is relatively inaccessible (e.g., trapped in an automobile) and neither LMA nor Combitube are available.

Oral intubation via direct laryngoscopy is also an acceptable method for the unresponsive patient and is the method of choice if the patient's jaw is not clenched. In the case of the unresponsive patient, intubation proceeds exactly as described previously in discussions of the crash airway scenario. Direct laryngoscopy is performed, and the tracheal tube is placed under direct vision. If direct laryngoscopy is unsuccessful in visualizing the vocal cords, then a drug-assisted intubation is required. In some settings, drug-assisted intubation will include both induction (sedative) agent and neuromuscular blockade. In other settings, where neuromuscular blockade is not permitted, drug-assisted intubation will be done with sedation (at times to the point of induction of general anesthesia) alone. In either case, drug-assisted intubation may be preferable to blind nasotracheal intubation, even in the clenched jaw patient.

If the patient is conscious and combative and requires intubation, then drug-assisted intubation is indicated. At the outset, though, the benefits and risks of intubation should be weighed against the benefits, and risks of rapid transport without intubation. Combative or uncooperative behavior is a strong relative contraindication to blind nasotracheal intubation (NTI) because of the increased risk of complications in attempting to insert the tube in a patient who is resisting. If the patient is not frankly comatose and is not uncooperative or combative, then assessment must be made as to whether the patient would tolerate laryngoscopy. If the patient is sufficiently cooperative or sufficiently obtunded to permit oral laryngoscopy without medications, then NTI may be attempted. Again, preference is expressed for oral intubation over nasal intubation except in circumstances in which the jaw is clenched preventing oral access. Even in such cases, oral intubation with medication may be preferable to blind nasotracheal intubation.

Blind nasotracheal intubation is discussed in detail in Chapter 9. In general, although blind nasotracheal intubation has been widely used in prehospital care, it has declined in popularity as medications are being introduced to facilitate intubation in the prehospital setting. Blind nasotracheal intubation has two main indications. First, in circumstances in which direct laryngoscopy and visualization of the glottis are impossible, blind nasotracheal intubation may be the method of choice. An example is the patient who is trapped in the automobile after a motor vehicle crash and requires intubation before extrication can be accomplished. In such cases, blind nasotracheal intubation may be the only method that can be used by an operator either from inside or outside the vehicle. The second circumstance is the patient with a clenched jaw. A small number of patients will have increased masseter tone and hence a clenched mandible, even when they are deeply unconscious and breathing inadequately. In such cases, the choice is between administering medications for oral intubation or performing blind nasotracheal intubation. Even though RSI is clearly the method of choice under these circumstances, many prehospital care providers do not have this option, and blind nasotracheal intubation may be preferable or may be the procedure of choice for the individual operator.

In general, blind nasotracheal intubation should not be performed in patients with asthma, chronic obstructive pulmonary disease, or pulmonary edema unless drug-assisted intubation is impossible. In such patients, prolonged attempts at nasotracheal intubation impair oxygenation and can worsen existing hypoxemia and lead to respiratory arrest. Again, this is a judgment call, and an individual provider might choose to attempt nasotracheal intubation on the patient with status asthmaticus; however, great caution must be exercised because prolonged or traumatic attempts may significantly worsen the patient's condition.

The prehospital environment is unique in that a provider may be far from assistance and rescue airway techniques, and devices have an important role. Although several new devices have been developed that may be useful for airway management in the prehospital setting, providers should become very facile with one or perhaps two rescue techniques and devices:

1. *LMA.* The LMA is described in detail in Chapter 10. The LMA is rapidly becoming the rescue device of choice for many prehospital systems and has gained some traction as a primary airway device in lieu of BMV for BLS providers and ETI for ALS providers. The LMA is inserted blindly through the oropharynx, and the skill is fairly easy to acquire. Although the LMA does not protect the airway against aspiration, it does provide effective ventilation in virtually every patient into whom it is placed properly. In certain circumstances, the patient can be intubated through the LMA. The standard LMA is available in both reusable and disposable models for prehospital systems. The disposable model is preferable because the LMA will likely stay with the patient once the patient arrives in the receiving hospital. Although the disposable LMA (LMA Unique) is available only in adult sizes, the reusable LMA (LMA Classic) has sizes ranging from neonate to large adult.

2. *Combitube.* The Combitube is widely used both as a rescue device and for elective anesthesia. The insertion technique is described in Chapter 10. The Combitube is also relatively easily learned, has a high ventilation success rate, and can be inserted into a patient in difficult circumstances, such as from the outside of a vehicle. The Combitube should not be confused with the esophageal obturator airway, which is a dangerous device that has no place in modern airway management.

3. *Continuous positive airway pressure.* Noninvasive ventilatory support (NVS) is addressed in detail in Chapter 38. NVS, specifically continuous positive airway pressure (CPAP), is slowly becoming more common in the out-of-hospital setting, especially in ground or air critical care transport. CPAP is most useful in treating patients who require minimal to moderate additional ventilatory support, such as those with congestive heart failure or an exacerbation of chronic obstructive pulmonary disease.

Failed Intubation

Occasionally, the prehospital provider will be faced with a failed intubation. The potential for a failed intubation in the field should be heralded by the evaluation of the patient for difficult airway attributes, as discussed in Chapter 7. If a difficult airway is anticipated, it may be most prudent to transport the patient rapidly to the ED for definitive care rather than attempting to intubate in the field, consuming valuable time and perhaps ending in a failed intubation and further damaging the airway, making intubation ultimately more difficult. Transport time should also be considered when determining whether it is appropriate to perform drug-assisted intubation. Again, in many settings, especially urban systems with short transport times, transport to the ED may be preferable to struggling with a difficult airway in the prehospital setting.

Traditionally, the primary rescue device for failed intubation has been BMV, although the thinking on this is evolving as described previously. Nonetheless, prehospital providers must be expert at BMV using both one-handed and two-handed techniques, supplemented by oral and nasal pharyngeal airways. If BMV is inadequate at providing effective oxygenation, the patient should be repositioned, the jaw thrust should be applied vigorously, oral and nasal airways should be placed (if not already), a two-handed technique should be used to seal the mask to the patient, and any other steps should be taken that the operator determines might be helpful (see Chapter 5). A subjective sense that BMV is inadequate or failing should motivate the immediate placement of an EGD. Again, meticulous BMV and rapid transport might be the appropriate action if oxygenation is adequate and intubation appears difficult or impossible.

If intubation is unsuccessful, it is important to try to determine why. Chapter 6 describes the sequence of steps involved in successful direct laryngoscopy. Repositioning of the patient, a change in equipment, or even a change in operator may help. In addition, prehospital providers should be familiar with techniques such as the Backward, Upward, Rightward Pressure (BURP) maneuver that may facilitate direct laryngoscopy and intubation, and with the use of routine intubation aids such as the Eschmann introducer, also known as the "gum elastic bougie."

When laryngoscopy fails, digital or tactile intubation may be an option (Chapter 9). This is a blind technique that uses anatomical landmarks to guide the placement of one's fingers and maneuver an endotracheal tube into the glottis by sliding the tube along the tongue to the undersurface of the epiglottis and then through the glottic opening. By palpating the epiglottis with the index and long fingers, the epiglottis can be picked up by the long finger and directed anteriorly. The tube is then guided by the index finger under the epiglottis and into the trachea. A stylet bent at a 90-degree angle 4 to 6 cm from the tip of the tube should be used to assist in placement. Although exceedingly rare, some advantages of digital intubation include relatively rapid placement even with experienced providers, no need for special equipment, no requirement to visualize the glottis, and no movement of the head and neck. The major significant limitations are the size of the operator's hands relative to the patient's oral cavity and that the patient must be unconscious.

Some systems allow cricothyrotomy to be performed in the prehospital setting. If this is the case, adequate training and skill maintenance are important. Cricothyrotomy in the field should be an exceedingly rare event. Cricothyrotomy accounts for only approximately 1% of all ED intubations, and although use has varied in reports among various systems, one might anticipate a similar or lower percentage in the field.

DRUG DOSAGE AND ADMINISTRATION

The evidence addressing the use of RSI by EMS personnel is discussed in detail in Chapter 25. The use of RSI, neuromuscular blockade, and sedatives is highly variable from one EMS system to another. Even though an ever-growing number of prehospital systems are using neuromuscular blockade to facilitate intubation in the field, many EMS systems have not instituted RSI for myriad reasons, including training and skill retention issues, short transport times, medical oversight and adequacy of quality management systems, and the failure of the literature to consistently identify clear benefits.

Medication administration for prehospital airway management can occur in two forms: (a) sedation alone (e.g., nonparalytic RSI), and (b) sedation with neuromuscular blockade (e.g., paralytic RSI).

HEMS services and critical care and specialized transport teams are usually trained and experienced in the use of neuromuscular blockade for intubation and encounter sufficient numbers of cases to maintain skills and knowledge (see Chapter 25). Field protocols for sedation or sedation with neuromuscular blockade vary from system to system. In general, sedation is used when the patient is not sufficiently cooperative for intubation, when mandibular relaxation is believed to be inadequate, or when the jaw is clenched. In such cases, sedative agents such as midazolam, diazepam, lorazepam, or others are administered and

> **BOX 23-1** Simplified Rapid Sequence Intubation for Prehospital Care
>
> 1. Prepare equipment, and ensure that the patient is in an appropriate area for intubation.
> 2. Preoxygenate the patient with nonrebreather mask or BMV for at least 3 minutes, if possible.
> 3. Pretreatment drugs—infrequently used. Suggestion: lidocaine 1.5 mg/kg intravenously for head injury, reactive airways disease.
> 4. Paralysis with sedation—administer sedative drug in adequate dose (e.g., midazolam 0.2 mg/kg) and neuromuscular blocking agent (e.g., succinylcholine 1.5 mg/kg).
> 5. Protection—wait 20 seconds. Apply Sellick's maneuver.
> 6. Placement—45 seconds after drugs are given, intubate. Confirm endotracheal tube placement, secure tube, transport patient.

titrated until the patient can be intubated. Some systems permit induction doses of medications to be used, particularly etomidate. In systems using neuromuscular blockade, a protocol typically dictates both the indications for and the manner of administration of neuromuscular blockade. In such cases, it is almost always mandatory to administer a sedative agent along with the neuromuscular blocking agent to ensure that the patient is optimized for intubation and that there is no undue physiological or psychological stress from the intubation attempts. Prehospital sequences are typically much simpler than those used in the ED in that pretreatment agents are rarely used. A typical prehospital, drug-assisted intubation protocol using neuromuscular blockade is shown in Box 23-1.

The sequence is simplified in the prehospital setting because the medication options are fewer. Prehospital providers rarely carry a wide array of induction agents, and the circumstances are less controlled.

POSTINTUBATION MANAGEMENT

Most commonly in the prehospital environment, after securing an airway, the patient is bag ventilated rather than placed on a mechanical ventilator, although the latter is preferable if available. Because airway management is often a high-intensity situation, it is important to attempt to control respiratory rate and tidal volume, which are often inappropriately elevated because of the provider's excitement. As interfacility critical care and specialized care transport become more common, transport ventilators permitting postintubation ventilation will become more prevalent in the pre- or interhospital environment.

TIPS AND PEARLS

- Always weigh the risks and benefits of intubation in the prehospital setting against transport to the ED. In many circumstances, rapid transport might be the best way of managing the airway.
- Master BMV. There are few airway emergencies in the prehospital setting that will not be temporized or managed adequately with proper BMV until the patient can be transported to the hospital, particularly when transport times are short.
- If transport times are long, especially in systems with high rates of trauma, consider introducing neuromuscular blockade into the prehospital setting. This approach requires a comprehensive program, including quality oversight.

- Newer devices, such as the LMA and Combitube, have a vitally important role in prehospital care.
- All prehospital intubations should have their airway reassessed on arrival at the ED. Even though prehospital providers are extensively trained in acute airway management and are comfortable caring for patients in respiratory distress, up to 25% of prehospital intubations are found to be esophageal on arrival at the ED. Confirmation of endotracheal tube placement with an end-tidal carbon dioxide detector should be a first priority both in the field and on arrival.
- Air medical, critical care, and specialized transport programs are frequently asked to transport patients from a community hospital ED or intensive care unit to a tertiary care facility. These teams are occasionally confronted with the situation in which a patient has not had his or her airway definitively managed, but it is needed for safety in transport. It is always preferable to manage these airways while still in the sending health care facility as opposed to en route in an ambulance or helicopter.

EVIDENCE

The evidence base on which important decisions relating to airway management in prehospital care are based is growing and is presented in Chapters 7 and 25. However, several important issues need to be resolved:

- Are EGDs more effective than BMV in unresponsive patients in the hands of BLS personnel, and do the outcomes reflect that fact?
- Are the outcomes of unresponsive patients managed with EGDs rather than ETI by ALS personnel improved?
- How should ALS providers manage the airway in responsive patients that require airway management?
- Does ETI by ALS personnel improve outcomes generally and in specific subpopulations of patients?
- What factors are critical to ensuring that RSI is performed safely in EMS?
- Is there evidence that airway intervention improves outcome (e.g., cardiac arrest)?

1. **Is there evidence in the EMS literature to suggest that intubation success rates employing "nonparalytic RSI" are as high as with "paralytic RSI"?** It is well established in the anesthesia literature that the use of an induction agent alone provides poorer intubating conditions than when a neuromuscular blocking agent is coupled with the induction agent. Bozeman, Kleiner, and Huggett (1) compared two groups in a HEMS system, one using etomidate alone and the other employing neuromuscular blockade (RSI group). The view of the larynx (laryngeal view grade) was significantly better in the RSI group, as was the intubation success rate (92% success with paralytic RSI vs. 25% in the nonparalytic RSI group). Sonday et al. (2), in contrast, found little difference, whereas Kociszewski et al. (3) found that the neuromuscular agent significantly improved the ease and success of intubation over induction alone.

2. **Is there any evidence that intubation training of paramedics on high-fidelity patient simulators is as good as training on live patients in the operating room (OR)?** Hall et al. (4) studied 36 paramedic students that had never intubated before. He randomized them into two groups. Both groups received didactic instruction and manikin training. Then half went to the OR to intubate 15 patients, while the other group received 10 hours of training on a high-fidelity simulator. The entire group was then tested on 15 live intubations. Overall success rates, success on first attempt, and complication rates were similar in both groups.

Interestingly, simulation has also been shown to be a valid evaluation tool for emergency airway management skills. Overly, Sudikoff, and Shapiro (5) evaluated the acute airway management skills of 16 pediatric residents and found that high-fidelity patient simulation was useful in evaluating not only the individual's skill set, but also the quality of the training program that produced the resident. Rosenthal et al. (6) had similar findings in the training and evaluation of interns.

REFERENCES

1. Bozeman WP, Kleiner DM, Huggett V. A comparison of rapid-sequence intubation and etomidate-only intubation in the prehospital air medical setting. *Prehosp Emerg Care* 2006; 10:8–13.

2. Sonday CJ, Axelband J, Jacoby J, et al. Thiopental vs. etomidate for rapid sequence intubation in aeromedicine. *Prehospital Disaster Med* 2005;20:324–326.

3. Kociszewski C, Thomas SH, Harrison T, et al. Etomidate versus succinylcholine for intubation in an air medical setting. *Am J Emerg Med* 2000;18:757–763.

4. Hall RE, Plant JR, Bands CJ, et al. Human patient simulation is effective for teaching paramedic students endotracheal intubation. *Acad Emerg Med* 2005;12:850–855.

5. Overly FL, Sudikoff SN, Shapiro MJ. High-fidelity medical simulation as an assessment tool for pediatric residents' airway management skills. *Pediatr Emerg Care* 2007;23:11–15.

6. Rosenthal ME, Adachi M, Ribaudo V, et al. Achieving housestaff competence in emergency airway management using scenario based simulation training: comparison of attending vs. housestaff trainers. *Chest* 2006;129:1453–1458.

24

Alternative Devices for EMS Airway Management

Charles N. Pozner and Stephen J. Nelson

INTRODUCTION

Airway evaluation and management is the first priority of health care providers in an emergency, regardless if it occurs in or out of the hospital. The austere environment in which prehospital providers must function (e.g., poor positioning and lighting, disruptive surroundings, limited assistance) demands that airway care be carried out both thoughtfully and skillfully to ensure the best outcomes.

The gold standard of airway management is the assurance of adequate oxygenation and minute ventilation. Every prehospital provider must acquire and maintain the necessary skills to ensure that this goal can be achieved until arrival at the hospital, regardless of the device used or the technique employed.

Endotracheal intubation has evolved to become the most common *advanced* airway procedure to be employed in the prehospital setting. The incidence of difficult intubation in emergency medical services (EMS) is 11%. Studies of prehospital endotracheal intubation have reported success rates from as high as 96.6% to less than 75%. This highly variable success rate, coupled with the dire consequences of failure, has been the foundation of much discussion concerning the range of airway interventions necessary to optimize patient outcome in the prehospital setting.

The approach to airway management in EMS is no different than the ED or the OR. Chapters 1 to 3, and particularly Chapter 2, provide the framework with which to approach airway management in the prehospital setting. In this chapter, we introduce alternative airway devices available for prehospital use. These devices can be either primary airway management tools or rescue devices when endotracheal intubation cannot be performed or has failed. In 2006, the National Association of EMS Physicians published a position statement on the use of alternative airways in the prehospital setting. We discuss the devices available and their prehospital use. For discussion of surgical airways, refer to Chapter 16.

THE CLINICAL CHALLENGE

The goal of airway management is to establish and maintain optimal minute ventilation and oxygenation, and to minimize the risk of aspiration throughout the course of care. When a patient is conscious and spontaneously breathing, close monitoring may be all that is necessary to accomplish this goal. It is the role of the EMS provider to immediately intervene when the patient can neither maintain nor protect his or her airway, or when the patient needs assistance with oxygenation and/or ventilation.

Historically in EMS, mouth-to-mouth ventilation or placement of an oro- or nasopharyngeal airway coupled with bag-mask ventilation (BMV) have been the initial and primary methods of providing oxygenation and ventilation to the patient who is unable to sustain adequate gas exchange. Failing access to and training with more sophisticated devices and techniques, these are the only options available until either advanced providers arrive on-scene or the patient reaches the hospital.

With adequate training, placement of an endotracheal tube has traditionally been considered the next procedure attempted. In the event that a patient is not a candidate for intubation or that intubation is unsuccessful, bag-mask ventilation (BMV) retains its primary role in assisted ventilation.

The introduction of medication-assisted intubation (e.g., rapid sequence intubation [RSI]) has led EMS systems to ensure that their advanced providers are trained in the use of alternative airway devices, in addition to BMV, as a means to rescue the airway in the event intubation following paralysis and/or sedation is unsuccessful. The growth of experience with and research in the prehospital use of these alternative airway devices has led EMS medical directors to examine the use of these devices as an alternative to endotracheal intubation for advanced providers and as an alternative to BMV for basic-level providers. In their 2005 guidelines, The European Resuscitation Council recommends that if ventilation cannot be provided through an endotracheal tube, alternative airway devices should be employed for ventilation in the management of cardiac arrest. The American Heart Association guidelines are less directive, stating that their use appears to be safe.

ALTERNATIVE AIRWAY DEVICES

Bag-mask Ventilation

Although there is a proclivity toward the use of alternative airway devices for assisted ventilation at all EMS provider levels, expertise with BMV is essential, despite the fact that it is a difficult technique to master. In fact, proper BMV coupled with oro- and/or nasopharyngeal airways and cricoid pressure is capable of providing adequate minute ventilation in the majority of circumstances in which assisted or artificial ventilation is required, and provides a measure of protection against gastric insufflation and the aspiration of gastric contents. Improper use can increase the risk of gastric insufflation, regurgitation, and aspiration of stomach contents. More in-depth discussion of the BVM can be found in Chapter 5.

Extraglottic Devices

Supraglottic Device Class

LMA Type

Introduced in 1981 and approved for use in the United States in 1992, Brain developed the first supraglottic airway device, the laryngeal mask airway (LMA). This blindly inserted device has several advantages over mask ventilation, including ease of use and the ability to provide an airtight seal without head or mandibular manipulation.

Typical of all extraglottic devices (EGDs), supraglottic airways transfer the mask seal from the face to a supraglottic location. (Refer to Chapter 10 for details on insertion.) Although ventilation is facilitated, protection from aspiration is not as reliable as with a cuffed endotracheal tube in the trachea. Some have found that although the application of cricoid pressure after insertion of the LMA decreased gastric insufflation, it tended to hinder ventilation. Finally, improper placement resulting in inadequate mask seal and ventilation is not uncommon, particularly as facility with these devices is acquired.

Since its introduction, modifications of the LMA-type design, the introduction of other innovative EGDs (see Chapter 10) and the provision of single-use devices have broadened the opportunity for their use in EMS. For instance, Brain introduced the intubating LMA (ILMA) in 1997, a supraglottic device (SGD) that not only permitted one to rescue gas exchange, but also reliably facilitated blind intubation through the device. (See Chapter 10 for details on insertion.)

In the event that the ILMA provides adequate gas exchange in the field and transport times are short (e.g., urban EMS systems), many believe that intubation through the device should not be performed in the field and that the decision as to how best to achieve a definitive airway should be deferred to hospital arrival.

The ProSeal laryngeal mask airway (PLMA), a modification of the LMA-type design, is designed to minimize the risk of aspiration if regurgitation occurs and improve mask seal. This device incorporates a tube that passes through the mask to permit the insertion of a gastric tube to decompress the stomach and aspirate regurgitated gastric contents. Designed with a larger mask and a softer wedge-shaped cuff, it facilitates a better fit in the pharynx, and its deeper bowl provides an enhanced cuff seal due to its more anterior position. Unfortunately, the device is much more difficult to insert than other SGDs. This has prompted the introduction of a similar, yet disposable device called the LMA Supreme. This device has superior insertion and seal characteristics, and has the potential to be a substantial advance on other SGD designs (see Chapter 10, Fig. 10-3).

In summary, although the LMA was embraced more slowly by emergency medicine than anesthesia, it is now being widely employed in both emergency medicine and the pre-hospital setting. The American Heart Association, the American Society of Anesthesiologists, and others have advocated the use of the LMA as a rescue device in the setting of failed intubation. Refer to Chapter 10 for a list of available SGDs.

Retroglottic Device Class

Esophageal Obturator Airway

The first extraglottic airway device to be used in the prehospital setting was the esophageal obturator airway, and it is of historical interest only. Introduced in the late 1970s, this blindly inserted device, when properly positioned, placed a cuffed obturator into the esophagus. A face mask was then applied to the device to permit BMV. This device and a subsequent version, the esophageal gastric tube airway, were widely used as both primary and rescue airway devices. Many complications were reported, including esophageal rupture, aspiration, and inadvertent tracheal occlusion by the obturator. Because of its complication profile, difficulty in placement, and failure to provide adequate gas exchange, continued use of either device in modern EMS systems is to be condemned.

Esophageal Tracheal Combitube

In 1987, Frass introduced the esophageal tracheal Combitube (ETC; see Chapter 10). It is a blindly inserted, double-lumen tube with balloon cuffs to be positioned below (esophageal) and above (hypopharyngeal) the glottis, permitting ventilation through periglottic fenestrations located between the proximal and distal cuffs. Ventilation is also possible if the device is inadvertently inserted into the trachea (<5% of insertions; see Chapter 10, Fig. 10-20). Since its introduction, the ETC has become a common alternative airway device employed in EMS as both a primary and a rescue airway device because of its ease of placement, the preferred neutral cervical positioning for placement in trauma patients, and a perceived benefit of the cuffed esophageal tube in the unfasted patient. Complications associated with the use of the ETC include aspiration, pneumothorax, pneumomediastinum, airway injuries, and esophageal lacerations and perforations. Some authors recommend employing laryngoscopy to avoid trauma to the airway.

King LT airway (Laryngeal Tube Airway in Europe)

The King LT, approved for use in the United States in 2003, has been introduced into the armamentarium of airway devices available to prehospital providers. See Chapter 10 for a detailed description of this device and a discussion of the evidence with respect to its use. This device is an airway tube with a small distal balloon at the tip and a larger balloon at the midportion of the tube. Both balloons are inflated simultaneously, employing a single syringe. Like the ETC, when positioned properly, the distal balloon is located in the upper esophagus and the proximal balloon in the hypopharynx (see Chapter 10, Fig. 10-21). The King LT differs from the ETC in that it possesses superior insertion characteristics and has a single pilot balloon to be inflated, conferring an ease of use. Its disadvantage is that inadvertent tracheal placement does not permit ventilation, and there is a paucity of published evidence regarding success and complication rates.

Although there have been other devices developed, the ETC and the King LT remain the most commonly deployed EGDs in the prehospital setting in the Untied States.

EVIDENCE

1. **How common is the difficult and failed airway in EMS?** As mentioned previously, the incidence of difficult or failed intubation in the operating room (OR) setting is 1.1% to 3.8% and 0.13% to 0.3% of cases, respectively (1). So, it is not uncommon to see a difficult airway even in the OR. The incidence of difficult intubation in EMS, not surprisingly, is three to ten times that seen in the OR at 11% (2). Studies of prehospital endotracheal intubation have reported success rates ranging from less than 75% to as high as 96.6% (3,4). It is this variation that has called into question the advisability of prehospital care personnel performing endotracheal intubation in general, and RSI in particular (see Chapter 25).

2. **Is there a statement that identifies the most appropriate airway management devices for prehospital care workers?** In 2006, the National Association of EMS Physicians published a position statement on the use of alternative airways in the prehospital setting (5).

3. **How easy is it to learn how to use these devices?**
   BVM
   Although it is often difficult to adequately ventilate patients with a BVM in the controlled environment of a hospital, it still remains the most commonly used emergency ventilation device in both the hospital and the prehospital setting. As early as 1986, Cummins et al. (6) reported that maintenance of an adequate mask seal is difficult and often requires more than one person to be effective; a luxury often not readily available in the prehospital setting. A study of emergency nurses reported a 25% skill retention rate 6 months after training (7).

   Supraglottic Airways
   The LMA has been found to be relatively easy to place by paramedics and other allied health professionals (8,9). Prehospital placement of an LMA in pediatric populations has also been shown to be straightforward. Although median insertion times were longer with the LMA as compared to BVM (30 seconds vs. 4 seconds), this was not considered to represent a clinically significant difference (10). In 2000, in a study of the ILMA, Levitan et al. (11) reported a 97% success rate, with a mean time to ventilation of 18 seconds and a mean time to intubation of 17 seconds in a variety of providers, including medical nonintubators and nonmedical personnel after a 60-minute training session. Dries et al. (12) reported similar ease of use in the aeromedical setting. In a review of PLMA literature, insertion success rates have ranged between 90% and 100%; however, studies included in this review were not in the prehospital environment (13).

   Retroglottic Airways
   Successful placement of the ETC in the prehospital setting as a primary airway device is reported to be 71% to 98%, and 64% to 100% as a rescue airway (14–16). In a retrospective analysis of ETC placement for failed endotracheal intubation in the prehospital setting, Calkins, Miller, and Langdorf (15) reported a success rate of 70%, and 16% of placements were tracheal. The King LT has been shown to be relatively easy to place. In a study by Russi, Wilcox, and House (17), paramedics with no previous exposure or training were able to place the King LT with 100% success in simulated trauma and medical cases. Again, the paucity of literature on the King LT obviates the possibility of discussing hazards and complications of the device.

4. **Although these devices *provide* an adequate airway, do they *protect* the airway?**
   Supraglottic Airways
   Although definitive airway protection from regurgitation and aspiration must never be assumed when employing an LMA, rates of aspiration in the anesthesia literature have been reported to be as low as 0.02%, likely related to the fasted state of operative patients (18). Stone, Chantler, and Baskett (19), in their study of 713 cardiac

arrest patients undergoing assisted ventilation, reported a lower incidence of regurgitation with the LMA than with BVM (LMA 3.5%, BVM 12.4%, respectively). The design characteristics of the PLMA (e.g., tighter seal, esophageal drainage tube) have resulted in a decreased incidence of aspiration in studies comparing it to the LMA. Unfortunately, because these data are derived from animal, cadaver, or OR studies, the advantages of the PLMA in the prehospital setting can only be considered theoretical (20).

Extraglottic Airways

In Quebec, where ETC is performed as a basic-level procedure for all cardiac arrests, Vézina et al. (21) reported an aspiration rate of 17%. Although it is generally believed that the esophageal balloon confers an element of protection against aspiration, there is good evidence that the risk of aspiration with use of the ETC is at least that of the LMA. There is no literature on the aspiration rate of the King LT to permit comparisons or compute risk.

5. **Can these devices be employed in trauma patients?** Use of the LMA in the management of prehospital trauma patients has undergone limited study. There are conflicting reports on the safe use of the LMA in patients with cervical spine trauma. Keller, Brimacombe, and Keller (22), in a study using pressure sensors attached to the vertebrae in a stable cadaveric cervical spine model reported unacceptable posterior vertebral displacement when an LMA was employed. However, Brimacombe and Berry (23), in a fluoroscopically assessed cadaveric model using a destabilized cervical spine, reported no difference in displacement between the LMA and direct laryngoscopy. In a difficult trauma airway algorithm developed by Ollerton et al. (24), they found that placement of an LMA can be performed both effectively and safely. Although the PLMA would theoretically have an advantage over the LMA in trauma patients due to its tighter seal and esophageal drainage tube, it is best placed in the sniffing positions.

   In a study of 420 head trauma patients, the Combitube was used as a rescue airway when endotracheal intubation was unsuccessful (15% of all cases). ETC insertion and ventilation were successful at a rate of 95% when employed as a rescue airway (25).

6. **Are there certain situations where I should use a specific device over another?** The majority of the literature addressing the use of EGDs in the prehospital environment concerns the LMA and the ETC. There is a paucity of data specific to the prehospital environment related to other devices to scientifically guide one with respect to device selection. However, most experts agree that systems ought to (a) seriously evaluate whether to promote EGD-based ventilation as a first-line device in unresponsive, apneic patients and relegate BMV to a subsidiary role; and (b) ensure that advanced life support providers have proficiency and the immediate availability of an EGD in the event that neither BMV nor endotracheal intubation is possible, particularly if medications are employed to facilitate airway management.

REFERENCES

1. Crosby ET, Cooper RM, Douglas MJ, et al. The unanticipated difficult airway with recommendations for management. *Can J Anaesth* 1998;45:757–776.

2. Adnet F, Jouriles NJ, Le Toumelin P, et al. Survey of out-of-hospital emergency intubations in the French prehospital medical system: a multicenter study. *Ann Emerg Med* 1998;32:454–460.

3. Jacobs LM, Berrizbeitia LD, Bennett B, et al. Endotracheal intubation in the prehospital phase of emergency medical care. *JAMA* 1983;250:2175–2177.

4. Krisanda TJ, Eitel DR, Hess D, et al. An analysis of invasive airway management in a suburban emergency medical services system. *Prehospital Disaster Med* 1992;7:121–126.

5. Guyette FX, Greenwood MJ, Neubecker D, et al. Alternate airways in the prehospital setting (resource document to NAEMSP position statement). *Prehosp Emerg Care* 2007;11:56–61.

6. Cummins RO, Austin D, Graves JR, et al. Ventilation skills of emergency medical technicians: a teaching challenge for emergency medicine. *Ann Emerg Med* 1986;15:1187–1192.

7. De Regge M, Vogels C, Monsieurs KG, et al. Retention of ventilation skills of emergency nurses after training with the SMART BAG compared to a standard bag-valve-mask. *Resuscitation* 2006;68:379–384.

8. Deakin CD, Peters R, Tomlinson P, et al. Securing the prehospital airway: a comparison of laryngeal mask insertion and endotracheal intubation by UK paramedics. *Emerg Med J* 2005; 22:64–67.

9. Martin P, Cyna A, Hunter W, et al. Training nursing staff in airway management for resuscitation: a clinical comparison of the face mask and laryngeal mask. *Anesthesia* 1993;48:33–37.

10. Guyette FX, Roth KR, LaCovey DC, et al. Feasibility of laryngeal mask airway use by prehospital personnel in simulated pediatric respiratory arrest. *Prehosp Emerg Care* 2007;11: 245–249.

11. Levitan RM, Ochroch EA, Stuart S, et al. Use of the intubating laryngeal mask airway by medical and nonmedical personnel. *Am J Emerg Med* 2000;18:12–16.

12. Dries D, Frascone R, Molinari P, et al. Does the ILMA make sense in HEMS? *Air Med J* 2001;20:35–37.

13. Cook TM, Lee G, Nolan JP. The ProSeal laryngeal mask airway: a review of the literature. *Can J Anaesth* 2005;52:739–760.

14. Atherton GL, Johnson JC. Ability of paramedics to use the Combitube in prehospital cardiac arrest. *Ann Emerg Med* 1993;22:1263–1268.

15. Calkins TR, Miller K, Langdorf MI. Success and complication rates with prehospital placement of an esophageal-tracheal Combitube as a rescue airway. *Prehospital Disaster Med* 2006;1(Suppl 2):97–100.

16. Rabitsch W, Schellongowski P, Staudinger T, et al. Comparison of a conventional tracheal airway with the Combitube in an urban emergency medical services system run by physicians. *Resuscitation* 2003;57:27–32.

17. Russi CS, Wilcox CL, House HR. The laryngeal tube device: a simple and timely adjunct to airway management. *Am J Emerg Med* 2007;25:263–267.

18. Brimacombe J, Berry A. The incidence of aspiration associated with the laryngeal mask airway—a meta-analysis of published literature. *J Clin Anesth* 1995;7:297–305.

19. Stone BJ, Chantler PJ, Baskett PJ. The incidence of regurgitation during cardiopulmonary resuscitation: a comparison between the bag valve mask and laryngeal mask airway. *Resuscitation* 1998;38:3–6.

20. Cook TM, Lee G, Nolan JP. The ProSeal laryngeal mask airway: a review of the literature. *Can J Anaesth* 2005;52:739–760.

21. Vézina MC, Trépanier CA, Nicole PC, et al. Complications associated with the esophageal-tracheal Combitube in the pre-hospital setting. *Can J Anaesth* 2007;54:124–128.

22. Keller C, Brimacombe J, Keller K. Pressures exerted against the cervical spine by the standard and intubating laryngeal mask airway. *Anesth Analg* 1999;89:1296–1300.

23. Brimacombe J, Berry A. Laryngeal mask airway insertion. *Anesthesiology* 1993;48:670–671.

24. Ollerton JE, Parr MJA, Harrison K, et al. Potential cervical spine injury and difficult airway management for emergency intubation of trauma adults in the emergency department—a systematic review. *Emerg Med J* 2006;23:3–11.

25. Davis DP, Valentine C, Ochs M, et al. The Combitube as a salvage airway device for paramedic rapid sequence intubation. *Ann Emerg Med* 2003;42:697–704.

25

Controversies in EMS Airway Management

Michael F. Murphy

OVERVIEW OF THE ISSUES

Although the training and credentials of those performing airway evaluation, management, and rescue may vary widely around the world, the *issues* related to prehospital emergency airway management demonstrate consistent themes, such as the following:

- Intubation of patients in the field
- Extraglottic devices versus endotracheal intubation (ETI)
- Use of neuromuscular blocking drugs in prehospital airway management
- Verification of intratracheal placement of the endotracheal tube

Airway management in an emergency situation is stressful and anxiety provoking. Crucial decisions must be made rapidly and often without the benefit of a detailed history or physical examination. The environment of care is therefore "error prone." Strategies designed to minimize error must do so reproducibly in a time-sensitive fashion. Clear definitions and simple evaluation and management memory tools, including mnemonics and algorithms, represent such strategies. Identifying the difficult airway, managing the failed airway, and performing a cricothyrotomy are no different prehospital than they are in-hospital. Thus, the "thinking" and "doing" in the prehospital environment is identical to that which occurs in an emergency department or operating room. However, the environment of care is much different in the prehospital arena and often presents unique features. At times, alternate and innovative methods must be employed in these unique situations.

DELEGATED MEDICAL ACTS AND STANDARDIZED MEDICAL PROTOCOLS

In most North American systems, prehospital care providers perform delegated medical acts based on pre-established, standardized medical protocols. Although protocols ought to reflect best clinical evidence, they are limited from a practical perspective by cost, training, competency maintenance, and space constraints.

Which equipment is available to medics in the field is driven by the protocols approved by the emergency medical services (EMS) system medical director. The type and range of equipment available for managing the *difficult airway* in the prehospital setting is limited compared to most emergency departments and operating rooms. Even basic equipment such as the Eschmann introducer (commonly known as the "gum elastic bougie"), laryngoscope blades, and endotracheal tubes in an array of types and sizes may be limited in availability. Alternate intubating devices, such as the intubating laryngeal mask airway (ILMA or LMA Fastrach) or light wands (e.g., Trachlight), are often not available due to cost and skills maintenance issues. Rescue devices such as the Combitube, laryngeal mask airway (LMA), and disposable extraglottic devices, such as the LMA Unique, LMA Supreme, Ambu LMA and the King LT airway, are becoming more popular because they are relatively inexpensive, effective, and easy to use, and they do not require access to sterilization facilities. However, as nontracheal ventilation devices, they may not be appropriate in some clinical situations, particularly if adequate ventilation calls for an increase in peak airway pressure beyond the seal capabilities of the device, if the patient is sufficiently responsive to reject the device or if protection against aspiration is mandatory. Surgical airway management devices must be available in any system considering rapid sequence intubation (RSI).

CONTROVERSIES IN PREHOSPITAL AIRWAY MANAGEMENT

Inadequate ventilation and oxygenation have been identified as primary contributors to preventable mortality, both in hospital and out of hospital. It would seem intuitive that successful ETI ought to mitigate these deaths, and because of this thinking, ETI became the gold standard in prehospital airway management. However, there has been considerable controversy as to whether patients requiring ETI should have tracheal intubation performed in the field or deferred until hospital arrival. There is ample evidence that ETI is not a benign intervention in the hands of inexperienced personnel who employ the technique infrequently. Studies have identified that intubation in the field may delay transport to higher echelons of care, injure airways, and lead to poorer outcomes.

The *Recommended Guidelines for Uniform Reporting of Data from Out-of-Hospital Airway Management* identifies four methods constituting "advanced airway management": direct oral laryngoscopy and intubation, nasotracheal intubation, oral rescue techniques (bag-mask ventilation [BMV], Combitube), and surgical rescue techniques (transtracheal jet ventilation and cricothyrotomy). These four methods may each be modified by five variables:

1. Oral approach: no facilitating sedative drugs or paralytics
2. Nasal approach: no facilitating sedative drugs or paralytics
3. Sedation-facilitated intubation
4. RSI (i.e., the use of paralytics ± induction agents)
5. Other intubation technique (e.g., digital, lighted stylet)

The *actual* number of alternatives available in an EMS system is limited by protocols, training, and equipment.

New, simple-to-use devices such as the LMA and the Combitube have been introduced successfully in the prehospital care setting. These devices may be employed as an alternative to ETI in the cardiac arrest (or deeply comatose) patient by basic life support providers or as a rescue device in the setting of failed intubation by advanced life support (ALS) or critical care providers.

An emerging alternative to ETI in the respiratory failure patient is prehospital noninvasive ventilation. Several case series have shown continuous positive airway pressure or bilevel ventilation to be feasible and potentially beneficial in the prehospital setting, although further study is necessary to validate its effectiveness and safety.

EVIDENCE

1. **Should tracheal intubation be performed in the field at all?** There are several dimensions to this controversy:
   - *Trauma victims:* There continues to be skepticism as to whether the intubation of trauma victims in the prehospital care environment improves survival. During the 1980s, it was generally believed that ETI by EMS personnel had the potential to delay transport and was ineffective in improving survival in urban environments, but might be effective in longer transport environments (1). Many studies with conflicting results populated the literature during the 1990s (2–7). The lack of clarity led some to speculate that for selected subsets of the trauma patient population, ETI might be of benefit. It seemed logical to analyze patients with acute, severe head injury. Early studies provided no clear direction (8–14), and a recent large trauma registry study found that prehospital intubation was associated with adverse outcomes after severe head trauma (8). There was a subset of air medical transport patients in this study that may have benefited from ETI in the field, although an accompanying editorial maintained that this factor reflected a retrospective association rather than causation (15). In summary, the question as to whether ETI in trauma victims improves outcome is unresolved, although serious questions as to its benefits have been raised.

- *Cardiac arrest:* In cardiac arrest patients, the issue of efficacy remains unresolved (16–20). In fact, one study of hospital cardiac arrest victims showed that patients who received only cardiopulmonary resuscitation with chest compressions had comparable survival outcome to those who received chest compression and mouth-to-mouth ventilation (21). Furthermore, a large prospective before/after study to determine the incremented benefit to introducing ALS (including intubation) to a previously optimized system did not show a mortality benefit in cardiac arrest patients (22). The issue as to the effect of oxygenation and ventilation on mortality in cardiac arrest victims in the prehospital arena remains unresolved.
- *Children:* Early studies showed that tracheal intubation in children by paramedics was associated with higher failure and complication rates than in adults (23). Subsequent studies have tended to confirm this early finding (5,24–28). The only prospective, pseudorandomized trial to investigate the effectiveness of ground paramedics in performing tracheal intubation in children showed that there was no demonstrable advantage in survival outcome following ETI compared to groups with BMV (24). This same study revealed concerns about ETI displacement and lack of recognition thereof. Finally, for a subpopulation of patients where ETI might be expected to show a benefit, children with acute severe head injuries, the issue remains unresolved (29,30). A pervasive critique of these studies is that the results reflect a deficiency in pediatric ETI training for the EMS personnel. In the final analysis, the emergency intubation of children is an uncommon and anxiety-provoking event for most ALS providers. Both factors are likely to increase performance stress and failure rates, compared to the intubation of adults.

2. **Is there evidence to support RSI by ALS prehospital providers?** The evidence in the EMS literature supporting the use of RSI is, until most recently, nonsupportive except in specific circumstances. For ground EMS systems, several recent well-designed studies have consistently shown suboptimal outcomes, or no difference in outcome, in patients suffering acute severe head injury where RSI was used to facilitate ETI (8,9,31,32). Head injury was deliberately chosen in these studies because prior studies have suggested that optimal oxygenation and ventilation of these patients improve outcomes. Therefore, it was assumed that successful ETI would demonstrate benefit (33).

   There have been attempts to determine the reasons for the poor outcomes associated with RSI in ground EMS services. These explanations have included
   - Increased on-scene time (average 15 minutes in one study) (34)
   - Lack of adequate training of the paramedics (8,13,32)
   - Inappropriate hyperventilation and nonrecognition of hypoxia during induction (35)
   - Patient paralysis and multiple attempts at intubation (35)

   Despite recent studies showing the lack of efficacy of RSI in the ground EMS systems, a distinct pattern of improved outcomes has emerged in the subpopulation of those patients where air medical transport had been used (8,36–39).

SUMMARY

It is unclear at present whether ETI by prehospital care providers improves outcome for specific populations. What *is clear* is that active medical direction, intense quality oversight and maintenance of competency programs, and high-quality airway management training are features of EMS systems that have high advanced airway management success rates and improved outcomes. Other issues such as equipment availability, the air versus ground environment, and the logistics associated with rural versus urban critical care transport/EMS suggest that a single, rigid approach to EMS airway management is inappropriate and cannot be supported.

REFERENCES

1. Pepe PE, Stewart RD, Compass MK. Prehospital management of trauma: a tale of three cities. *Ann Emerg Med* 1986;15:1484–1490.

2. Ruchholtz S, Waydhas C, Ose C, et al. Working Group on Multiple Trauma of the German Trauma Society. Prehospital intubation in severe thoracic trauma without respiratory insufficiency: a matched-pair analysis based on the Trauma Registry of the German Trauma Society. *J Trauma* 2002;52:879–886.

3. Karch SB, Lewis T, Young S, et al. Field intubation of trauma patients: complications, indications, and outcomes. *Am J Emerg Med* 1996;14:617–619.

4. Frankel H, Rozycki G, Champion H, et al. The use of TRISS methodology to validate prehospital intubation by urban EMS providers. *Am J Emerg Med* 1997;15:630–632.

5. Eckstein M, Chan L, Schneir A, et al. Effect of prehospital advanced life support on outcomes of major trauma patients. *J Trauma* 1996;48:643–648.

6. Adnet F, Lapostolle F, Ricard-Hibon A, et al. Intubating trauma patients before reaching hospital—revisited. *Crit Care* 2001;5:290–291.

7. Liberman M, Mulder D, Sampalis J. Advanced or basic life support for trauma: meta-analysis and critical review of the literature. *J Trauma* 2000;49:584–599.

8. Wang HE, Peitzman AB, Cassidy LD, et al. Out-of-hospital endotracheal intubation and outcome after traumatic brain injury. *Ann Emerg Med* 2004;44:439–450.

9. Bochicchio GV, Ilahi O, Joshi M, et al. Endotracheal intubation in the field does not improve outcome in trauma patients who present without an acutely lethal traumatic brain injury. *J Trauma* 2003;55:1184.

10. Garner A, Rashford S, Lee A, et al. Addition of physicians to paramedic helicopter services decreases blunt trauma mortality. *Aust N Z J Surg* 1999;69:697–701.

11. Garner A, Crooks J, Lee A, et al. Efficacy of prehospital critical care teams for severe blunt head injury in the Australian setting. *Injury* 2001;32:455–460.

12. Murray JA, Demetriades D, Berne TV, et al. Prehospital intubation in patients with severe head injury. *J Trauma* 2000;49:1065–1070.

13. Ochs M, Davis DP, Hoyt DB. Lessons learned during the San Diego paramedic RSI Trial. *J Emerg Med* 2003;24:343–344.

14. Winchell RJ, Hoyt DB. Endotracheal intubation in the field improves survival in patients with severe head injury. Trauma Research and Education Foundation of San Diego. *Arch Surg* 1997;132:592–597.

15. Zink BJ, Maio RF. Out-of-hospital endotracheal intubation in traumatic brain injury: outcomes research provides us with an unexpected outcome. *Ann Emerg Med* 2004;44:451–453.

16. Rainer TH, Marshall R, Cusack S. Paramedics, technicians, and survival from out of hospital cardiac arrest. *J Accid Emerg Med* 1997;14:278–282.

17. Mitchell RG, Guly UM, Rainer TH, et al. Can the full range of paramedic skills improve survival from out of hospital cardiac arrests? *J Accid Emerg Med* 1997;14:274–277.

18. Eisen JS, Dubinsky I. Advanced life support vs basic life support field care: an outcome study. *Acad Emerg Med* 1998;5:592–598.

19. Bissell RA, Eslinger DG, Zimmerman L. The efficacy of advanced life support: a review of the literature. *Prehospital Disaster Med* 1998;13:77–87.

20. Adnet F, Jouriles N, Le Toumelin P, et al. Survey of out-of-hospital emergency intubations in the French prehospital medical system: a multicenter study. *Ann Emerg Med* 1998;32: 454–460.

21. Hallstrom A, Cobb L, Johnson E, et al. Cardiopulmonary resuscitation by chest compression alone or with mouth-to-mouth ventilation. *N Engl J Med* 2000;342:1546–1553.

22. Stiell IG, Wells GA, Field B, et al. Advanced cardiac life support in out-of-hospital cardiac arrest. *N Engl J Med* 2004;351:647–656.

23. Aijian P, Tsai A, Knopp R, et al. Endotracheal intubation of pediatric patients by paramedics. *Ann Emerg Med* 1989;18:489–494.

24. Gausche M, Lewis RJ, Stratton SJ, et al. Effect of out-of-hospital pediatric endotracheal intubation on survival and neurological outcome: a controlled clinical trial. *JAMA* 2000;283: 783–790.

25. Vilke GM, Steen PJ, Smith AM, et al. Out-of-hospital pediatric intubation by paramedics: the San Diego experience. *J Emerg Med* 2002;22:71–74.

26. Brownstein D, Shugerman R, Cummings P, et al. Prehospital endotracheal intubation of children by paramedics. *Ann Emerg Med* 1996;28:34–39.

27. Su E, Mann NC, McCall M, et al. Use of resuscitation skills by paramedics caring for critically injured children in Oregon. *Prehosp Emerg Care* 1997;1:123–127.

28. Boswell WC, McElveen N, Sharp M, et al. Analysis of prehospital pediatric and adult intubation. *Air Med J* 1995;14:125–128.

29. Suominen P, Baillie C, Kivioja A, et al. Intubation and survival in severe paediatric blunt head injury. *Eur J Emerg Med* 2000;7:3–7.

30. Cooper A, DiScala C, Foltin G, et al. Prehospital endotracheal intubation for severe head injury in children: a reappraisal. *Semin Pediatr Surg* 2001;10:3–6.

31. Dunford J, Davis D, Ochs M, et al. Incidence of transient hypoxia and pulse rate reactivity during paramedic rapid sequence intubation. *Ann Emerg Med* 2003;42:721–728.

32. Davis DP, Hoyt DB, Ochs M, et al. The effect of paramedic rapid sequence intubation on outcome in patients with severe traumatic brain injury. *J Trauma* 2003;54:444–453.

33. Chesnut RM, Marshall LF, Klauber MR, et al. The role of secondary brain injury in determining outcome from severe head injury. *J Trauma* 1993;34:216–222.

34. Ochs M, Davis D, Hoyt D, et al. Paramedic-performed rapid sequence intubation of patients with severe head injuries. *Ann Emerg Med* 2002;40:159–167.

35. Dunford JV, Davis DP, Ochs M, et al. Incidence of transient hypoxia and pulse rate reactivity during paramedic rapid sequence intubation. *Ann Emerg Med* 2003;42:721–728.

36. Ma OJ, Atchley RB, Hatley T, et al. Intubation success rates improve for an air medical program after implementing the use of neuromuscular blocking agents. *Am J Emerg Med* 1998;16:125–127.

37. Murphy-Macabobby M, Marshall WJ, Schneider C, et al. Neuromuscular blockade in aeromedical airway management. *Ann Emerg Med* 1992;21:664–668.

38. Sing RF, Rotondo MF, Zonies DH, et al. Rapid sequence induction for intubation by an aeromedical transport team: a critical analysis. *Am J Emerg Med* 1998;16:598–602.

39. Slater EA, Weiss SJ, Ernst AA, et al. Preflight versus en route success and complications of rapid sequence intubation in an air medical service. *J Trauma* 1998;45:588–592.

26

RSI Using Nondepolarizing Agents

Ron M. Walls

THE CLINICAL CHALLENGE

Succinylcholine is the preferred agent for rapid sequence intubation (RSI) in the emergency department (ED), but certain patients have contraindications to its use, principally related to the risk of hyperkalemia for patients with certain pre-existing conditions or, rarely, to known prior adverse reactions. These are discussed in detail in Chapter 19. This chapter addresses the approach to patients for whom an alternative neuromuscular blocking agent (NMBA) is required for RSI.

APPROACH TO THE AIRWAY

Of the nondepolarizing NMBAs, two have pharmacokinetic properties that support use during RSI: rocuronium (Zemuron) and vecuronium (Norcuron). Of these, rocuronium is clearly superior for emergency intubation because of its consistently rapid onset; it has been shown to produce intubating conditions almost identical to succinylcholine 60 seconds after administration when used with an adequate dose of an effective sedative induction agent. Rocuronium does not release histamine, is not a ganglionic blocking agent, and is devoid of cardiac muscarinic blocking effects, so it is virtually free of adverse effects. The biggest drawback to rocuronium, when compared to succinylcholine, is its relatively longer duration, which averages approximately 45 minutes when used in the recommended 1 mg/kg RSI dose. Sugammadex, the first of a novel class of reversal agents for competitive NMBAs, specifically reverses rocuronium. Unlike traditional reversal regimens, sugammadex can be given before any spontaneous muscular recovery occurs. With adequate dosing of sugammadex, early evidence indicates that full neuromuscular paralysis with rocuronium can be reversed sufficiently to permit adequate spontaneous ventilations within approximately 1 minute.

Vecuronium is a reasonable alternative to rocuronium for RSI, although it is a bit more complicated to use. Vecuronium is also devoid of any clinically significant side effects, but the time to achieve intubation-level relaxation is somewhat longer than with rocuronium (count on 75–90 seconds), even when the priming technique (described below) is used. The duration of action of vecuronium is significantly greater than for rocuronium, and there is presently no rapid reversal agent available.

TECHNIQUE

When a nondepolarizing agent is used for RSI, the time to adequate relaxation for laryngoscopy and intubation is slightly prolonged when compared to that for succinylcholine. In general, time 45 seconds to begin laryngoscopy after succinylcholine, 60 seconds after rocuronium, and 75 to 90 seconds after vecuronium. One method to shorten the apparent time to paralysis for vecuronium is to reverse the order of administration of the induction agent and the NMBA, giving the vecuronium first, followed immediately by the induction agent. This approach is not necessary when rocuronium is used.

When vecuronium is used for RSI, its onset can be hastened by the administration of a small priming dose (0.01 mg/kg or one tenth of the paralyzing dose) 3 minutes before giving the large, intubating dose (0.15 mg/kg; almost twice the paralyzing dose). This is called the "priming principle," and the small dose is referred to as the priming dose. The small priming dose serves to bind a small percentage of the motor end plate acetylcholine (ACh) receptors, such that clinical weakness is not experienced by the patient, yet the onset of action of the subsequent intubating dose is hastened. Using the priming principle, intubation-level paralysis can be achieved with vecuronium in 75 to 90 seconds. As is the case with other NMBAs, the intubating dose of vecuronium (i.e., the dose needed to achieve rapid paralysis for intubation) is significantly greater than the paralyzing dose. When using the priming principle, it is recommended that the paralytic dose be increased from the typical dose of 0.1 mg/kg (two times the effective dose that results in paralysis of 95% of the population, or ED_{95}) to 0.15 mg/kg (three times the ED_{95}).

There is another method for hastening the onset of vecuronium, called the "timing" method, in which the vecuronium is administered first, but the induction agent is withheld until the first sign of clinical weakness (ptosis) is observed, at which time the induction agent is then rapidly pushed. This timing method is advocated on the basis that it better aligns the onset of paralysis and hypnosis, minimizing the period that the patient is unconscious (but not yet paralyzed or intubatable) and, therefore, the risk of aspiration. We do not recommend the timing method for emergency intubation because it has the potential to cause severe distress for the patient, who experiences the onset of paralysis while still awake. This method also requires a level of patient observation, timing, and sequencing of drugs not used in any other RSI protocol, so seems prone to error.

DRUG DOSAGE AND ADMINISTRATION

Much research has been done on rocuronium to determine the appropriate dose for the most rapid and consistent onset of paralysis for RSI. The ED_{95} of rocuronium is 0.3 mg/kg. Consequently, the most commonly studied dosages in the literature are multiples of that, namely, 0.6 mg/kg, 0.9 mg/kg, and 1.2 mg/kg. Pharmacokinetic studies have unequivocally identified 1.0 mg/kg as the best intubation dose for RSI. This dose allows for laryngoscopy and intubation to occur 45 to 60 seconds after administration and results in approximately 45 minutes of motor paralysis. Rocuronium is distributed as a solution in 50- and 100-mg vials, at a concentration of 10 mg/mL. Using the larger vial (100 mg) allows the dose for the average adult patient (70–80 mg) to be obtained from a single vial. Because reconstitution is not necessary, the drug can be drawn up and administered quickly during the RSI protocol. For RSI, rocuronium, 1.0 mg/kg, is simply substituted for succinylcholine 1.5 mg/kg. All other steps remain the same. The shelf-life of rocuronium at room temperature is only a month, and thus, refrigeration or active inventory control is required to avoid spontaneous degradation of the drug. A sample RSI using rocuronium is shown in Box 26-1.

Vecuronium is supplied as a lyophilized powder in 10-mg vials that must be reconstituted with normal saline before use. When the vial is mixed with 10 cc of saline, a solution

---

BOX 26-1 Rapid Sequence Intubation Using Rocuronium

Time	Action
Zero minus 10 minutes	Preparation
Zero minus 5 minutes	Preoxygenation
Zero minus 3 minutes	Pretreatment
	ABC as for all patients
Zero	Paralysis with induction
	Induction agent intravenous (IV) push
	Rocuronium 1 mg/kg IV push
Zero plus 30 seconds	Positioning; apply Sellick's maneuver, if desired
Zero plus 60 seconds	Placement with proof
Zero plus 90 seconds	Postintubation management
	Administer long-acting sedation (see Chapter 3) to supplement long-acting paralysis of rocuronium.

BOX 26-2 Rapid Sequence Intubation Using Vecuronium with the Priming Principle

Time	Action
Zero minus 10 minutes	Preparation
Zero minus 5 minutes	Preoxygenation
Zero minus 3 minutes	Pretreatment
	ABC as for all patients
	Vecuronium 0.01 mg/kg (priming dose)
Zero	Paralysis with induction
	Induction agent intravenous (IV) push
	Vecuronium 0.15 mg/kg IV push
Zero plus 30 seconds	Positioning; apply Sellick's maneuver, if desired
Zero plus 90 seconds	Placement with proof
Zero plus 120 seconds	Postintubation management
	Administer longer-acting sedation (see Chapter 3) to
	supplement long-acting paralysis of vecuronium.

---

of 1 mg/mL vecuronium is produced. When performing RSI using vecuronium, the priming principle should be used. This involves the administration of a small, nonparalyzing dose of vecuronium, followed a few minutes later by a larger, paralyzing dose to hasten onset of intubation-level paralysis. Many variations of priming dose, interval, and intubating dose have been studied and recommended. On balance, to achieve intubating conditions as consistently as possible in the emergency situation, we recommend that the patient receive 0.01 mg/kg (usually rounded to a full 1 mg in most adult patients of average weight), concordant with the pretreatment phase of RSI, followed 3 minutes later by 0.15 mg/kg of vecuronium, given by rapid intravenous administration, immediately before or after the sedative (induction) agent. In most circumstances, laryngoscopy can be initiated in 75 to 90 seconds. Because of the larger intubating dose, the duration of paralysis will be prolonged (approximately 40 minutes). When using the priming principle, the operator must be extremely vigilant of the patient because an elderly or severely debilitated patient or a patient with respiratory failure may experience significant motor paralysis after the priming dose alone and require bag-mask ventilation and accelerated movement to the paralysis/induction step of RSI. A sample RSI using vecuronium with the priming principle is shown in Box 26-2.

POSTINTUBATION MANAGEMENT

Postintubation management after RSI with a nondepolarizing NMBA is comparable to that of conventional RSI with succinylcholine, with an obvious exception. The duration of action of succinylcholine is so short that spontaneous recovery of neuromuscular function can be anticipated within 10 minutes. Paralysis with a competitive NMBA will be much longer, as described previously, necessitating appropriate use of generous doses of sedatives and analgesics (see Chapter 3) to ensure that the patient is not "paralyzed but awake."

TIPS AND PEARLS

- When succinylcholine is contraindicated, rocuronium is the preferred NMBA for RSI because it provides an earlier onset of paralysis than vecuronium.

- Rocuronium substitutes easily for succinylcholine in the RSI protocol, and it is supplied in solution, like succinylcholine, so it does not need to be reconstituted. It is neither advisable nor necessary to use the priming principle with rocuronium.

EVIDENCE

1. **What is the correct dose of rocuronium for RSI, and how fast does it work?** Many studies performed in the operating room have shown that rocuronium can produce excellent intubating conditions within 60 seconds. The best analysis is that of Kirkegaard-Nielsen, et al. (1), who were able to use pharmacokinetic measurements to calculate the optimal intubating dose of rocuronium for RSI at 1.04 mg/kg. This dose provided for intubation at 60 seconds in 95% of patients with a 46-minute duration of action. This result strongly supports the use of 1.0 mg/kg of rocuronium for RSI, rather than the frequently recommended 0.6 mg/kg.

   Perry, Lee, and Wells (2) performed a detailed meta-analysis of 26 randomized clinical trials, including 1,606 patients undergoing RSI with succinylcholine versus rocuronium and found that there was a statistically significant relative risk (0.87) of less favorable intubating conditions with rocuronium. In a subgroup analysis, when propofol was used as the induction agent, intubation conditions were found to be the same between succinylcholine and rocuronium. These data support the widely held notion that using a potent induction agent can significantly improve the intubation conditions during RSI. This is likely because when intubation is attempted, the NMBA has not reached its peak effect, and the additional relaxation produced by the induction agent thus further optimizes the intubation conditions. However, the differences between succinylcholine and rocuronium depend on the definitions and outcomes used, and much of the apparent superiority of succinylcholine over rocuronium depends on narrow definitions of "excellent" intubating conditions. Success rates were comparable in the two groups.

   Studies have fairly consistently shown that succinylcholine is more rapid and of shorter duration than rocuronium, but many of these have not replicated true RSI conditions, and doses of both rocuronium and succinylcholine have varied (3). Nevertheless, for now, succinylcholine remains the drug of choice for emergency RSI.

   Rocuronium does not require priming when used in the 1 mg/kg dose. A recent study in children found that 0.6 mg/kg of rocuronium resulted in much more rapid intubating conditions when it was divided, with 10% given as a priming dose and the remaining 90% given a minute later (4). However, this study also did not replicate true RSI conditions, and the duration of action was over 40 minutes, comparable to that when 1.0 mg/kg of rocuronium is used. As expected, priming does not prolong the action of rocuronium.

2. **Are there any studies of rocuronium in the ED?** Unfortunately, few ED-based studies exist because of the practical difficulties involved in carrying out pharmacological intubation studies in an uncontrolled setting on unstable patients with unplanned intubations. Over a 6-month period, Sakles et al. (5) studied 58 patients who received rocuronium for RSI in the ED, and found that a mean dose of 1.0 ± 0.2 mg/kg of rocuronium was used for intubation and that etomidate was the most frequently used induction agent. The time from rocuronium administration to the initiation of laryngoscopy was able to be timed in 34 patients and averaged 45 ± 15 seconds (range 20–90 seconds). Laurin et al. (6) studied 520 ED intubations in which succinylcholine or rocuronium was used for RSI over a 1-year period. In the 382 patients receiving succinylcholine, the mean onset time of paralysis was 39 ± 13 seconds, and in the 138 patients receiving rocuronium, the onset time was 44 ± 20 seconds. This difference has no statistical or clinical significance.

3. **What is all the interest in sugammadex?** There is a new class of drugs, called the selective relaxant binding agents (SRBAs), which are designed to reverse the effects of the competitive aminosteroid NMBAs. Each drug in this class is specific to a particular aminosteroid NMBA, and sugammadex, which encapsulates and disables rocuronium, is the first agent to come to clinical trials. Traditional reversal methods for competitive NMBA involve administration of a cholinesterase inhibitor, which greatly increases acetylcholine concentrations, allowing effective competition with the NMBA at the neuromuscular junction. The reversal is not effective, however, until significant spontaneous recovery has occurred, and the excess of acetylcholine causes muscarinic effects that require the concomitant administration of an antimuscarinic agent, such as atropine. SRBAs hold the promise of immediate (within a minute or two) reversal of aminosteroid NMBA without any prior recovery, so that even a long-acting NMBA could be quickly reversed, if necessary. Initial studies appear to demonstrate both safety and tolerance for sugammadex (7). Doses up to 16 mg/kg of sugammadex have been well tolerated by healthy adults (8), and Groudine et al. (9) recently demonstrated reversal of paralysis approximately 1 minute after administration of 8 mg/kg of sugammadex to healthy adult patients fully paralyzed with 1.2 mg/kg of rocuronium. Although additional studies are needed, sugammadex and its fellow SRBAs hold the promise of rapid reversal of competitive NMBA, which could open the door for widespread adoption of an aminosteroid NMBA, likely rocuronium, as the agent of choice for emergency RSI. With rapid reversal possible, rocuronium would have the advantages of succinylcholine (fast, consistent, effective, brief duration of action) without the potentially serious adverse effects, especially hyperkalemia, associated with succinylcholine in certain patients.

REFERENCES

1. Kirkegaard-Nielsen H, Caldwell JE, Berry PD. Rapid tracheal intubation with rocuronium: a probability approach to determining dose. *Anesthesiology* 1999;91:131–136.
2. Perry JJ, Lee J, Wells G. Are intubation conditions using rocuronium equivalent to those using succinylcholine? *Acad Emerg Med* 2002;9:813–823.
3. Sluga M, Ummenhofer W, Studer W, et al. Rocuronium versus succinylcholine for rapid sequence induction of anesthesia and endotracheal intubation: a prospective, randomized trial in emergent cases. *Anesth Analg* 2005;101:1356–1361.
4. Bock M, Haselmann L, Böttiger BW, et al. Priming with rocuronium accelerates neuromuscular block in children: a prospective randomized study. *Can J Anesth* 2007;54:538–543.
5. Sakles JC, Laurin EG, Rantapaa AA, et al. Rocuronium for rapid sequence intubation of emergency department patients. *J Emerg Med* 1999;17:611–616.
6. Laurin EG, Sakles JC, Panacek EA, et al. A comparison of succinylcholine and rocuronium for rapid sequence intubation of emergency department patients. *Acad Emerg Med* 2000;7:1362–1369.
7. Sorgenfrei IF, Norrild K, Larsen PB, et al. Reversal of rocuronium-induced neuromuscular block by the selective relaxant binding agent sugammadex: a dose-finding and safety study. *Anesthesiology* 2006;104:667–674.
8. Gijsenbergh F, Ramael S, Houwing N, et al. First human use of Org 25969, a novel agent to reverse the action of rocuronium bromide. *Anesthesiology* 2005;103:695–703.
9. Groudine SB, Soto R, Lien C, et al. A randomized, dose-finding, phase II study of the selective relaxant binding drug. Sugammadex, capable of safely reversing profound rocuronium-induced neuromuscular block. *Anesth Analg* 2007;104(3):555–562.

27

Trauma

Ron M. Walls

THE CLINICAL CHALLENGE

The trauma patient poses several unique challenges with respect to airway management. Conflicting priorities may arise because of multiple system injuries, and resuscitation often requires a team response. Success demands excellent assessment skills, an understanding of the physiology of injury, a thorough knowledge of airway pharmacology, and strong leadership. Fundamentally, though, the principles of trauma airway management are no different than those applied to management of the airway in other complex medical situations. A consistent approach and a reproducible thought process help create a successful outcome.

APPROACH TO THE AIRWAY

Although many trauma intubations turn out to be straightforward and routine, systematic application of the airway algorithms and difficult airway mnemonics is essential. At the outset, all intubations performed in the injured patient should be considered at least *potentially* difficult. During the primary survey, the presence of multiple severe injuries can combine with distracting presentations (external hemorrhage, combative behavior) to create information overload for the treating clinician, impeding data gathering and impairing decision making. This underscores the importance of applying the main airway algorithm (see Chapter 2) and using the difficult airway mnemonics (LEMON, MOANS, SHORT, and RODS; see Chapter 7) in orderly fashion while assessing the patient:

1. **L**: Look externally: Injury to the face, mouth, or neck may distort anatomy or limit access, making the process of intubation difficult or impossible. The integrity of the mask seal may be impaired by facial hair, external bleeding, pre-existing physiognomy, or anatomical disruption (**M**OANS). Injury to the anterior neck, such as by a clothesline mechanism or hematoma, may preclude successful cricothyrotomy (**SH**ORT) or extraglottic device (EGD) placement (RO**D**S).
2. **E**: Evaluate 3-3-2. In blunt trauma, the cervical spine is immobilized, and a cervical collar is usually in place at the time that airway decisions must be made. A cervical collar is not particularly effective at limiting cervical spine movement during intubation, but greatly impairs mouth opening, limiting both laryngoscopy and insertion of an EGD (**R**ODS). The front portion of the collar should be opened to facilitate the primary survey and removed entirely during intubation. Other injuries, such as mandibular fractures, may either facilitate or impair oral access, and mouth opening should be assessed as carefully as possible.
3. **M**: Mallampati. The trauma patient is rarely able to cooperate with a formal Mallampati assessment, but the airway manager should open the patient's mouth as widely as possible and inspect the oral cavity for access, using a tongue blade, or the laryngoscope blade, which has the advantage of illumination. At this time, potential hemorrhage or disruption of the upper airway may also be evident (RO**D**S).
4. **O**: Obstruction, Obesity. Obstruction, usually by hemorrhage or hematoma, can interfere with laryngoscopy, BMV (M**O**ANS), or EGD placement (R**O**DS). Obesity in the trauma patient presents the same challenges as for the nontrauma patient.
5. **N**: Neck mobility. The majority of trauma patients, including all those with blunt trauma and certain patients with penetrating trauma, require manual inline stabilization to prevent cervical spine movement during intubation. The role of cervical spine immobilization during penetrating injury is controversial. Spinal instability caused by penetrating injury (usually gunshot wounds) is extremely rare in a patient presenting without neurological deficit. In other words, when these high-energy injuries create spinal instability, they also cause injury to the spinal cord or emerging nerve roots. Therefore, cervical spine immobilization in such patients is based on the

location and mechanism of the wound, the physical (especially neurological) findings on examination, and the urgency and difficulty of the airway intervention. Patients with penetrating injury can be subjected to secondary injury, as from falling down a flight of stairs, and these patients should be immobilized as for their blunt injury. Patients with gunshot injury to the head and neck may have brain injury that confounds spinal assessment. In general, though, an intact neurological examination in the context of penetrating injury argues strongly against the possibility of spinal instability. If spine immobilization is preventing successful intubation, it is advisable to relax the spine immobilization to permit completion of the intubation. This may expose the patient to a tiny risk of spinal cord injury, but the likelihood of brain injury from hypoxemia because of the failed intubation is many-fold greater. Similarly, even for blunt injury with intact neurological examination, if strict cervical spine immobilization is preventing intubation and hypoxemia is developing, judicious relaxation of the degree of immobilization to an extent just sufficient to permit intubation may be necessary, depending on the judgment of the airway manager.

6. Other factors: Pre-existing comorbidities and certain other injuries can complicate both the decision making and execution of trauma airway management:
   a) A patient with heart failure or chronic obstructive pulmonary disease, for example, may desaturate rapidly, requiring bag-mask ventilation during rapid sequence intubation (RSI).
   b) Injuries to the chest may create conflicting priorities between tube thoracostomy and intubation.
   c) Hypotension or marginal hemodynamic stability may influence the choice of pretreatment and sedative agents for RSI. For example, the brain injured patient with hypotension is not a good candidate for fentanyl pretreatment, despite the presence of central nervous system injury or presumed elevated intracranial pressure (ICP), because of the likelihood of further lowering the mean arterial blood pressure. Similarly, the patient's circulatory status may influence selection of the sedative agent, with etomidate and ketamine providing much greater hemodynamic stability than propofol or midazolam, for example.
   d) Specific illness or injury may require consideration as for the uninjured patient. For example, the trauma patient with asthma may receive lidocaine pretreatment.

Evaluation of the trauma patient follows the primary/secondary survey as described within the Advanced Trauma Life Support course. During the "A" phase of the primary survey, assess the integrity of the airway by observing the patient's air movement during respiration; quickly inspect and palpate the anterior neck (with cervical collar open); have the patient phonate ("What is your name?"); and inspect the oral cavity for disruption, dental or tongue injury, hemorrhage, or pooling secretions. A patient whose eyes are open and who is phonating (even nonsensically) likely has an adequate airway at that moment in time. If an oral or nasal airway is required to maintain airway patency, the patient is likely not able to protect the airway, and early (but not necessarily immediate) intubation is indicated. Next, inspect and feel the chest wall for injury, and listen for breath sounds. Although much is made about palpating the trachea to ensure it is in the midline, this is not a reliable finding for pneumothorax, and the presence or absence of tracheal deviation should not be considered to diagnose or exclude pneumo- or hemothorax. Careful palpation for subcutaneous air in the red alerts the examiner to the possibility of direct airway violation, which may render tracheal intubation difficult and BMV ineffective.

During this phase of examination, the pulse oximetry, blood pressure, and pulse are assessed in concert with auscultation of the chest. Presence of suspected pneumo- or hemothorax with hemodynamic compromise can create a dilemma with respect to the sequence of tube thoracostomy versus intubation. On the one hand, the patient may be so critically ill that immediate intubation seems necessary. Consideration of the effects of the hypotensive effect of the sedative agent and positive-pressure ventilation, however, may argue strongly for tube thoracostomy before intubation, in hopes that relief of the pneumothorax will improve the blood pressure. In general, if the airway is patent and functioning (i.e., immediate intubation is not required), and patient factors do not prevent insertion of a chest tube, it is preferable to perform tube thoracostomy first and then to intubate. The improved hemodynamics after tube thoracostomy may expand the choices for RSI drugs and also improve the safety of the intubation. However, the patient may be restless or combative, and thoracostomy may be difficult unless it is delayed until after the patient is sedated and paralyzed. Striking the right balance can be challenging and is one of the most difficult decisions facing the trauma leader. Options include (a) when a trauma team is present, the patient may be induced for RSI, and then the tube thoracostomy is performed by one team member while another intubates; or (b) when resuscitation is by a single provider or small team, a needle thoracostomy may be performed, followed immediately by intubation, and then by tube thoracostomy.

SPECIFIC CLINICAL CONSIDERATIONS

The trauma airway is one of the most challenging clinical circumstances in emergency care. It requires knowledge of a panoply of techniques, guided by a reproducible approach (the airway algorithms), sound judgment, and technical expertise. The principles common to the various clinical scenarios in trauma airway management are discussed previously. In this section, we describe the considerations unique to certain specific presentations.

Cervical Spine Injury

All severely injured blunt trauma patients have cervical spine injury until proven otherwise. In the vast majority of cases, the patient will be immobilized by prehospital providers in the field. Although this step is essential to prevent further spinal injury, it can create several problems as well. Intoxicated or head injured patients typically become agitated and difficult to control when strapped down on a backboard. Physical and chemical restraint may be required. Aspiration is a significant risk in the supine patient with traumatic brain injury or vomiting. In this position, ventilation may be impaired, especially in the presence of chest injury. High-flow oxygen should be provided to all patients, and suction must be immediately available.

If urgent airway management is needed, there is no purpose served by obtaining a crosstable-lateral cervical spine x-ray before intubation. This single view is inadequate to exclude injury, with a sensitivity of 80% at best, even with a technically perfect film. Waiting for the x-ray will expend precious time and give the operator a false sense of security when the film is interpreted as "normal." Instead, all patients must be assumed to have cervical injury, and inline stabilization must be maintained at all times. The preintubation neurological status of the patient and the use of inline manual immobilization of the cervical spine during intubation should be clearly documented in the medical record. The intubation itself is performed as gently as possible, with inline cervical stabilization by a second provider and optimal preoxygenation. Although most trauma intubations present some degree of difficulty, as described previously, RSI is often the best method for intubation, provided that the operator is confident about the likelihood of success and of the effectiveness of bag-mask ventilation or EGD placement, if intubation is unsuccessful. As experience with video laryngoscopy increases, it is likely that these devices will provide superior glottic views with less cervical stress than is possible by conventional laryngoscopy.

Disrupted Airway Anatomy

Here, the very condition that mandates intubation may also render it much more difficult and prone to failure. Direct airway injury may be the result of

- Maxillofacial trauma
- Blunt or penetrating anterior neck trauma
- Caustic ingestion

In cases of distorted anatomy, the approach must be one that minimizes the potential for catastrophic deterioration. Although some authors recommend a period of expectant observation, waiting to see if the nearly obstructed airway becomes completely obstructed can be disastrous. Theoretically, a short period of observation determines that the situation is deteriorating, and intubation is then undertaken. It is often not possible, however, to determine whether the airway threat is increasing; for example, expansion of a deep hematoma may not be clinically obvious. In such cases, deterioration may not be evident until a crisis occurs, at which time the patient's airway is nearly or completely obstructed, hypoxemia rapidly ensues, and intubation is difficult or impossible because of the extreme anatomical distortion. In these cases, neither bag-mask ventilation nor insertion of an EGD is possible, and the window of opportunity for cricothyrotomy has also often passed, with devastating consequences.

Airway disruption may be marginal or significant, real or potential. In either case, the guiding principle is to secure the threatened airway early, while more options are preserved, and the patient's stability permits a more deliberate approach. As for any other anatomically distorted airway, application of the difficult airway algorithm will often lead to a decision to perform an awake intubation. In patients with signs of significant airway compromise (e.g., stridor, drooling, respiratory distress, voice distortion), both the urgency of the intubation and the risk of using neuromuscular blockade are high. When symptoms are more modest, there is more time to plan and execute the airway intervention, but in neither case is delay advisable. Application of the difficult airway algorithm will lead the clinician through the evaluation of the patient's oxygenation (i.e., "Is there time?"), and then help determine whether RSI is advisable, possibly under a double setup, even though the airway is difficult. This will depend on the clinician's confidence about the likelihood of success of bag ventilation and intubation by direct laryngoscopy (see Chapters 2 and 7). Often, the best approach is to attempt awake intubation by fiberoptic laryngoscopy with sedation and topical anesthesia (see Chapters 8 and 12). This permits both examination of the airway and careful navigation through the injured area, even when the airway itself has been violated. When the airway is disrupted and the scope is used to traverse the disruption, the endotracheal tube should be as small as possible so it closely follows the fiberoptic scope when advanced, minimizing the likelihood of catching on the pathological breach in the airway. No other method of intubation allows the airway to be visualized both above and below the glottis. Although "awake" direct laryngoscopy is also a reasonable technique, using either a conventional or a video laryngoscope, this does not permit visualization of the airway beyond the glottis, so the intubation itself is "blind" with respect to the infraglottic trachea.

Smoke Inhalation

Smoke inhalation can present on a spectrum from mild smoke exposure to complete airway obstruction with death. Exposure to the toxic products of combustion usually does not cause direct thermal injury to the airway, and the ensuing edema is caused by tissue toxicity of the constituents of the smoke. Initially, the patient presents with evidence of smoke exposure (history of closed space fire) and physical findings suggestive of inhalation (singed nasal hairs, perinasal or perioral soot, carbon deposits on the tongue, hoarse voice, carbonaceous sputum.) When evidence of airway involvement is present, direct examination of the airway, often with intubation, is mandatory. This is usually, and best, done with fiberoptic laryngoscopy, which permits evaluation of the airway and simultaneous intubation, if indicated. Identification of supraglottic edema should be considered an indication for intubation, even if the edema is mild, because progression can be both rapid and occult. If examination of the upper airway identifies that the injury is confined to the mouth and nose, and the supraglottic area is spared (and normal), then intubation in not indicated, and subsequent examination can be at the discretion of the operator. If erythema or edema is identified, gentle intubation, either by direct laryngoscopy or over the fiberoptic scope, is indicated. The patient may well be extubated 24 or even 12 hours later without any evidence of intervening airway swelling, but that cannot be predicted at the time of initial examination, except by the presence of a normal upper airway. If doubt exists, the patient can be observed, but with a plan for a repeated upper airway examination in 30 minutes, even if symptoms do not develop or worsen. Observation in lieu of airway examination can be hazardous because the airway edema can worsen significantly without any external evidence, and by the time the severity of the situation is apparent, intubation is both immediately required and extremely difficult or impossible.

Chest Trauma

Chest injury, such as pneumothorax, hemothorax, flail chest, pulmonary contusion, or open chest wound, impairs ventilation and oxygenation. Preoxygenation may be difficult or impossible in these patients, and rapid desaturation following paralysis is the rule. In addition, the positive pressure delivered via the endotracheal tube may convert a simple pneumothorax to a tension pneumothorax. Refer to the previous discussion in this chapter regarding the clinical dilemma that often ensues when a patient has evidence of severe chest injury with hemo- or pneumothorax and is in need of immediate intubation.

Hypotension

Patients suffering significant injury may have obvious or occult hypotension from many different sources. Shock in the multiply injured patient can be broadly classified as *hemorrhagic* (e.g., external, intrathoracic, intra-abdominal, retroperitoneal, long bone) or *nonhemorrhagic* (e.g., tension pneumothorax, pericardial tamponade, myocardial contusion, spinal shock). As the causes of shock are elucidated and corrected, airway management choices must consider the loss of hemodynamic reserve in these patients. Mechanical causes of shock, such as tension pneumothorax or hemothorax, are addressed early and almost simultaneously with airway management (see previous discussion). Pericardial tamponade is rare in blunt trauma, but may be the most critical element destabilizing the patient with penetrating thoracic or upper abdominal trauma. Induction, intubation, and initiation of positive-pressure ventilation in a patient with untreated pericardial tamponade may precipitate cardiovascular collapse and arrest. Accordingly, the tamponade must be relieved before intubation. If this is not possible, a minimal dose of the most hemodynamically stable induction agent should be used (e.g., 0.5 mg/kg of ketamine). Rapid fluid administration is used to maximize filling pressure. The heart rate is maintained, and minimum effective tidal volumes are used to mitigate the inhibition of venous return to the thorax. Redistributive shock (spinal shock) is treated with fluids and, as necessary, pressors, with the constant caveat that spinal shock, in isolation, is not to be diagnosed until hemorrhagic shock has been excluded. Administration of crystalloid and blood will improve the hemodynamic tolerance for intubation and mechanical ventilation in patients with blood loss.

Traumatic Brain Injury

The principles of management of the patient with traumatic brain injury (TBI) fall within those discussed in Chapter 28 for patients with elevated ICP. The technique chosen is one that will optimize cerebral perfusion pressure by preserving systemic mean arterial blood pressure and minimize the extent and duration of hypoxemia. In the past, aggressive hyperventilation was advocated as a means to reduce ICP, and this, in itself, was considered an indication for intubation. This approach has long since been discredited, and hyperventilation is now known to worsen, not improve, the outcome in severe TBI. Hypercapnia is undesirable, however, because it causes cerebral vasodilation, and Pco_2 should be maintained at 35 torr. Certain sedative induction agents are believed to be more "cerebroprotective" because of their ability to decrease cerebral blood flow or oxygen demand. Etomidate, because of its balance of preservation of hemodynamics and modest cerebroprotective properties, is often the agent of choice. Formerly, it was widely believed that ketamine was contraindicated in head injury, but the evidence in this regard is scant and contradictory. Ketamine may be the drug of choice in the hypotensive TBI patient, as an alternative to etomidate. Because of its tendency to release catecholamines, ketamine is not advised for normotensive or hypertensive TBI patients.

TECHNIQUE

Paralysis versus Rapid Tranquilization of the Combative Trauma Patient

The combative trauma patient presents a series of conflicting problems. The causes of combative behavior in the trauma patient are numerous and include head injury, drug or ethanol intoxication, pre-existing medical conditions (diabetes, in particular), hypoxemia, shock, anxiety, personality disorder, and others. The priority is to rapidly control the patient so that potentially life-threatening causes can be identified and corrected. Controversy exists as to whether such patients ought to undergo rapid tranquilization with a neuroleptic agent or sedative, or whether immediate intubation with neuromuscular blockade is appropriate. Rapid tranquilization using haloperidol is well established as a safe and effective means for gaining control of the combative trauma patient who cannot be settled by other means. Haloperidol can be used intravenously in 5- to 10-mg increments every 5 minutes until a sufficient clinical response is achieved. There is extensive literature supporting the safety of this approach. Recently, concerns have been raised about the potential for intravenous haloperidol to worsen QT prolongation or cause Torsades Des Pointes. If possible, obtain a pre-administration monitor strip to assess QT interval length, but the patient's behavior often precludes this. Haloperidol has minimal effect on the CO_2 response curve, so does not depress respirations, although, occasionally, the additive effect of haloperidol to another general anesthetic agent, such as ethanol, can cause hypoventilation. Opioids, such as morphine or fentanyl, although indicated for pain control, are not primary sedative agents, and should not be used for this purpose because of their profound respiratory depressant effects.

The decision to use rapid tranquilization rather than RSI with neuromuscular blockade depends on the nature of the patient's presentation and injuries. If intubation is required based on the patient's injuries, independent of the combative behavior, then immediate intubation is indicated. If, however, the patient is presenting primarily with control problems and does not appear have injuries that would mandate intubation, then rapid tranquilization is appropriate. In many situations, the decision will not be clearcut, and judgment will be required. In either situation, control of the patient is an essential step in overall management, whether this is achieved through intubation with sedation and paralysis or through rapid tranquilization.

Choice of Pretreatment Agents

Pretreatment agents for the multiply injured patient are the same as those for other patients requiring intubation (see previous discussion), with a few important caveats. Fentanyl is indicated when the catecholamine surge, which accompanies intubation, is undesirable, such as in traumatic cerebral hemorrhage and penetrating injury, particularly involving a great vessel. In the trauma patient, however, sympathetic tone is often maximized to preserve blood pressure in the face of blood loss, and administration of an agent to reduce sympathetic tone is not desirable. In such patients, although there may be a theoretical reason to administer fentanyl, it should not be given because of the potential to greatly worsen hemodynamic compromise. In cases of isolated head injury without hypotension, though, fentanyl is indicated, as is lidocaine. There are no particular traumatic contraindications to lidocaine, when it is otherwise indicated for pretreatment (see Chapter 17).

Choice of Neuromuscular Blocking Agent

Succinylcholine (SCh) is the drug of choice for RSI in the trauma patient because of its rapid, reliable onset and brief duration of action. Although patients with spinal cord injury, extensive burns, or severe crush injuries are at risk for SCh-induced hyperkalemia, the receptor upregulation that causes the hyperkalemia takes several days to develop and is not an issue in the context of acute injury. SCh is contraindicated in these patients beginning 5 days post injury, though, and extending for 6 months or until the burns are healed (see Chapter 19).

SCh also has been implicated in the elevation of ICP in the patient with traumatic brain injury. We no longer recommend the use of a defasciculating agent in this setting, however, and elevated ICP is neither an absolute nor relative contraindication to the use of SCh (see Chapters 19 and 28). SCh's short duration of action permits ongoing postintubation sedation using a propofol infusion, without paralysis, in many cases of traumatic brain injury, thus facilitating ongoing neurological evaluation.

Choice of Sedative Induction Agent

Table 27-1 provides a summary of recommendations for RSI sedative induction agent selection based on the particular clinical situation. In most circumstances, etomidate is the drug of choice, based on its hemodynamic stability and familiarity. The controversy regarding the use of etomidate in shock, related to suppression of the adrenal axis, is discussed in Chapter 18. This controversy has related primarily to septic shock, and there is currently no evidence to support abandoning this reliable, proven, and hemodynamically stable agent in trauma. Overall, the preservation of hemodynamic status and cerebral perfusion pressure outweighs considerations of theoretical transient suppression of the adrenal axis.

Failed Airway

When a failed airway situation develops in the trauma patient, the failed airway algorithm is followed, just as for the nontrauma patient. The trauma patient has a higher incidence of upper airway distortion that may render oral approaches impossible, necessitating cricothyrotomy, and cricothyrotomy is required over four times more often in trauma than in

TABLE 27-1
RSI Sedative Induction Agent Selection in the Trauma Patient

Clinical scenario	First choice	Alternatives
No brain injury		
Hemodynamically stable	Etomidate	Propofol, thiopental, midazolam
Shock	Ketamine	Etomidate[a]
Brain injury		
Hemodynamically stable	Etomidate	Thiopental, propofol
Shock	Etomidate[a]	Ketamine[a,b]
Profound shock	Ketamine[a]	None

[a]In the presence of shock, reduce the dose by 25% to 50%.
[b]Hemodynamic considerations outweigh intracranial pressure controversy.

medical cases. Careful application of the LEMON, MOANS, RODS, and SHORT mnemonics during the preintubation assessment will ensure that the devices chosen are appropriate for the patient's particular injuries, and that transition from the primary method selected (e.g., RSI) to the rescue technique (e.g., intubating LMA [ILMA]) in the event of a failed airway is as smooth as possible. Cricothyroidotomy equipment should always be readily available, and the operator must be familiar with both the technique and the cricothyroidotomy kit contents.

TIPS AND PEARLS

1. Most considerations related to intubation of the multiply injured patient follow the same principles as for the medical patient, and the primary challenge for the intubator is to avoid being distracted by the patient's obvious external injuries, combative behavior, or the intrinsic anxiety that accompanies care of the severely injured, often young, trauma patient.
2. Resist the temptation to observe the patient with upper airway injury or smoke inhalation. Delay can lead to disaster, and, at the least, the upper airway should be examined fiberoptically to ensure that there is adequate airway patency and time.
3. The hemodynamically compromised trauma patient may be much more severely injured than is apparent. Young patients, in particular, can preserve a reasonably normal blood pressure in the face of significant blood loss. The occult hypotension may be suddenly unmasked by the administration of sedative agents, initiation of positive-pressure ventilation, or both.

EVIDENCE

1. **Are there any large series of intubation of trauma patients?** In an evidence-based literature review, Dunham et al. (1) provided a comprehensive overview (demographics, airway management techniques, success rates) of trauma patients requiring emergency airway management. Although most of these patients were critically ill, the degree of injury was highly variable; the mean Injury Severity Score was 29 (range 17–54), and the mean Glasgow Coma Scale was 6.5 (range 3–15). On average, 41% of patients died (range 2%–100%). They reported death more frequently when airway management was delayed, difficult, or unsuccessful, but a lack of randomization makes these findings difficult to interpret. In the multicenter National Emergency Airway Registry (NEAR) project, analysis of more than 2,000 trauma intubations identified head trauma as the single largest indication. RSI was the most common airway management method used, and the RSI success rate was more than 97% (2). Cricothyrotomy is required in approximately 2.5% of all trauma patients, almost always as a secondary, or "rescue," technique (3). Cricothyrotomy, when required, has a high success rate and a low rate of adverse events (3). More detailed analysis of trauma intubations by the NEAR investigators is forthcoming.
2. **Has inadequate or inappropriate airway management been linked to preventable death?** When 629 trauma deaths in the state of Montana were reviewed to determine the rate and cause of preventable mortality and "inappropriate" care by a panel of physicians and prehospital care providers, the overall preventable death rate was judged to be 13%. The most common cause of inappropriate care was inadequate management of the airway in either the prehospital setting (6.8% of cases) or emergency department (5.4% of cases) (4). This argues for proper airway training, as well as the availability of adequate equipment and drugs for trauma airway management, in the context of a comprehensive quality program.

3. **Is oral endotracheal intubation safe in cervical spine injury?** A prospective study of airway management practice and associated neurological outcome in 150 patients subsequently diagnosed with cervical spine injury used a standardized neurological examination that was performed before and after intubation, which was performed using inline stabilization. Twenty-six (32%) of 81 patients without a neurological deficit required intubation on presentation, and none manifested a subsequent neurological deficit. Twenty-nine (42%) of 69 additional patients with high cervical injury required intubation, and no patient exhibited neurological deterioration (5). A retrospective review was conducted of 150 patients with known cervical spine injuries who were electively intubated: 50 patients (33%) had preoperative neurological deficit, 83 patients (55%) were intubated after induction of general anesthesia, and 67 patients (45%) were intubated awake. Cervical immobilization with inline stabilization was documented in 86 patients (57%). Two patients (1.3%) developed new neurological deficits. The study size was insufficient to determine whether awake intubation versus general anesthesia conferred any potential benefit (6). A retrospective study of 73 out of 393 patients with traumatic cervical spine injuries who underwent RSI with inline stabilization within 30 minutes of presentation (36 patients) or between 30 minutes and 24 hours (37 patients) found no neurological sequelae as a result of the intubation (7).

A retrospective analysis of patients undergoing tracheal intubation for surgical fixation of cervical spine injuries compared results when awake fiberoptic intubation was used with those obtained using general anesthesia and neuromuscular blockade. Sixteen of the 45 patients had preoperative neurological deficit. Cervical traction was used to stabilize the spine for all intubations. None of the 45 patients sustained a new or worsened neurological injury (8). A similar retrospective review of 113 patients with cervical spine fractures requiring operative repair, of whom 33 (30%) had a partial neurological deficit, found no new neurological deficits among the 86 (76%) who underwent nasal intubation or the 27 (24%) who underwent oral intubation with inline stabilization (9).

There are no guarantees that any particular approach is safe, but there is solid evidence that a controlled intubation using manual inline cervical stabilization protects the patient against neurological injury.

4. **Are the ILMA and Combitube safe in cervical spine injury?** A prospective study of radiographs taken before, during, and after intubation using the ILMA versus direct laryngoscopy in patients with normal cervical spines found that the ILMA intubation took about twice as long (39 seconds vs. 21 seconds), but that the cervical spine movement was significantly less with the ILMA ($p < .008$) (10).

Although the Combitube (CT) airway has been recommended as a device for airway rescue when RSI fails, it may be more difficult to place in patients with immobilized cervical spines. When CT placement was attempted in 15 patients (mean age, 32 years) with Philadelphia collars on during anesthesia for elective surgery, blind insertion was possible in only 5 patients; in the remaining 10, the investigators were unable to advance the device through the mouth into the hypopharynx and required laryngoscopy. Once placed, the CT functioned effectively. These results cast doubt on the use of the CT in the immobilized trauma patient (11).

5. **Do alternative methods create more or less cervical spine movement than direct laryngoscopy?** In a study of cervical spine movement during intubation in 24 healthy volunteers, the Shikani optical stylet (see Chapter 13) caused 55% less cervical spine movement in three of the four cervical spine segments studied than did intubation with the MacIntosh laryngoscope. Intubation took an average of 28 seconds with the SOS versus 17 seconds with the MacIntosh (12). The same researchers subsequently compared intubations with the lighted stylet, GlideScope, and MacIntosh laryngoscope in 36 elective anesthesia patients (13). Compared with direct Macintosh laryngoscopy, the Trachlight (see Chapter 11) reduced motion by 49%, 72%, 64%, and 41% at four studied cervical segments, and the GlideScope reduced

motion by 50% at the C2–C5 segment, but did not affect other levels. Time to successful intubation was similar with the Trachlight and MacIntosh laryngoscope (14 and 16 seconds), but was significantly longer with the GlideScope (27 seconds). (See also Chapters 14 and 15.)

REFERENCES

1. Dunham MC, Barraco RD, Clark DE, et al. Guidelines for emergency tracheal intubation immediately after traumatic injury. *J Trauma* 2003;55:162–179.

2. Brown CA, Walls RM. National Emergency Airway Registry (NEAR III): an initial report of 3,342 emergency department intubations [abstract]. *Acad Emerg Med* 2004;11(5):491.

3. Collins JJ, Brown CA, Walls RM. Surgical airways in emergency department patients: a report of 75 cases from the National Emergency Airway Registry (ii) [abstract]. *Acad Emerg Med* 2004;11(5):522–523.

4. Esposito TJ, Sanddal ND, Hansen JD, et al. Analysis of preventable trauma deaths and inappropriate trauma care in a rural state. *J Trauma* 1995;39(5):955–962.

5. Shatney CH, Brunner RD, Nguyen TQ. The safety of orotracheal intubation in patients with unstable cervical spine fracture or high spinal cord injury. *Am J Surg* 1995;179:676–679.

6. Suderman VS, Crosby ET, Lui A. Elective oral tracheal intubation in cervical spine-injured adults. *Can J Anaesth* 1992;39:516–517.

7. Criswell JC, Parr MJ, Nolan JP. Emergency airway management in patients with cervical spine injuries. *Anaesthesia* 1994;49(10):900–903.

8. McCrory C, Blunnie WP, Moriarty DC. Elective tracheal intubation in cervical spine injuries. *Irish Med J* 1997;90:234–235.

9. Holly J, Jorden R. Airway management in patients with unstable cervical spine fractures. *Ann Emerg Med* 1988;18:1237–1239.

10. Walti B, Melischek M, Schuschig C, et al. Tracheal intubation and cervical spine excursion: direct laryngoscopy vs. intubating laryngeal mask. *Anaesthesia* 2001;56:221–226.

11. Mercer MH, Gabbott DA. Insertion of the Combitube airway with the cervical spine immobilized in a rigid cervical collar. *Anaesthesia* 1998;53(10):971–974.

12. Turkstra TP, Pelz DM, Shaikh AA, et al. Cervical spine motion: a fluoroscopic comparison of Shikani optical stylet vs MacIntosh laryngoscope. *Can J Anesth* 2007;54(6):441–447.

13. Turkstra TP, Craen RA, Pelz DM, et al. Cervical spine motion: a fluoroscopic comparison during intubation with lighted stylet, GlideScope, and MacIntosh laryngoscope. *Anesth Analg* 2005;101(3):910–915.

28

Elevated Intracranial Pressure

Andy S. Jagoda and John J. Bruns, Jr.

THE CLINICAL CHALLENGE

Elevated intracranial pressure (ICP) poses a direct threat to the viability and function of the brain. In head trauma, elevated ICP has been clearly associated with worse outcomes. The problems associated with elevated ICP may be compounded by many of the techniques and drugs used in airway management because they may cause further elevations of ICP. In addition, victims of multiple trauma may present with hypotension, thus limiting the choice of agents and techniques available. This chapter provides the basis for an understanding of the problems of increased ICP and the optimal methods of airway management in this patient group.

When increased ICP occurs as a result of an injury or medical catastrophe, the brain's ability to regulate blood flow (autoregulation) over a range of blood pressures is often lost. In general, the ICP is maintained through a mean arterial pressure (MAP) range of 80 to 180 mm Hg. When the ICP becomes elevated, autoregulation often, but not always, has been lost. In this setting, excessively high or excessively low blood pressure could aggravate brain injury by promoting cerebral edema or ischemia. Hypotension, even for a very brief period, is especially harmful, and along with hypoxia, has been shown to be an independent predictor of mortality and morbidity in patients with traumatic brain injury (TBI).

Cerebral perfusion pressure (CPP) is the driving force for blood flow to the brain. It is measured by the difference between the MAP and the ICP, expressed as the formula:

$$CPP = MAP - ICP$$

It is clear from this formula that excessive decreases in MAP, as might occur during rapid sequence intubation (RSI), would decrease CPP and contribute to cerebral ischemia. Conversely, increases in MAP, if not accompanied by equivalent increases in ICP, may be beneficial because of the increase in the driving pressure for oxygenation of brain tissue. It is generally recommended that the ICP be maintained below 20 mm Hg, the MAP between 100 to 110 mm Hg, and the CPP near 70 mm Hg. There are a number of confounding elements that may increase ICP during airway management.

Reflex Sympathetic Response to Laryngoscopy

The reflex sympathetic response to laryngoscopy (RSRL) is stimulated by the rich sensory innervation of the supraglottic larynx. Use of the laryngoscope, and particularly the attempted placement of an endotracheal tube, results in a significant afferent discharge that increases sympathetic activity to the cardiovascular system mediated through direct neuronal activity and release of catecholamines. More prolonged or aggressive attempts at laryngoscopy and intubation result in greater sympathetic nervous system stimulation. This catecholamine surge leads to increased heart rate and blood pressure, which significantly enhances cerebral blood flow (CBF) at the apparent expense of the systemic circulation through redistribution. These hemodynamic changes may contribute to increased ICP, particularly if autoregulation is impaired; therefore, it is desirable to mitigate this RSRL. Gentle intubation techniques that minimize airway stimulation and pharmacological adjuncts (e.g., beta blockade, lidocaine, synthetic opioids) have been studied to accomplish this mitigation.

Evidence is mixed regarding the use of lidocaine to blunt the hemodynamic response to laryngoscopy. Studies in patients without cardiovascular disease have failed to show effect, and other studies have shown variable results with respect to hemodynamic protection, with some appearing to demonstrate benefit and others showing none. As a result, lidocaine cannot be recommended at the present time for mitigation of the RSRL associated with emergency intubation.

The short-acting beta-blocker esmolol, in contrast, has consistently demonstrated the ability to control both heart rate and blood pressure responses to intubation. A dose of 2 mg/kg given 3 minutes before intubation has been shown to be effective. Unfortunately, in the emergency situation, the administration of a beta-blocking agent, even one that is short acting, may be problematic by causing or exacerbating hypotension in a trauma patient, or by confounding interpretation of a decrease in the blood pressure changes immediately following intubation. For these reasons, although esmolol is consistent and reliable for mitigation of RSRL in elective anesthesia, it is generally not used for this purpose for emergency intubation.

Fentanyl at doses of 3 to 5 μg/kg has also been shown to attenuate the RSRL associated with intubation. Although a full sympathetic blocking dose of fentanyl is 9 to 13 μg/kg, the recommended pretreatment dose of fentanyl for emergency RSI is 3 μg/kg and should be administered as a single pretreatment dose over 60 seconds. This technique permits effective mitigation of the RSRL, with greatly reduced chances of apnea or hypoventilation before sedation and paralysis.

Several studies have investigated the potential advantages of fiberoptic or lighted stylet intubation over direct laryngoscopy, working on the premise that these techniques minimize tracheal stimulation and thus the RSRL. Results of these studies are mixed and do not permit any conclusions recommending one technique over the other. In a controlled operating room setting, the insertion of the endotracheal tube into the trachea is more stimulating than a routine laryngoscopy.

At present, based on the best available evidence, it seems advisable to administer 3 μg/kg of fentanyl intravenously (IV) as a pretreatment agent 3 minutes before administration of the induction and neuromuscular blocking agents to mitigate the RSRL. Fentanyl should not be administered to patients with incipient or actual hypotension or to those who are dependent on sympathetic drive to maintain an adequate blood pressure for cerebral perfusion. In such cases, the ensuing hypotension may cause further central nervous system injury. In addition to pharmacological maneuvers to reduce RSRL, intubation should be performed in the gentlest manner possible, limiting both the time and intensity of laryngoscopy.

Reflex ICP Response to Laryngoscopy

Laryngoscopy may also increase the ICP by a direct reflex mechanism not mediated by sympathetic stimulation of the blood pressure or heart rate. The details of this reflex are poorly elucidated. Insertion of the laryngoscope or endotracheal tube may, therefore, further elevate ICP, even if the RSRL is blunted. It would seem desirable to blunt this ICP response to laryngoscopy in patients at risk for having elevated ICP. The literature related to the use of lidocaine to blunt ICP response to laryngoscopy and intubation is discussed in Chapter 17. In patients with elevated ICP, lidocaine should be administered as a pretreatment drug in the dose of 1.5 mg/kg IV 3 minutes before the induction agent and succinylcholine (SCh) to mitigate the ICP response to laryngoscopy and intubation.

ICP Response to Succinylcholine

SCh itself may be capable of causing a mild and transient increase in ICP. Studies have shown that this increase is temporally related to the presence of fasciculations in the patient, but is not the result of synchronized muscular activity leading to increased venous pressure. Rather, there appears to be a complex reflex mechanism originating in the muscle spindle and ultimately resulting in an elevation of ICP. One recent study challenged the claim that SCh causes an elevation of ICP, and SCh remains the drug of choice for management of patients with elevated ICP because of its rapid onset and short duration. Although we recommended in former editions of this manual the routine use of a defasciculating agent when SCh is administered to a patient with elevated ICP, we no longer advocate this practice. There is insufficient evidence to support the use of a defasciculating agent, and it adds unnecessary complexity.

Choice of Induction Agent

When managing the patient with potential brain injury, it is important to choose an induction agent that will not adversely affect CPP. Ideally, one would like to choose an induction agent that is capable of improving or maintaining CPP and providing some cerebral protective effect. Sodium thiopental is an ultra short-acting barbiturate induction agent. Thiopental confers some cerebroprotective effect because it decreases the basal metabolic rate of oxygen utilization of the brain ($CMRO_2$). This effect can be likened to decreasing myocardial oxygen demand in the ischemic heart. In addition, sodium thiopental decreases CBF, thus decreasing ICP. This combination of characteristics, the decrease in ICP and the decrease in $CMRO_2$, make thiopental a desirable agent for use in patients with elevated ICP and a normal or high blood pressure. However, thiopental is a potent venodilator and negative inotrope. Therefore, it has a tendency to cause significant hypotension and thus reduce CPP, even in relatively hemodynamically stable patients. In the hemodynamically unstable patient, this hypotensive effect can be profound. A single episode of hypotension significantly increases mortality in acute, severe head injury. Therefore, although thiopental is a desirable agent for management of patients with elevated ICP, its hemodynamic instability relegates it to an alternative role, with etomidate being the agent of choice. When the circulating blood volume is known to be normal, and hemodynamic stability is preserved, however, thiopental remains an appropriate choice as the induction agent.

Etomidate is a short-acting imidazole derivative that has a similar profile of activity to thiopental, but without the tendency to cause hemodynamic compromise. In fact, etomidate is the most hemodynamically stable of all commonly used induction agents except ketamine (see Chapter 18). Its ability to decrease $CMRO_2$ and ICP in a manner analogous to that of sodium thiopental and its remarkable hemodynamic stability make it the drug of choice for patients with elevated ICP. Recently, the use of etomidate in patients with elevated ICP has been challenged on the basis of evidence from animal studies. This preliminary evidence, which is addressed in Chapter 18, does not justify avoidance of etomidate, with its excellent hemodynamic profile, in patients with elevated ICP.

Ketamine, in general, has been avoided in patients with known elevations in ICP because of the belief that it may elevate the ICP further. The evidence regarding this phenomenon is mixed, however, and is discussed in Chapter 18. In patients with elevated ICP and hypotension, ketamine's superior hemodynamic stability, on balance, argue for its use.

APPROACH TO THE AIRWAY

RSI is the preferred method for patients with suspected elevated ICP because it provides protection against the reflex responses to laryngoscopy and rises in ICP. The presence of coma should not be interpreted as an indication to proceed without pharmacological agents or to administer only a neuromuscular blocking agent without a sedative induction drug. Although the patient may seem unresponsive, laryngoscopy and intubation will provoke the reflexes described previously, if appropriate pretreatment and induction agents are not used. Following appropriate assessment and preparation, as described in Chapter 3, the sequence in Box 28-1 is recommended for patients with elevated ICP.

INITIATING MECHANICAL VENTILATION

Mechanical ventilation in the patient with elevated ICP should be predicated on two principles: (a) optimal oxygenation, and (b) avoidance of ventilation mechanics (e.g., positive end-expiratory pressure, high peak inspiratory pressure) that would increase venous congestion in the brain.

There is no scientific basis for the use of "therapeutic" hyperventilation, with good evidence that it promotes worse outcomes rather than better. The Brain Trauma Foundation Guidelines for the Management of Severe Traumatic Brain Injury recommend that prophylactic hyperventilation be avoided and that patients with severe TBI be ventilated in such a way as to target the lower limits of normocapnia ($PaCO_2$ of 35–40 mm Hg). A similar

BOX 28-1 Rapid Sequence Intubation for Patients with Elevated Intracranial Pressure

Time	Action
Zero minus 10 minutes	**P**reparation
Zero minus 5 minutes	**P**reoxygenation
Zero minus 3 minutes	**P**retreatment:
	Lidocaine 1.5 μg/kg intravenously (IV)
	then
	Fentanyl 3 μg/kg (over 1 minute; if hemodynamically stable)
Zero	**P**aralysis with induction:
	Etomidate 0.3 mg/kg IV
	Succinylcholine 1.5 mg/kg IV
Zero plus 30 seconds	**P**ositioning
Zero plus 45 seconds	**P**lacement with proof: intubate, confirm placement
Zero plus 60 seconds	**P**ostintubation management

approach seems prudent in patients with medically induced elevations of ICP (e.g., cerebral hemorrhage).

Hyperventilation to a $PaCO_2$ of 30 mm Hg should be used only as a temporizing measure in patients demonstrating clinical signs of herniation (blown pupil or decerebrate posturing) and when osmotic agents, cerebrospinal fluid drainage, or both are not effective in managing an acute rise in ICP accompanied by patient deterioration. Normal initial physiological ventilation parameters are described in Chapter 37. Initial inspired fraction of oxygen (F_IO_2) should be 1.0 (100%). F_IO_2 can later be decreased according to pulse oximetry, as long as 100% oxygen saturation is maintained. Carbon dioxide tension can be followed with arterial blood gases or, preferably, continuous capnography, the first assessment of which should occur approximately 10 minutes after initiation of steady-state mechanical ventilation. To permit early and frequent neurological examinations (e.g., by a neurosurgeon to decide whether there is sufficient persisting neurological functioning to warrant an attempt at surgical evacuation of a massive subdural hematoma), long-term sedation is best accomplished by using a propofol infusion, which can be terminated as needed with prompt patient recovery. Deep sedation is desired, however, to permit effective controlled mechanical ventilation and other necessary interventions, while mitigating the stimulating effects of the tube in the trachea and eliminating any possibility of the patient coughing or bucking. An analgesic, such as fentanyl, is used to improve endotracheal tube tolerance and reduce stimulation and responsiveness.

TIPS AND PEARLS

RSI is clearly the desired method for tracheal intubation in patients with suspected elevation of ICP. The technique allows control of various adverse effects and optimal control of ventilation after intubation. However, the use of neuromuscular blockade in patients with potential neurological deficit carries the responsibility of performing a detailed neurological evaluation on the patient before initiation of neuromuscular blockade. The patient's ability to interact with the surroundings, spontaneous motor movement, response to deep pain, response to voice, localization, pupillary reflexes, and other pertinent neurological details must be assessed carefully before administration of neuromuscular blockade. The careful recording of these findings will be invaluable for the ongoing evaluation of the patient.

If the patient's ventilatory status is severely compromised by the head injury or by concomitant injuries, positive-pressure ventilation with bag and mask may be required throughout the intubation sequence. In such circumstances, one is trading off the increased risk of aspiration against the hazard of inadequate oxygenation and rising $PaCO_2$ during the intubation sequence. When such a tradeoff arises, it should be resolved in favor of oxygenation over the risk of aspiration.

EVIDENCE

Evidence-based recommendations depend on a careful analysis of the methodology used in the studies reviewed and an understanding of the outcome measure, which must be sound to make the study clinically relevant. In this light, it becomes challenging to make evidence-based recommendations regarding airway management in the patient with a brain injury. Regarding methodology, most of the studies of the effect of interventions discussed in this chapter were performed on stable patients in the operating room setting; others were performed on deeply anesthetized patients in the intensive care unit during tracheal suctioning. It is difficult to extrapolate the findings in these patient groups to critical patients undergoing emergency intubation. In addition, the timing and dosing of pharmacological interventions varied significantly, making it difficult to compare one study with another. For example, in one study lidocaine was found effective when given 3 minutes before intubation and ineffective if given at 4, 2, or 1 minute before (1). There is only one randomized double-blind interventional study identified that was performed in the ED on patients with head injury (2). This prospective double-blind study found that esmolol and lidocaine had similar efficacy in attenuating the hemodynamic response to intubation of patients with isolated head injury.

Regarding outcome, there is no study in the literature that compares airway interventions with a functional outcome measure, that is, disability or death. Rises in heart rate, blood pressure, and ICP are the commonly measured parameters comparing one technique or pharmacological intervention with the other because these affect CPP. However, there is no evidence that these are valid surrogates for more meaningful outcome measures such as disability, nor is there evidence that transient rises in any of the previously mentioned measures have any meaningful impact on morbidity or mortality. That said, there is no evidence that the interventions presented in this chapter do harm, and pending more direct evidence, it does seem intuitive that minimizing adverse changes in ICP, blood pressure, and heart rate can only contribute to maximizing good outcomes.

1. Should premedication(s) be used when RSI is performed on patients with elevated ICP? The choices of RSI premedications for patients with elevated ICP include lidocaine, fentanyl, esmolol, and a defasciculating dose of a nondepolarizing agent. Evidence for the use of lidocaine, 1.5 mg/kg IV, and fentanyl, 3 μg/kg IV, 3 minutes before induction, is discussed in Chapter 17. In summary, there is insufficient evidence that lidocaine can mitigate the RSRL, but it appears somewhat effective in limiting the intracranial response to upper airway stimulation, which is not mediated by catecholamines. Fentanyl, however, is known to blunt the reflex sympathetic response to upper airway manipulation, mitigating the extent of catecholamine release and, therefore, rise in MAP (see Chapter 17).

Esmolol has been studied as a premedication to blunt the RSRL through its beta-blocking properties. In one randomized double-blind, placebo-controlled study, esmolol, 2 to 3 mg/kg IV, provided better control of heart rate and blood pressure than either lidocaine or fentanyl (3). Of note, fixed doses of drugs were used, and the lidocaine and fentanyl were given only 2 minutes before intubation. Similar results were reported in another randomized double-blind study using 1.4 mg/kg (4) and 2 mg/kg (5). In a randomized double-blind study comparing the hemodynamic response of esmolol and lidocaine, both were found equally effective (2).

There is some controversy, but no evidence, whether the increase in ICP caused by SCh is clinically significant, and whether a defasciculating dose of a competitive neuromuscular blocking agent is capable of mitigating this response. On balance, we no longer recommend the use of a defasciculating dose (one-tenth of the paralyzing dose) of a competitive neuro-muscular blocking agent such as vecuronium (0.01 mg/kg) or rocuronium (0.06 mg/kg) 3 minutes before SCh is given. Based on the best evidence available at this time, the fol-lowing recommendations can be made regarding the pharmacological mitigation of exacer-bations of elevated ICP during emergency intubation:

- Administer lidocaine, 1.5 mg/kg, 3 minutes prior to airway manipulation to mitigate the raise in ICP from laryngoscopy.
- In patients without compensated or decompensated shock, administer fentanyl, 3 μg/kg, 3 minutes prior to airway manipulation in order to mitigate raises in ICP from RSRL.
- When patients with elevated ICP are paralyzed with SCh, use of a defasciculating dose of nondepolarizing paralytic agent is no longer recommended.
- Esmolol is an effective agent in mitigating raises in ICP from RSRL; however, because of its potential to cause or aggravate hypotension, especially in patients with hypovolemia, it is not recommended for routine use in emergency intubation.

2. Is hyperventilation (ETCO$_2$ <30–35 mm Hg) recommended in the management of the TBI patient with suspected ICP? Hyperventilation can be defined as a PaCO$_2$ <35 or an ETCO$_2$ <30–35: the correlation between the two measures is generally good in patients who are normotensive (6). It causes vasoconstriction and thus reduces ICP (7). Unfortunately, hyperventilation will also cause a reduction in CBF. Because CBF is reduced by almost 50% in the first days after TBI, hyperventilation poses a risk of exacerbating ischemia (8). In a randomized, controlled trial, Muizelaar et al. (9) found that patients with an initial Glasgow Coma Scale score of 4 to 5 who were hyperventilated to a PaCO$_2$ of 25 mm Hg during the first days after head injury had significantly worse outcomes than patients kept at a PaCO$_2$ of 35 mm Hg.

Despite observations that hyperventilation reverses the clinical signs of herniation, there is no evidence that hyperventilation improves outcomes (10). In an observational study, 59 adult severe TBI patients who required RSI for intubation were matched to 177 historical nonintubated controls (11,12). The study used ETCO$_2$ monitoring and found an association between hypocapnia and mortality, and a statistically significant association between venti-latory rate and ETCO$_2$. Both the lowest and final ETCO$_2$ readings were associated with increased mortality versus matched controls. Although the study did not specifically iden-tify which if any of the patients demonstrated signs of herniation, it contributes to the grow-ing body of evidence arguing against hyperventilation under any circumstance in TBI patients, and this is likely analogous to patients with medically caused elevated ICP.

Based on the best available evidence, the following recommendations can be made:

- Hyperventilation (ETCO$_2$ <30–35) should be carefully avoided in patients with medical intracranial catastrophe or TBI who do not demonstrate signs of increased ICP ("blown pupil" or extensor posturing).
- There is no evidence that hyperventilation improves outcome in patients with ele-vated ICP, and there is some evidence that it causes harm. If hyperventilation is con-sidered, it should only be used briefly, as a temporizing measure, in the management of patients exhibiting signs of increased ICP who have failed to respond to osmotic agents.
- Intubated patients with TBI should have continuous ETCO$_2$ monitoring in order to avoid inadvertent hypocapnia (ETCO$_2$ <35).

There is a clear need for a well-controlled comparative study using a meaningful outcome measure to determine which, if any, of these interventions will decrease morbidity or mortality in patients with elevated ICP undergoing emergency RSI. Pending such a study, which will likely never be done because of logistical challenges, the approach outlined in Box 28-1 seems rational. Management of the patient at risk for elevated ICP should ensure cerebral perfusion and oxygenation. When intubation is indicated, pretreatment should be provided using lidocaine 1.5 mg/kg and fentanyl 3 μg/kg. There is insufficient evidence to support the use of a defasciculating agent. Once the patient is intubated, continuous ETCO$_2$ should be provided to safeguard against inadvertent hypocapnia and its associated increase in mortality.

REFERENCES

1. Abou-Madi MN, Keszler H, Yacoub JM. Cardiovascular reactions to laryngoscopy and tracheal intubation following small and large intravenous doses of lidocaine. *Can Anaesth Soc J* 1977;24:12–19.

2. Levitt M, Dresden G. The efficacy of esmolol versus lidocaine to attenuate the hemodynamic response to intubation in isolated head trauma patients. *Acad Emerg Med* 2001;8:19–24.

3. Helfman SM, Gold MI, DeLisser EA, et al. Which drug prevents tachycardia and hypertension associated with tracheal intubation: lidocaine, fentanyl, or esmolol? *Anesth Analg* 1991;72:482–486.

4. Singh H, Vichitvejpaisal P. Comparative effects of lidocaine, esmolol, and nitroglycerin in modifying the hemodynamic response to laryngoscopy and intubation. *J Clin Anesth* 1995;7:5–8.

5. Feng CK, Chan KH, Liu KN, et al. A comparison of lidocaine, fentanyl, and esmolol for attenuation of cardiovascular response to laryngoscopy and tracheal intubation. *Acta Anaesthesiol Sin* 1996;34:61–67.

6. Yosefy C, Hay E, Nasri Y, et al. End tidal carbon dioxide as a predictor of the arterial P$_{CO_2}$ in the emergency department setting. *Emerg Med J* 2004;21:557–559.

7. Raichle M, Plum F. Hyperventilation and cerebral blood flow. *Stroke* 1972;3:566–575.

8. Marion D, Darby J, Yonas H. Acute regional cerebral blood flow changes caused by severe head injuries. *J Neurosurg* 1991;74:407–414.

9. Muizelaar J, Marmarou A, Ward J, et al. Adverse effects of prolonged hyperventilation in patients with severe head injury: a randomized clinical trial. *J Neurosurg* 1991;75:731–739.

10. Brain Trauma Foundation. Guidelines for the management of severe traumatic brain injury, third edition. *J Neurotrauma* 2007;24(Suppl 1):S1–S108.

11. Davis DP, Dunford JV, Poste JC, et al. The impact of hypoxia and hyperventilation on outcome after paramedic rapid sequence intubation of severely head-injured patients. *J Trauma* 2004;57:1–10.

12. Davis DP, Dunford JV, Ochs M, et al. The use of quantitative end-tidal capnometry to avoid inadvertent severe hyperventilation in patients with head injury after paramedic rapid sequence intubation. *J Trauma* 2004;56:808–814.

29

Reactive Airways Disease

Bret P. Nelson and Andy S. Jagoda

THE CLINICAL CHALLENGE

There are a number of confounders that make airway management of the patient with asthma or chronic obstructive pulmonary disease (COPD) challenging. These patients often have difficult anatomy, are hypoxic, desaturate quickly, and can be hemodynamically unstable. Unlike many other clinical conditions, intubation itself does not resolve the primary problem, which is obstruction of the small airways. The actual intubation may be the easiest part of the resuscitative sequence because postintubation ventilation may be extremely difficult with persistent or worsening respiratory acidosis, barotrauma, or worsening hypotension caused by high intrathoracic pressures with diminished venous return. Thus, the decision to intubate must be made carefully, and the appropriate technique must be chosen to facilitate the best possible outcome.

Severe asthma often presents one of the most difficult airway management cases encountered in the emergency department. Diaphoresis is a particularly ominous sign, and the diaphoretic asthmatic patient who cannot speak full sentences, appears anxious, or is sitting upright and leaning forward to augment the inspiratory effort must not be left unattended until stabilized.

Standard initial management of acute severe asthma exacerbation includes reversal of dynamic bronchospasm using continuous beta$_2$-agonist nebulization therapy (albuterol 15–20 mg/hour) and anticholinergic nebulization therapy (ipratropium bromide 0.5 mg per dose). In addition, oral or intravenous (IV) steroids are indicated for the treatment of the inflammatory component. If the patient is severely bronchospastic and cannot comply with a nebulized treatment, subcutaneous epinephrine or terbutaline 0.2 to 0.5 mg may be of benefit. The use of IV terbutaline is controversial; however, if selected, it should be initiated in the adult at 4 μg/kg over 10 minutes followed by a continuous infusion of 0.1–0.4 μg/kg/min, and in the child at 10 μg/kg over 30 minutes followed by a continuous infusion of 0.1 μg/kg/minute. IV albuterol can be administered at 3 μg/kg over 10 minutes followed by an infusion of 0.04 to 0.2 μg/kg/minute in the adult. The addition of inhaled or IV anticholinergic agents (atropine or glycopyrrolate), IV magnesium sulfate, IV ketamine, or inhalational helium/oxygen mixture is controversial but may be of benefit (Fig. 29-1).

In COPD, much of the obstruction is fixed, comorbidity (especially cardiovascular disease) plays a greater role, and the prognosis (even with short-term mechanical ventilation) is worse. In the patient with COPD, anticholinergic therapy may be as important as beta$_2$-agonist therapy. Steroids are again important to attenuate underlying inflammation. Noninvasive ventilation (bilevel positive airway pressure [BL-PAP]) is of proven value in certain COPD patients and may help avoid intubation (see Chapter 38). By the time COPD patients have tired and require intubation, they have usually exhausted their catecholamine stores, are usually more hypoxic than one suspects clinically, and, like the asthmatic patient, present significant clinical challenges after intubation. There are recent reports in the literature of COPD patients in extremis who shortly after intubation became bradycardic and asystolic, and were unable to be resuscitated. The physiological explanation is not apparent. It is proposed that these patients are profoundly hypoxic before intubation, are volume depleted because of their work of breathing and their asthenic body habitus, and experience a relative sympathectomy after intubation. This condition vasodilates them globally, contributing to a decrease in cardiac output, which eventually results in cardiac arrest. These case reports, although of concern, do not reflect experience with the many COPD patients who are intubated annually and do not constitute scientific evidence regarding the incidence, cause, or treatment of this uncommon occurrence. As in the asthmatic patient, it is recommended that empiric incremental infusions of 500 mL of normal saline to a maximum of 1 to 2 L be started as soon as intubation is contemplated, and that atropine and catecholamine infusions be available before intubation.

There is no role for IV aminophylline in the management of either acute severe asthma or acute severe COPD exacerbation.

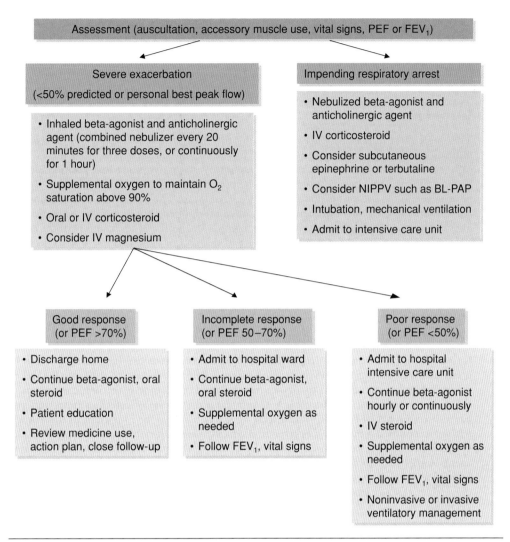

Figure 29-1 ● Approach to the Patient with Severe Asthma Exacerbation. *Source:* Adapted from National Heart, Lung, and Blood Institute, National Institutes of Health, National Asthma Education and Prevention Program. *Expert panel report 2: guidelines for the diagnosis and management of asthma.* NIH publication no. 97-4051. Bethesda, MD: U.S. Department of Health and Human Services; July 1972, and from the *Global Strategy for Asthma Management and Prevention*, Global Initiative for Asthma (GINA) 2006. Available from: http://www.ginasthma.org.

APPROACH TO THE AIRWAY

Despite this vast array of noninvasive treatment modalities, 1% to 3% of acute severe asthma exacerbations will require intubation. These patients are usually fatigued and have reduced functional residual capacity, so it is difficult (if not impossible) to preoxygenate them optimally, and rapid desaturation must be anticipated. Because most of these patients have been struggling to breathe against severe resistance, usually for hours, they have little if any residual physical reserve, and mechanical ventilation will be required. In fact, the need for mechanical ventilation is the indication for tracheal intubation; the airway itself is almost invariably patent and protected. This fact argues strongly against awake intubation techniques, such as blind nasotracheal intubation, which take longer, exacerbate hypoxemia, and carry higher complication rates and lower success rates than rapid sequence intubation (RSI).

Technique

The single most important tenet in managing the status asthmaticus patient who requires intubation is to take total control of the airway as expeditiously as possible. Patients typically adopt an upright posture as their respiratory status worsens; this position should be maintained as much as possible during the preintubation period. Preoxygenation should be achieved to the greatest extent possible (see Chapter 3). The RSI drugs chosen should be administered to the patient in their position of comfort, often sitting upright. As the patient loses consciousness, place the patient supine, position the head and neck, and perform laryngoscopy and intubation, preferably with an 8.0- to 9.0-mm endotracheal tube to decrease resistance and facilitate aggressive pulmonary toilette. If bag-mask ventilation is required because of desaturation before intubation is achieved, Sellick's maneuver may help prevent the passage of air down the esophagus, particularly in these patients, who have high pulmonary resistance to ventilation.

Drug Dosing and Administration

If time permits, patients with reactive airways disease or obstructive lung disease should be pretreated with 1.5 mg/kg of IV lidocaine 3 minutes before induction to attenuate the reflexive bronchospasm in response to airway manipulation. Ketamine is the induction agent of choice in the asthmatic patient because it stimulates the release of catecholamines and also has a direct bronchial smooth muscle relaxing effect that may be important in this clinical setting. Ketamine 1.5 mg/kg IV is given immediately before the administration of 1.5 mg/kg of succinylcholine. If ketamine is not available, any of the other commonly used induction agents (propofol, etomidate, midazolam) may be used, but the barbiturates should be avoided as they release histamine. For COPD patients, who often have concommitant cardiovascular disease, etomidate may be preferred to avoid the catecholanine stimulation of ketamine.

POSTINTUBATION MANAGEMENT

After the patient is successfully intubated and proper tube position has been confirmed, sedation, paralysis if needed (see Chapter 3), and meticulous ventilator management are critical in improving patient outcome. Continuous profound sedation (and amnesia) with an appropriate benzodiazepine, accompanied by fentanyl, in analgesic doses (4–6 μg/kg, repeated as necessary) may permit optimal ventilation of the patient. For many patients, paralysis using a competitive muscle relaxant for at least the first 4 to 6 hours will prevent asynchronous respirations, promote total relaxation of fatigued respiratory muscles, decrease the production of carbon dioxide, and allow optimum ventilator settings. Additional ketamine, as well as continuous inline albuterol and other pharmacological adjuncts, may also be given.

Mechanical Ventilation

All asthmatic patients have obstructed small airways and dynamic alveolar hyperinflation with varying amounts of end-expiratory residual intra-alveolar gas and pressure (auto-positive end expiratory pressure [PEEP] or intrinsic PEEP). Elevations in auto-PEEP increase the risk for baro/volutrauma. Reversal of airflow obstruction and decompression of end-expiratory filled alveoli are the primary goals of early mechanical ventilation in the asthmatic. The former requires prompt administration of IV steroids and continuous inline nebulization with beta$_2$-agonists until reversal is objectively measured (decrease in peak and plateau airway pressures) or unacceptable side effects are produced. Safe, uncomplicated alveolar decompression requires prolonged expiratory time (inspiration/expiration [I/E] ratio of 1:4–1:5), which is achieved by using smaller tidal volumes than usual, with a high inspiratory flow rate to shorten the inspiratory cycle time, permitting a longer expiratory phase. A general discussion of ventilation parameters can be found in Chapter 37.

The initial goal of ventilator therapy in the asthmatic patient is to improve arterial oxygen tension to adequate levels without inflicting barotrauma on the lungs or increasing auto-PEEP. Initial tidal volume should be reduced to 6 to 8 mL/kg to avoid barotrauma and air trapping. The speed at which a mechanical breath is delivered in liters per minute, typically 60 L/minute, is called the *inspiratory flow* (IF) *rate*. In asthma, the initial IF should be increased to 80 to 100 L/minute with a decelerating flow pattern. Pressure control is preferred to volume control because of the lower risk of barotrauma. If volume control is used, the operator should select the flow waveform to use ramp (decelerating) instead of square (constant). The ventilation rate should be determined in conjunction with the tidal volume, and an initial rate of 8 to 10 breaths per minute (bpm) with a high IF rate promote a prolonged expiratory phase that allows sufficient time for alveolar decompression. It is acceptable to permit the maintenance or gradual development of hypercapnia through reduced minute ventilation (the product of tidal volume and ventilatory rate) in the asthma or COPD patient because this approach reduces peak inspiratory pressure and thus minimizes the potential for barotrauma. High intrathoracic pressure may compromise cardiac output and produce hypotension; therefore, it is to be avoided.

The highest measured pressure at peak inspiration is the peak inspiratory pressure (PIP). The patient's lungs, chest wall, endotracheal tube, ventilatory circuit, ventilator, and mucus plugs all contribute to the PIP. This reading has an inconsistent predictive value for baro/volutrauma, but ideally should be kept under 50 cm H_2O. A sudden rise in PIP should be interpreted as indicating tube blockage, mucous plugging, or pneumothorax until proven otherwise. A sudden, dramatic fall in PIP may indicate extubation.

The measured intra-alveolar pressure during a 0.2- to 0.4-second end-inspiratory pause is referred to as the *plateau pressure* (P$_{plat}$). Values <30 cm H_2O are best and are not usually associated with baro/volutrauma. Measurement and trending of P$_{plat}$ is an excellent objective tool to confirm optimal ventilator settings and the patient's response, as well as the reversal of airflow obstruction. If initial ventilator settings disclose a P$_{plat}$ of more than 30 cm H_2O, consider lowering minute ventilation and increasing IF, both of which will prolong expiratory time and attenuate hyperinflation. If P$_{plat}$ is unavailable, PIP may be used as a surrogate.

Most status asthmaticus patients who require intubation are hypercapnic. The concept of controlled hypoventilation (permissive hypercapnia) promotes *gradual* development (over 3–4 hours) and maintenance of hypercapnia (P$_{CO_2}$ up to 90 mm Hg) and acidemia (pH as low as 7.2). This treatment is done primarily to decrease the risk of ventilator-related lung injury and prevent hemodynamic compromise as a result of increasing intrathoracic pressure from auto-PEEP or intrinsic PEEP. Permissive hypercapnia is usually accomplished by reducing minute ventilation, increasing inspiratory flow rate to 80 to 120 L/minute, and heavily sedating (and usually paralyzing) patients who otherwise would not tolerate these settings. Permissive hypercapnia may be instrumental in promoting prolonged expiratory times and reducing auto-PEEP.

Summary for Initial Ventilator Settings

1. Determine the patient's ideal body weight.
2. Set a tidal volume of 6 to 8 mL/kg with a F$_I$O$_2$ of 1.0 (100% oxygen).
3. Set a respiratory rate of 8 to 10 bpm.

4. Set an inspiratory-to-expiratory (I/E) ratio of 1:4 to 1:5. Pressure control is preferred. If using pressure control, the I/E ratio is adjusted directly by the I/E ratio parameter or by adjusting the inspiratory time parameter. If using volume control, the I/E ratio can be adjusted by increasing the peak flow rate, and the ramp inspiratory waveform should be selected. Peak inspiratory flow can be as high as 80 to 100 L/minute.

5. Measure and maintain the plateau pressure at <30 cm H_2O; try to keep PIP at <50 cm H_2O.

6. Focus on the oxygenation and pulmonary pressures initially. If necessary, allow maintenance or gradual development of hypercapnia to avoid high plateau pressures and increasing auto-PEEP.

7. Ensure continuous sedation and analgesia with a benzodiazepine and a nonhistamine releasing opioid, such as fentanyl, and consider paralysis with a nondepolarizing muscle relaxant if it is difficult to achieve ventilation goals (see Chapter 3).

8. Continue inline beta$_2$-agonist therapy and additional pharmacological adjunctive treatment based on the severity of the patient's illness and objective response to treatment.

Complications of Mechanical Ventilation

Two of the more common complications seen in mechanically ventilated asthmatic patients are lung injury (baro/volutrauma) and hypotension. Lung injury is exemplified by tension pneumothorax. In those patients without tension pneumothorax, hypotension is usually related to either absolute volume depletion or relative hypovolemia caused by decreased venous return from increasing auto-PEEP and intrathoracic pressure. The inherent risks of developing either one of these complications are directly related to the degree of pulmonary hyperinflation. Of the two, hypotension occurs much more frequently than tension pneumothorax. Most asthmatic patients will have intravascular volume depletion because of the increased work of breathing, decreased oral intake following the onset of asthmatic exacerbation, and generalized increased metabolic state. It is appropriate for these reasons to infuse up to 2 L of normal saline (NS) either before the initiation of RSI or early during mechanical ventilation.

The differential diagnosis for hypotension in the mechanically ventilated patient is discussed in Chapter 3. A trial of hypoventilation (apnea test) may be used to distinguish tension pneumothorax from volume depletion. The patient is disconnected from the ventilator and allowed to be apneic up to 1 minute as long as adequate oxygenation is ensured by pulse oximetry. In volume depletion, the mean intrathoracic pressure will fall quickly, blood pressure should begin to rise, pulse pressure will widen, and pulse rate will fall within 30 to 60 seconds. If auto-PEEP is high, reductions in tidal volume and increases in inspiratory flow and I/E times will be required to reduce auto-PEEP. If auto-PEEP is not an issue, then an empiric volume infusion of 500 mL NS should be instituted and may be repeated based on the patient's response to the additional volume. With tension pneumothorax, cardiopulmonary stability will not correct during the apnea time. This result should prompt the immediate insertion of bilateral chest tubes and re-evaluation of the patient. Obviously, lower ventilatory pressure settings will be required thereafter. The initial ventilator settings and potential ventilator complications of the asthma patient are shared by the COPD patient.

EVIDENCE

1. **Does lidocaine improve clinical outcomes when patients with status asthmaticus are intubated?** Intravenous lidocaine has been recommended in the literature to attenuate airway reflexes during intubation in patients with reactive airway disease (1,2). Stimulation of the airway in asthmatic patients is reported to result in bronchoconstriction, which is believed to be mediated via the vagus nerve (3). The recommendation to use IV lidocaine in RSI protocols for the severe asthmatic is extrapolated from the results

of studies using healthy volunteers with a history of bronchospastic disease (4–6). In one double-blind, placebo-controlled randomized study, volunteers who had a demonstrated decrease in forced expiratory volume (FEV_1) in response to histamine inhalation were shown to have a significant attenuation of response when pretreated with IV lidocaine (5). Unfortunately, there is also evidence that IV lidocaine does not protect against intubation-induced bronchoconstriction in asthma. In a prospective randomized double-blind, placebo-controlled trial of 60 patients, lidocaine and placebo groups were not different in their transpulmonary pressure and airflow immediately after intubation and at 5-minute intervals (7). The same study evaluated inhaled albuterol (four puffs from a metered dose inhaler [MDI] 20 minutes before intubation), which showed significant mitigation of intubation-induced bronchospasm. There are no studies that have demonstrated that premedicating with IV lidocaine in RSI changes outcome; conversely, there is no evidence that premedication with IV lidocaine is harmful. Until better data are available, it seems reasonable to minimize the risk of intubation-induced bronchoconstriction by using lidocaine premedication in the asthmatic.

2. **Do inhaled anticholinergics improve outcomes in acute reactive airways disease when compared to inhaled beta-agonists alone?** The bronchodilatory effects of anticholinergic agents are well known, but there has been controversy over whether these agents act synergistically with beta-agonists in the setting of acute bronchospasm. A recent meta-analysis of the role of ipratropium bromide in the emergency management of acute asthma exacerbation concluded that there is a modest benefit when it is used in conjunction with beta-agonists (8). Thirty-two randomized controlled trials enrolling 3,611 subjects were included. The use of inhaled anticholinergics was associated with reduced hospital admissions in adults and children, as well as improved spirometric parameters within 2 hours of treatment. For severe asthma exacerbations, the number needed to treat to prevent one admission was 7 for adults and 14 for children. The meta-analysis recommended the use of inhaled ipratropium bromide because the benefit appears to outweigh any risks. In addition, pooled data suggest that multiple doses convey more benefit than single-dose regimens. A recent prospective, double-blind, randomized controlled trial examined the benefit of adding continuous nebulized ipratropium bromide to a continuous albuterol nebulization (9). In this study, the addition of ipratropium bromide was not found to improve peak expiratory flow rate (PEFR) or admission rates compared to albuterol alone in a total of 62 enrolled patients. Theoretically, in status asthmaticus where inhaled agents have limited delivery, IV anticholinergic agents may have benefit (10). However, other than case reports, there is no evidence at this time supporting their use. There is strong evidence for the long-term use of anticholinergic agents in the routine management of COPD (11–14). Use in acute exacerbations has been less well studied; a Cochrane Database review summarized four studies comparing inhaled albuterol with ipratropium bromide in the setting of acute COPD exacerbation (15). Pooled data from these studies (129 total patients) demonstrated no difference in FEV_1 at 1 hour or 24 hours between the albuterol and ipratropium bromide groups. The addition of ipratropium bromide to albuterol did not yield any benefit over albuterol alone. Despite this relative paucity of evidence, the American Thoracic Society and European Respiratory Society (16) and the Global Initiative for Chronic Obstructive Lung Disease (17) advocate the use of inhaled ipratropium in acute COPD exacerbations. Thus, based on available evidence, anticholinergic agents should be used in acute asthmatic patients as standard therapy and should be considered in the treatment of acute COPD exacerbations, especially when little improvement is seen with beta-agonists alone.

3. **Does the use of IV magnesium improve outcomes in patients with acute asthma?** Magnesium plays a role in smooth muscle relaxation, and recent research has focused on the role of this medication in alleviating bronchospasm. Several meta-analyses have examined the role of magnesium in acute asthma (18,19). Pooled data do not demonstrate significant improvement in PEFR or admission rates with the

administration of IV magnesium. However, in a subgroup analysis of patients with severe asthma (defined as PEFR of 25% to 30% of predicted for adults or failure to improve beyond 60% predicted after 1 hour of care for children), IV magnesium improved PEFR by 9.8% predicted and reduced hospital admission rates. There is no good evidence that in severe asthma, magnesium decreases the need for intubation. Recently, a systematic review examining the role of nebulized magnesium demonstrated a benefit in pulmonary function in severe asthma (20). No benefit (vs. standard therapy) was seen in less severe cases, and no subgroup experienced a decreased rate of hospital admission. Based on these data, IV magnesium therapy should be considered as adjunctive therapy only in selected cases of severe asthma.

4. **Are there any noninvasive ventilatory strategies that may improve respiratory status in acute asthma?** Noninvasive positive-pressure ventilation has demonstrated a bronchodilatory effect in methacholine-induced bronchospasm (21,22), and it has been postulated that the addition of positive pressure may offset intrinsic PEEP and decrease work of breathing. However, few studies have examined the role of noninvasive positive-pressure ventilation in the setting of acute asthma. In a prospective, randomized cross-over study of 20 pediatric intensive care unit (ICU) admissions, BL-PAP use for 2 hours decreased respiratory rate, accessory muscle use, wheeze, and dyspnea (23). A 2003 emergency department study randomized 15 adult patients to BL-PAP and 15 to standard therapy for a 3-hour treatment period (24). The BL-PAP group demonstrated fewer hospital admissions, improved respiratory rate, and improved PEFR and FEV_1. There were no cases in either study of pneumothorax. Based on these limited data, it would be reasonable to consider BL-PAP for more severe cases of acute asthma, when immediate intubation does not appear to be required.

5. **Is there a role for heliox in the management of acute asthma or COPD exacerbations?** In obstructive lung disease with bronchospasm, increased turbulent flow through proximal airways decreases airflow and may contribute to increased work of breathing. Heliox, with a lower density than air-oxygen mixtures, has been believed to decrease turbulent flow and could increase carriage of nebulized medications to distal airways. A recent systematic review examined controlled studies of acute asthma and COPD exacerbations (25). For asthma, heliox-driven nebulizers improved PEFR in pooled data from two studies. No differences in admission rates were found. Heliox was found in a single study to improve PEFR when used as a breathing gas in intubated asthmatics. In COPD, heliox-driven nebulizers did not change PEFR compared with controls. When used in conjunction with noninvasive ventilation, heliox did not improve Pco_2, change intubation rates, or decrease length of stay in the ICU. There was a decreased overall hospital length of stay in the heliox group, however. In intubated COPD patients, heliox used as a breathing gas demonstrated a reduction in intrinsic PEEP of 2.2 cm H_2O compared to controls and improved work of breathing, but did not affect other outcomes. There is one case series of seven intubated patients with elevated airway pressures who had remarkable improvement with a 60 to 40 helium/oxygen mixture; however, this is a case series and thus suffers from inherent bias, precluding recommendations (26). At this time, there is insufficient evidence of outcome benefit to justify the cost and complexity of heliox administration.

6. **Is IV ketamine of benefit in severe asthma?** Theoretically, ketamine is a logical choice in managing the airway of the severe asthmatic because it increases circulating catecholamines, it is a direct smooth muscle dilator, it inhibits vagal outflow, and it does not cause histamine release (27). However, there are no good controlled studies demonstrating the benefit of IV ketamine in the management of the nonintubated asthmatic. Case reports of dramatic improvement in pulmonary function with ketamine have driven its popularity (28,29), but no randomized studies have been performed to demonstrate ketamine's superiority over other agents. In a case series, 19 of 22 actively wheezing

asthmatics had a decrease in bronchospasm during ketamine-induced anesthesia (30). In one prospective double-blind, placebo-controlled trial of 14 mechanically ventilated patients with bronchospasm, the 7 patients treated with ketamine (1 mg/kg) had a significant improvement in oxygenation but no improvement in Pco_2 or lung compliance. Outcome (discharge from the ICU) was the same in both groups. The study population was heterogeneous, making conclusions of the benefit of ketamine difficult at best (31). A randomized double-blind, placebo-controlled trial of low-dose IV ketamine, 0.2 mg/kg bolus, followed by an infusion of 0.5 mg/kg/hour in nonintubated adult patients with acute asthma failed to demonstrate a benefit from IV ketamine (32). The incidence of dysphoric reactions led the investigators to decrease the bolus to 0.1 mg/kg. Recently, a double-blind, placebo-controlled study randomized 33 pediatric asthma patients to ketamine infusion (0.2 mg/kg bolus, followed by 0.5 mg/hour for 2 hours) and 35 patients to placebo (33). Each group also received albuterol, ipratropium bromide, and glucocorticoids. No significant difference in pulmonary index scores (comprised of respiratory rate, wheeze, I/E ratio, accessory muscle use, and oxygen saturation) were found between the two groups. No difference in hospitalization rate was noted. At the present time, based on its mechanism of action and safety profile, ketamine appears to be the best agent available for RSI in the asthmatic. In the absence of ketamine, other agents may be used. There is insufficient evidence to support the use of IV ketamine as adjunctive therapy in nonventilated patients.

REFERENCES

1. Walls RM. Lidocaine and rapid sequence intubation. *Ann Emerg Med* 1996;27:528–529.
2. Gal T. Bronchial hyperresponsiveness and anesthesia: physiologic and therapeutic perspectives. *Anesth Analg* 1994;78:559–573.
3. Gold M. Anesthesia, bronchospasm, and death. *Semin Anesth* 1989;8:291–306.
4. Groeben H, Foster W, Brown R. Intravenous lidocaine and oral mexiletine block reflex bronchoconstriction in asthmatic subjects. *Am J Respir Crit Care Med* 1997;156:1703–1704.
5. Groeben H, Silvanus M, Beste M, et al. Both intravenous and inhaled lidocaine attenuate reflex bronchoconstriction but at different plasma concentrations. *Am J Respir Crit Care Med* 1999;159:530–535.
6. Downes H, Gerber N, Hirshman C. IV lignocaine in reflex and allergic bronchoconstriction. *Br J Anaesth* 1980;52:873–880.
7. Maslow A, Regan M, Israel E, et al. Inhaled albuterol, but not intravenous lidocaine, protects against intubation-induced bronchoconstriction in asthma. *Anesthesiology* 2000;93:1198–1204.
8. Rodrigo GJ, Castro-Rodriguez JA. Anticholinergics in the treatment of children and adults with acute asthma: a systematic review with meta-analysis. *Thorax* 2005;60:740–746.
9. Salo D, Tuel M, Lavery R, et al. A randomized, clinical trial comparing the efficacy of continuous nebulized albuterol (15 mg) verus continuous nebulized albuterol (15 mg) plus ipratropium bromide (2 mg) for the treatment of asthma. *J Emerg Med* 2006;31(4):371–376.
10. Slovis C, Daniels G, Wharton D. Intravenous use of glycopyrrolate in acute respiratory distress due to bronchospastic pulmonary disease. *Ann Emerg Med* 1987;16:898–900.
11. Vincken W, van Noord JA, Greefhorst AP. Improved health outcomes in patients with COPD during 1 yr's treatment with tiotropium. *Eur Respir J* 2002;19:205–206.
12. Donohue JF, van Noord JA, Batemane ED, et al. A 6-month, placebo-controlled study comparing lung function and health status changes in COPD patients treated with tiotropium and salmeterol. *Chest* 2002;122:47–55.

13. Donohue JF, Menojoge S, Kesten S. Tolerance to bronchodilating effects of salmeterol in COPD. *Respir Med* 2003;97:1014–1020.

14. Ringback T, Viskum K. Is there any association between inhaled ipratropium and mortality in patients with COPD and asthma? *Respir Med* 2003;97:264–272.

15. McCrory DC, Brown CD. Anticholinergic bronchodilators versus beta$_2$-sympathomimetic agents for acute exacerbations of chronic obstructive pulmonary disease. *Cochrane Database Syst Rev* 2003;(1):CD003900.

16. Celli BR, MacNee W, ATS/ERS Task Force. Standards for the diagnosis and treatment of patients with COPD: a summary of the ATS/ERS position paper. *Eur Respir J* 2004;23(6): 932–946.

17. Global Strategy for Diagnosis, Management and Prevention of COPD – 2006 Executive Summary. Available from http://www.goldcopd.com.

18. Alter H, Koopsell T, Hilty W. Intravenous magnesium as an adjuvant in acute bronchospasm: a meta-analysis. *Ann Emerg Med* 2000;36:191–197.

19. Rowe B, Bretzlaff J, Bourdon C, et al. Intravenous magnesium sulfate treatment for acute asthma in the emergency department: a systemic review of the literature. *Ann Emerg Med* 2000;36:181–190.

20. Blitz M, Blitz S, Beasely R, et al. Inhaled magnesium sulfate in the treatment of acute asthma. *Cochrane Database Syst Rev* 2005;(4):CD003898.

21. Wang, CH, Lin, HC, Huang, TJ, et al. Differential effects of nasal continuous positive airway pressure on reversible or fixed upper and lower airway obstruction. *Eur Respir J* 1996;9:952–959.

22. Lin, HC, Wang, CH, Yang, CT, et al. Effect of nasal continuous positive airway pressure on methacholine-induced bronchoconstriction. *Respir Med* 1995;89:121–128.

23. Thill PJ, McGuire JK, Baden HP, et al. Noninvasive positive-pressure ventilation in children with lower airway obstruction. *Pediatr Crit Care Med* 2004;5(4):337–342.

24. Soroksky A, Stav D, Shpirer I. A pilot prospective, randomized, placebo-controlled trial of bilevel positive airway pressure in acute asthmatic attack. *Chest* 2003;123:1018–1025.

25. Colebourn CL, Barber V, Young JD. Use of helium-oxygen mixture in adult patients presenting with exacerbations of asthma and chronic obstructive pulmonary disease: a systematic review. *Anaesthesia* 2007;62:34–42.

26. Gluck E, Onorato D, Castriotta R. Helium-oxygen mixtures in intubated patients with status asthmaticus and respiratory acidosis. *Chest* 1990;98:693–698.

27. Huber F, Reeves J, Gutierrez J, et al. Ketamine: its effect on airway resistance in man. *South Med J* 1972;65:1176–1180.

28. Hommedieu C, Arens J. The use of ketamine for the emergency intubation of patients with status asthmaticus. *Ann Emerg Med* 1987;16:568–571.

29. Rock M, de la Roca S, Hommedieu C, et al. Use of ketamine in asthmatic children to treat respiratory failure refractory to conventional therapy. *Crit Care Med* 1986;14:514–516.

30. Corssen G, Gutierrez J, Reves J, et al. Ketamine in the anesthetic management of asthmatic patients. *Anesth Analg* 1972;51:588–596.

31. Hemmingsen C, Nielsen P, Odorica J. Ketamine in the treatment of bronchospasm during mechanical ventilation. *Am J Emerg Med* 1994;12:417–420.

32. Howton J, Rose J, Duffy S, et al. Randomized, double-blind, placebo-controlled trial of intravenous ketamine in acute asthma. *Ann Emerg Med* 1996;27:170–175.

33. Allen JY, Macias CG. The efficacy of ketamine in pediatric emergency department patients who present with acute severe asthma. *Ann Emerg Med* 2005;46(1):43–50.

30

Distorted Airways and Acute Upper Airway Obstruction

Michael F. Murphy and Richard D. Zane

THE CLINICAL CHALLENGE

Anatomically, the term *upper airway* refers to that portion of the anatomy that extends from the lips and nares to the first tracheal ring. Thus, the first portion of the upper airway is redundant: a nasal pathway and an oral pathway. However, at the level of the oropharynx, the two pathways merge and redundancy is lost. The most common, life-threatening causes of acute upper airway distortion and obstruction occur in the region of this common channel and are typically laryngeal. In addition, disorders of the base of the tongue and the pharynx can cause obstruction (Box 30-1). This chapter deals with problems that distort or obstruct the upper airway. Foreign bodies in the upper airway are dealt with in Chapter 36.

APPROACH TO THE AIRWAY

The signs of upper airway distortion and obstruction may be occult or subtle. Deadly deterioration may occur suddenly and unexpectedly. Seemingly innocuous interventions, such as small doses of sedative hypnotic agents to alleviate anxiety or the use of topical local anesthetic agents, may precipitate sudden and total airway obstruction. Rescue devices may not be successful and may even be contraindicated in some circumstances. The goal in these patients is to proceed rapidly in a sensible, controlled manner to manage the airway before complete airway obstruction occurs.

When should an Intervention be Performed?

Chapter 1 deals with the important question of when to intubate. If airway obstruction is severe, progressive, or potentially imminent, then immediate action (often cricothyrotomy) is required without further consideration of moving the patient to another venue (e.g., the operating room, another hospital). Failing such an indication for an *immediate* cricothyrotomy, the question becomes more difficult: What is the expected clinical course?

BOX 30-1 Causes of Upper Airway Obstruction

A. Infectious
   a. Viral and bacterial laryngotracheobronchitis (e.g., croup)
   b. Parapharyngeal and retropharyngeal abscesses
   c. Lingual tonsillitis (a lingual tonsil is a rare but real congenital anomaly and a well-recognized cause of failed intubation)
   d. Infections, hematomas, or abscesses of the tongue or floor of the mouth (e.g., Ludwig's angina)
   e. Epiglottitis (also known as supraglottitis)
B. Neoplastic
   a. Laryngeal carcinomas
   b. Hypopharyngeal and lingual (tongue) carcinomas
C. Physical and chemical agents
   a. Foreign bodies
   b. Thermal injuries (heat and cold)
   c. Caustic injuries (acids and alkalis)
   d. Inhaled toxins
D. Allergic/idiopathic: including angiotensin-converting enzyme inhibitor–induced angioedema
E. Traumatic: blunt and penetrating neck and upper airway trauma

Penetrating wounds to the neck and airway are notoriously unpredictable (see Chapter 27). Some advocate securing the airway regardless of warning signs, whereas others advocate expectant observation. There are substantial problems with the second strategy. The first is that the patient often remains relatively asymptomatic until they suddenly and unexpectedly totally obstruct, resulting in an airway (and patient) that cannot be rescued. The second is that unless fiberoptic scopes are used, the observer is only able to see the anterior portion of the airway and not the posterior and inferior parts where the obstruction will likely occur. In other words, when not using fiberoptics, one can see only "the tip of the iceberg."

Thus, for any condition where the obstruction may be progressive, silent, and unobservable externally (e.g., angioedema, vascular injuries in the neck, epiglottitis), acting earlier to secure the airway rather than later is the most prudent course.

There are three cardinal signs of acute upper airway obstruction:
- "Hot potato" voice: the muffled voice one often hears in patients with mononucleosis and very large tonsils
- Difficulty in swallowing secretions, either because of pain or obstruction; the patient is typically sitting up, leaning forward, and spitting or drooling secretions
- Stridor

The first two signs do not necessarily suggest that total upper airway obstruction is imminent; however, stridor does. The patient presenting with stridor has already lost at least 50% of the airway caliber and requires immediate intervention. In the case of children younger than 8 to 10 years with croup, medical therapy may suffice. In older children and adults, the presence of stridor typically mandates a surgical airway or, at the least, a double setup. This technique uses an awake attempt (e.g., using ketamine sedation) from above with the capability, prepared in advance, to move to a surgical airway if needed. Positive pressure by bag and mask or other noninvasive ventilatory devices has been described as one method to help open an obstructed airway and may buy some time; however, this technique should not be relied on as more than a temporizing maneuver.

What Options Exist if the Airway Deteriorates or Obstructs?

The answer to this question needs to incorporate the following when considering alternatives to cricothyrotomy:
- *Will rescue bag-mask ventilation (BMV) be possible?* Will a mask seal be possible to achieve, or is the lower face disrupted? Has a penetrating neck wound entered the airway rendering it incompetent to high airway pressures? As discussed in Chapter 5, the bag and mask devices most commonly used in resuscitation settings are capable of generating 50 to 100 cm of water pressure in the upper airway, provided that they do not have positive-pressure relief valves and that an adequate mask seal can be obtained. Pediatric and neonatal devices often incorporate positive-pressure relief valves that easily can be defeated if needed. This degree of positive pressure is often sufficient to overcome the moderate degree of upper airway obstruction caused by redundant tissue (e.g., the obese), edematous tissue (e.g., angioedema, croup, epiglottitis), or laryngospasm. Lesions that are hard and fixed, such as hematomas, abscesses, cancers, and foreign bodies, produce an obstruction that cannot be reliably overcome with bag-mask ventilation, even with high upper airway pressures.
- *Where is the airway problem?* If the lesion is at the level of the face or oral and nasal pharynx and orotracheal intubation is judged to be impossible (for whatever reason), but there is oral access, then supralaryngeal rescue devices such as laryngeal mask airways (LMAs), King LTs, and Combitubes may be considered and ought to be immediately at hand to attempt rescue of the airway.

What are the Advantages and Risks of an Awake Look?

In most instances, unless the patient is in crisis or deteriorating rapidly, an awake direct laryngoscopy is possible. If the tip of the epiglottis is visible without paralysis (grade 3 view) and is in the midline, orotracheal intubation employing rapid sequence intubation (RSI) is probably possible, especially when using a bougie, unless the working diagnosis is a primary laryngeal disorder. However, it has been shown that this maneuver is not failsafe in that the airway rarely may be more difficult to visualize in some patients after induction and paralysis. If a primary laryngeal disorder is suspected, complete visualization of the larynx is mandatory (e.g., fiber-optic visualization). Attempting direct laryngoscopy in an awake, uncooperative patient with a laryngeal disorder is potentially dangerous and ill advised.

Is RSI Reasonable?

If one is confident that orotracheal intubation is possible and highly confident that the patient can be successfully ventilated using BMV or some other device, then it is reasonable to proceed with RSI (e.g., early in the course of a penetrating neck injury). A double setup with readiness for a surgical airway is still advised. Even then, in patients with occult upper airway obstruction, some would say that RSI is not considered advisable, and a controlled, urgent surgical or fiber-optic airway is appropriate, especially if patient cooperation and time are limited. One's degree of confidence in being able to secure an airway is multifactorial and depends highly on experience, the clinical practice environment and armamentarium of airway devices. These airway problems underscore the importance of securing alternative airway devices, such as the fiberoptic bronchoscope or video laryngoscope, in addition to a conventional laryngoscope and bougie. Practicing alone off-hours with only a direct laryngoscope is obviously very different than having access to these advanced devices and consultative backup.

TIPS AND PEARLS

- Be reluctant to transfer patients with suspected acute upper airway obstruction and unsecured airways, even short distances. Always secure the airways of patients with significant acute penetrating neck wounds or blunt laryngeal trauma before transport.
- Angioedema involving the upper airway is a dangerous and unpredictable condition. The external examination of the lips, tongue, and pharynx tell you little of what is going on at the level of the airway. Intervention earlier rather than later is the most prudent course of action. Often, flexible fiberoptic nasopharyngoscopy will provide the additional information that is needed.
- The patient with acute upper airway obstruction, a disrupted airway, or a distorted airway who *can* protect and maintain the airway and *can* maintain oxygenation and ventilation should always be considered a *difficult airway*, and the difficult airway algorithm should be used.
- The patient with upper airway obstruction, a disrupted airway, or a distorted airway who *cannot* maintain oxygenation or ventilation should be considered a *failed airway*, and the failed airway algorithm should be used.
- Blind techniques (e.g., blind nasotracheal intubation) of airway management in these situations are contraindicated and should not be attempted.
- Bag-mask ventilation alone cannot be relied on to rescue the airway, particularly if the obstruction is caused by a fixed lesion.
- RSI is usually contraindicated unless the awake look proves otherwise or the RSI is done early after onset of the disease or injury.
- Contemplate a cricothyrotomy early and prepare for it before the awake look.
- Titrate ketamine rather than sedative/hypnotic drugs (e.g., midazolam, propofol, thiopental, etomidate) to get an adequate awake look. Topical anesthesia of the airway will not be particularly successful and will not be adequate unless accompanied by sedation.
- If the awake look indicates that orotracheal intubation is not possible or is equivocal, proceed directly to a cricothyrotomy or fiberoptic intubation.

- If the patient suddenly crashes and the lesion is above the level of the larynx, do two-handed BMV and try an extraglottic airway device while setting up for a cricothyrotomy. If the lesion is at the larynx, do two-handed bag-mask ventilation and proceed immediately to a cricothyrotomy.
- Heliox may buy time. Helium is less dense than nitrogen, reducing turbulent flow and resistance through tight orifices, as is the case with some causes of upper airway obstruction. The commercial preparations are usually 80% helium and 20% oxygen, and provided lung function is adequate, this mix will produce acceptable oxygen saturations. Other concentrations may be prepared.
- Crush injuries to the larynx and laryngeal fractures are best managed with tracheostomy rather than cricothyrotomy. Gently performed RSI or fiberoptic intubation may be advisable if circumstances permit.
- In the event of a tracheal separation (e.g., clothesline-type injury to the neck) when one is performing a surgical airway, grasp the distal stump with an instrument before opening the pretracheal fascia.
- The patient with a bulky pharyngeal or laryngeal tumor may be intubated using a fiberoptic technique. Although this technique typically requires more time to perform, it is preferable to surgically invading an airway that may hemorrhage or be subject to subsequent operative resection.

EVIDENCE

1. **Is there much in the way of evidence relating to the emergency management of patients with acute upper airway obstruction?** The evidence with respect to the emergency management of the patient with an airway that is potentially or actually disrupted, distorted, or obstructed is essentially anecdotal. Most of the information dealing with the topic comes either from the surgical or anesthesia literature: primarily small series or case reports. There are no controlled studies comparing intervention with expectant observation. In the surgical literature, cricothyrotomy, as might be expected, is typically overrecommended. In the anesthesia literature, intubation under deep inhalation anesthesia and spontaneous ventilation has been the standard and, as might be expected, cricothyrotomy is underrecommended. Despite the lack of scientifically sound studies, the following additional reading is recommended (1–5).

2. **How commonly does angiotensin-converting enzyme inhibitor (ACEI)–induced angioedema require intubation?** The clinical course of ACEI-induced angioedema is extremely unpredictable, and life-threatening presentations requiring airway interventions are reported in up to 20% of these patients (6–10). According to the literature, 0% to 22.2% of patients with angioedema will require intubation (11). It is extremely difficult to predict which patients who present with a stable airway will progress to a requirement for airway intervention. Researchers from Boston (11) retrospectively analyzed cases of ACEI-related angioedema and determined that increasing age and oral cavity/oropharyngeal involvement predicted the need for airway intervention. These predictors had a sensitivity of 65.2% and specificity of 83.7%. The clinical course of angioedema, especially ACEI induced, is unpredictable. It is recommended that these patients be admitted for close monitoring for at least 24 hours.

3. **Do adult patients who present with stridor secondary to epiglottitis require immediate airway management?** Since the advent of the *Haemophilus influenzae* vaccine, epiglottitis has now become a largely adult disease. Most cases of adult epiglottitis are secondary to other infectious etiologies (12), and many patients have an underlying anatomical abnormality such as cancer or surgery. Even though most adult patients with epiglottitis can be managed conservatively, the presence of stridor is ominous and is a predictor of the need for airway management (13).

REFERENCES

1. Crosby E, Reid D. Acute epiglottitis in the adult: is intubation mandatory? *Can J Anaesth* 1991;38:914–918.

2. Donald PJ. Emergency management of the patient with upper airway obstruction. *Clin Rev Allergy* 1985;3:25–36.

3. Halvorson DJ, Merritt RM, Mann C, et al. Management of subglottic foreign bodies. *Ann Otol Rhinol Laryngol* 1996;105:541–544.

4. Jacobson S. Upper airway obstruction. *Emerg Med Clin North Am* 1989;7:205–217.

5. Tong MC, Chu MC, Leighton SE, et al. Adult croup. *Chest* 1996;109:1659–1662.

6. Kaplan AP, Greaves MW. Angioedema. *J Am Acad Dermatol* 2005;23:373–388.

7. Kostis JB, Kim HJ, Rasnak J, et al. Incidence and characteristics of angioedema associated with enalapril. *Arch Intern Med* 2005;165:1637–1642.

8. Reid M. Angioedema. April 26, 2006. Available at: http://www.emedicine. com/med/topic135.htm.

9. Roberts JR, Wuerz RC. Clinical characteristics of angiotensin-converting enzyme inhibitor-induced angioedema. *Ann Emerg Med* 1991;20:555–558.

10. Thompson T, Frable MA. Drug-induced, life-threatening angioedema revisited. *Laryngoscope* 1993;103:10–12.

11. Zirkle M, Bhattacharyya N. Predictors of airway intervention in angioedema of the head and neck. *Otolaryngol Head Neck Surg* 2000;123:240–245.

12. Roscoe DL. Microbiologic investigations for head and neck infections. *Infect Dis Clin North Am* 2007;21(2):283–304.

13. Frantz TD. Acute epiglottitis in adults: analysis of 129 cases. *JAMA* 1994;272(17):1358–1360.

31

The Critically Ill Patient

Michael F. Murphy, Stephen Beed, and Ron M. Walls

THE CLINICAL CHALLENGE

Airway management of the critically ill patient, whether in the intensive care unit (ICU), the emergency department, or elsewhere is characterized by the following:

1. The physical environment often presents patient access and positioning challenges.
2. The airways of critically ill patients are frequently characterized as "difficult."
3. The patients have limited "physiological reserve"; they poorly tolerate airway manipulation and the medications employed to facilitate airway management.
4. Knowing when and how to extubate is challenging.
5. An array of routine and rescue airway management equipment is often unavailable.

Physicians who practice in the emergency department or ICU environment, or who respond to airway emergencies in inpatient units, must be prepared to deal with the challenges listed above. This chapter emphasizes the ICU environment, but the principles apply equally, regardless of the patient's physical location within the health care system.

APPROACH TO THE AIRWAY

The Physical Environment

The American College of Critical Care Medicine describes three echelons of ICUs, all of which demand expertise in airway management:

1. A level one center provides multidisciplinary, comprehensive care and is typically located in a large urban hospital environment affiliated with an academic medical center.
2. A level two center provides comprehensive care, although not all disciplines may be accessible.
3. A level three center provides limited intensive care support and stabilization of the critically ill patient.

In addition to the psychological stress associated with the "crisis-like atmosphere" that colors most airway management events in the ICU, the physical environment of the ICU presents additional challenges to the airway manager. For example, physical barriers, such as mechanical ventilators, monitors, infusion pumps, dialysis machines, and intravenous lines can make it difficult even to get to the head of the bed. Specialized apparatus for patient care (e.g., air beds, cervical spine collars, orthopedic frames) in an already overcrowded environment also contribute to the difficulty in accessing the airway or positioning the patient for airway management, particularly in an emergency. Space limitations may make it difficult for other members of the resuscitation team to access the patient. Finally, finding room for the equipment needed for airway management, such as the difficult airway cart and the bronchoscopy cart, can be a challenge.

Difficult Airways in the ICU

There are several dimensions to this issue:

- The skills and abilities of the practitioner as they relate to airway management
- The stress of the environment
- The physical barriers to care
- The effects of compromised physiological reserve on the choices of medications used in managing the airway
- An increased incidence of difficult mask ventilation, laryngoscopy and intubation, and cricothyrotomy; in addition, successful rescue with an extraglottic device is less likely

Although many intensive care practitioners have significant expertise in airway management, not all "intensivists" are airway experts. Varying routes of entry to critical care medicine (e.g., internal medicine, surgery, anesthesia, pediatrics, emergency medicine) result in intensivists with varying skill levels and comfort with airway management, especially for this challenging patient population.

Considered as a population, critically ill patients requiring airway management are prone to difficulty in each of the four dimensions of the difficult airway discussed in Chapter 7:

1. Bag-mask ventilation is more difficult due to several factors: upper airway edema associated with prior intubation or the underlying condition is more common, these patients tend to be older and more obese, and they suffer increased airways resistance and reduced pulmonary compliance.
2. Laryngoscopy and intubation difficulty may be encountered due to a limited capacity to preoxygenate; increased incidence of anatomical abnormalities such as airway edema as noted previously; and neck immobilization in the case of trauma victims.
3. Cricothyrotomy is made more difficult by the width of the ICU bed and, often, access to the neck or the ability to position the neck appropriately.
4. Rescue with extraglottic devices is more challenging due to a variety of factors, particularly increased airway resistance and reduced pulmonary compliance in these patient populations.

Physiological Reserve

As described in Chapters 4 and 8, the larynx is the most heavily innervated sensory structure in the body. Laryngoscopy and endotracheal intubation stimulate these sensory organs and produce adverse physiological effects. The intensity of these physiological responses is related to the intensity of stimulation, which in turn depends on the duration of laryngoscopy, the aggressiveness of laryngoscopy, the degree of attendant hypoxemia/hypercarbia, stimulation of the carina by the endotracheal tube (ETT), and the device used. These stimuli, if unchecked, have the potential to produce significant responses and, potentially, adverse end-organ consequences. Depending on which organ systems are involved in a particular critically ill patient, the following organ system responses to endotracheal intubation may be the most important to consider:

- Increased intracranial pressure (ICP) and cerebral blood flow, particularly if autoregulation is disturbed
- Increased airways resistance
- The autonomic nervous system
  - Adrenergic responses: Endotracheal intubation causes increased adrenergic activity with activation of the sympathetic nervous system and elevated circulating catecholamines. This in turn results in
    - An increased systolic blood pressure and mean arterial pressure (up to two times normal)
    - Increased diastolic blood pressure (up to 50% increase)
    - Increased heart rate (up to 50% increase)
    - Increased cardiac work and myocardial oxygen consumption
    - Ventricular dysrhythmias (increased automaticity/irritability due to increased circulating catecholamines and increased blood pressure)
    - Decreased gastric emptying (increased gastric volume and risk of aspiration)
    - Decreased gut motility (ileus)
  - Cholinergic responses:
    - Bronchoconstriction and bronchorrhea
    - Bradycardia: rarely but occasionally in children and infants, especially if hypoxemic

---

BOX 31-1 High-Risk Conditions

- Upper airway and respiratory system
  - Reactive airways disease
- Cardiovascular system
  - Major vessel aneurysm rupture (congenital, traumatic, or atherosclerotic)
  - Aortic or major vessel dissection and rupture
  - Ischemic heart disease
  - Left ventricular (LV) systolic or diastolic dysfunction ("failure") from any etiology (e.g., ischemic, hypertensive, congestive)
  - Valvular heart disease: stenotic lesions limit the heart's ability to provide an adequate cardiac output to meet the needs of the body; regurgitant lesions may see increased retrograde flow in the face of increased systemic vascular resistance (SVR)
  - L to R shunts (e.g., ventricular septal defect) will increase as SVR and LV systolic pressure increase
  - Cor pulmonale: the stress of intubation increases pulmonary vascular resistance and, in the face of cor pulmonale, may produce acute right heart failure
  - Ventricular and atrial arrhythmias may be induced
- Brain
  - Patients with intracranial hypertension or increased intracranial pressure

Box 31-1 lists the most important underlying conditions that place the patient at higher risk of adverse effects.

Both nonpharmacological and pharmacological approaches can be used to mitigate or prevent adverse physiological responses to intubation in these patients. The nonpharmacological methods include limiting the intensity (rigor) and duration of laryngoscopy, maintaining oxygen saturation and keeping the ETT off the carina. Some alternatives to direct laryngoscopy, such as use of the Trachlight, have been shown to reduce adrenergic responses.

Pharmacological interventions are a double-edged sword in the critically ill patient. Although they may mitigate many of the adverse effects outlined previously, the agents themselves may cause adverse effects, especially hypotension, respiratory depression (during the pretreatment interval), and hypercapnia. Consider the following:

- The additive or potentiating effects of one technique or drug on another (e.g., the obtunded overdose patient may need less induction agent)
- The patient's physiological reserve: Patients with reduced cardiac reserve [decreased left ventricular (LV) function and valvular heart disease] are more sensitive to myocardial depressants such as induction agents; as are patients who are hypovolemic, such as those with uncontrolled hypertension, blood loss, or dehydration.
- The potential of an adverse outcome related to the physiological response to intubation: The physiological response to intubation may be especially detrimental in patients with severe asthma, ischemic heart disease, elevated ICP, intracranial hemorrhage, and aneurysm rupture or major vessel dissection.
- Underlying sympathetic tone: If the sympathetic nervous system is already maximally stimulated (e.g., hemorrhagic shock) and the patient is barely compensated, one must be cautious with any drug that can reduce sympathetic tone. This potentially includes all sedative hypnotic agents (benzodiazepines, barbiturates), neuroleptics (haloperidol and droperidol), opioids, lidocaine, and any drugs that release histamine. Etomidate, ketamine, succinylcholine, vecuronium, and rocuronium are the most hemodynam-

ically stable drugs in their respective classes. For sedation, small titrated doses of ketamine or haloperidol are probably safer than benzodiazepines or barbiturates. Although still a good choice for induction, etomidate is avoided as an infusion because of its ability to suppress the adrenal axis.

When using medications to mitigate the adverse physiological responses to intubation in patients with marginal pulmonary or cardiovascular reserve (e.g., those who are critically ill), administer conservative doses and err on the side of too little rather than too much. If postintubation hypertension and tachycardia occur, they can be managed by administering small doses of the induction agent or by titrating a benzodiazepine and opioid (e.g., fentanyl).

SPECIFIC CLINICAL CONSIDERATIONS

Acute Pulmonary Edema

The patient with acute pulmonary edema due to LV failure who requires intubation presents several challenges to the physician performing the intubation: preoxygenation will provide little in the way of oxygen reserve because these patients have little or no functional residual capacity (FRC). Oxyhemoglobin desaturation will occur rapidly; the patient may be unable to lie flat and is often struggling and uncooperative, presenting airway access difficulties; foamy secretions may obscure visualization of the airway; high airway resistance and low pulmonary compliance are likely to render bag-mask ventilation difficult or ineffective; cardiac reserve varies such that the patient who is hypertensive is more likely to tolerate opioids and induction agents than one who is normotensive, who in turn is more likely to tolerate opioids and induction agents than a hypotensive patient. Finally, laryngoscopy and intubation are likely to exacerbate any element of bronchospasm.

All these points emphasize the fact that there is little margin for error in these patients and that intubation should be carefully planned. This argues strongly for the superior pharmacological and physiological control, and success rates provided by rapid sequence intubation (RSI). Even when a difficult airway is identified, other factors, especially the immediacy of the need for intubation and the inability of the patient to tolerate a sedated "awake look," may make RSI the best choice, although often with a double setup.

Patients in acute pulmonary edema are difficult to preoxygenate, although it should be attempted with 100% oxygen, even though it may not be as effective as in patients with normal lungs. Assist ventilation to maintain oxygen saturation if at all possible. Bilevel positive airway pressure has been used in many patients with heart failure and may be useful for optimizing preoxygenation, even if it is ultimately unsuccessful in averting intubation (see Chapter 38). Even after the best attempts at preoxygenation, the patient may require positive-pressure ventilation throughout the intubation sequence to maintain adequate oxygen saturation. The cardiovascular system will tolerate the procedure, medications, and ventilation better in the supine position, but the patient usually prefers to be erect. It may be best to administer drugs with the patient erect and then to place the patient in a supine position for intubation as consciousness is lost.

Patients who are hypertensive and hyperdynamic have the capacity to respond in exaggerated fashion to intubation and may require medications to attenuate this response. Use caution in patients who are normotensive and extreme caution in those who are hypotensive. Have both intravenous nitroglycerine and pressors, such as dobutamine or dopamine, available. Alpha agent pressors such as phenylephrine and methoxamine are inappropriate because they increase blood pressure at the expense of myocardial work. An exception is the patient with significant aortic or mitral stenosis and a fixed cardiac output, in which case alpha-adrenergic agonists may be preferable. The patient should be pretreated with lidocaine or fentanyl as for any other patient, but fentanyl is avoided when sympathetic tone is required to maintain cardiac output. Etomidate is probably the induction agent of choice, as is succinylcholine as a neuromuscular blocking agent.

If the intubation is anticipated to not be difficult, use the largest ETT possible to minimize resistance to ventilation and facilitate pulmonary toilette (8 mm inner diameter [ID] in an adult female; 9 mm ID in an adult male). If a difficult laryngoscopy is anticipated, a smaller tube may enhance success and minimize stimulation. Place a stylet in the tube.

Once the patient is intubated, initiate mechanical ventilation with caution because irreversible hypotension immediately following intubation and positive-pressure ventilation in this setting (and in patients with chronic obstructive pulmonary disease) is not uncommon. Immediately after intubation, bag ventilate the patient to assess compliance and resistance. Appreciate the time needed to complete expiration. Note the effect of positive-pressure ventilation on blood pressure. Obtain a chest x-ray and look especially carefully for a right mainstem intubation because one-lung ventilation is even less well tolerated when the patient has pulmonary edema. Set the inspired fraction of oxygen (F_io_2) at 100%. A tidal volume of 8 mL/kg at a rate of 12 to 14 breaths/minute, as usual, is a good place to start. An elevated mean intrathoracic pressure due to positive-pressure ventilation may impede venous return and improve LV function in the setting of acute LV failure, although peak airway pressures exceeding 35 to 40 cm of water pressure (CWP) are associated with an increased risk of pneumothorax. In the event that the lungs are stiff and high airway pressures are compromising venous return and cardiac output, faster rates at lower tidal volumes may be required. If there is significant bronchospasm, the rate may have to be decreased to extend the expiratory time and the tidal volume increased, if possible, to maintain minute volume. Positive end-expiratory pressure (PEEP) beginning at 5 CWP or other forms of pressure support may be introduced to enhance FRC and oxygenation if the cardiac output will tolerate it. Increase the PEEP as needed and as tolerated. Treat the pulmonary edema aggressively according to its cause.

Dramatic falls in blood pressure caused by drugs (especially nitrates and histamine releasers) and ventilation may provide clues to underlying significant valvular heart disease. The patient who has worrisome hypertension caused by the intubation will respond to small repeated doses of thiopental (25–50 mg) or propofol (10–20 mg), which may be used to both sedate and lower the blood pressure. However, postintubation hypertension that persists is the result of inadequate sedation and excessive sympathetic tone. Lorazepam, supplemented with fentanyl or morphine, constitutes a good approach (see Chapter 3). Nitrates may also be useful. Circulation times are slowed in these patients, and medication onset time may be considerably delayed.

Cardiogenic Shock

The patient in cardiogenic shock is gravely ill with a high mortality rate. This fact serves to emphasize the attention to detail that is required in managing the intubation. Provided the patient is not in pulmonary edema, the FRC is probably intact, and preoxygenation is useful. By definition, there is no cardiac reserve, and medications that reduce cardiovascular performance are contraindicated. Induction agents, in particular, must be carefully selected. An amnestic agent, such as midazolam 1 to 4 mg, may be well tolerated. Etomidate and ketamine in much-reduced doses (e.g., etomidate 0.1 mg/kg or ketamine 0.5 mg/kg) are also reasonable, although, as for midazolam, either may depress cardiac function. Long-term sedation with lorazepam in small titrated doses of 0.25 to 1 mg may be tolerated. Circulation times are prolonged, so drug effects are substantially delayed.

As with the patient in pulmonary edema, RSI is usually the safest, most controlled, and best approach. Be prepared to handle surges in blood pressure and myocardial oxygen demand after intubation, rather than pre-emptively. No pretreatment medications are indicated, and in fact, they are contraindicated. Depending on the patient's circulatory status, either no induction agent or a greatly reduced dose, such as 0.05 mg/kg of midazolam *or* 0.5 mg/kg of ketamine *or* 0.1 mg/kg of etomidate should be used. This is immediately followed by succinylcholine 1.5 mg/kg. When initiating mechanical ventilation, be cautious of impeding venous return and cardiac filling. Paralytic agents such as succinylcholine do not have substantial cardiovascular activity. Pancuronium has cardiac muscarinic blocking properties, so may exacerbate tachycardia, although this may be difficult to detect in the setting of cardiogenic shock, where sympathetic activity is already maximal. Histamine-releasing agents, such as sodium thiopental or the benzyl isoquinoline neuromuscular blocking agents, should be avoided.

Septic Shock

Septic shock may be hyperdynamic or hypodynamic; myocardial contractility and systemic vascular resistance are compromised. The challenge is to maintain cardiac output and oxygen delivery to the tissues. Any agent that may compromise myocardial contractility or systemic vascular resistance must be considered with great caution, and alternatives should be sought, if at all possible.

The approach to airway management in the patient with septic shock is no different from that in the patient in cardiogenic shock (see previously recommended sequence). Ventilation should be initiated at 8 mL/kg at 12 to 14 breaths/minute. However, as most patients in septic shock are also acidemic, consideration should be given to carefully increasing minute ventilation by 20% to 30%, if the cardiac output will tolerate it, until arterial blood gases can be obtained. However, be cautious with ventilation. Any reduction in venous return will not be tolerated. Pressure support may reduce shunt fraction and improve oxygenation, provided cardiac output is maintained. The use of etomidate in patients with sepsis is discussed in Chapter 18.

Anaphylaxis

The patient suffering from a systemic anaphylactic reaction demonstrates hypotension due to release of vasoactive mediators, intense bronchoconstriction, and upper airway edema. The patient may be profoundly acidemic (respiratory and metabolic). Orotracheal intubation may be difficult or impossible because of upper airway edema, so a small-diameter ETT and surgical airway equipment should be readily at hand. Transtracheal needle ventilation and other supralaryngeal rescue airway devices such as the Combitube or laryngeal mask airway will be ineffective because of the combination of upper airway obstruction and bronchospasm. Hypotension limits the spectrum of pharmacological options for sedation. Intense bronchospasm will challenge the ability to ventilate the patient effectively.

Intense bronchospasm and hypotension will limit the effectiveness of preoxygenation and gas exchange in the preintubation period. Therefore, expeditious intubation is desirable. Be prepared to perform a surgical airway. If you are confident in your ability to intubate the patient, maximize the success rate by using RSI, with cricothyroidotomy prepared as a backup. If severe upper airway edema or stridor is present, an awake technique or primary cricothyrotomy is recommended. Treat the anaphylaxis aggressively with intravenous epinephrine during preparation for intubation. Steroids and antihistamines may be helpful, but epinephrine is the primary agent. Ketamine provides the best blood pressure support and is a bronchodilator.

Pretreat with lidocaine 1.0 mg/kg, if time permits; induce with ketamine, 1 to 1.5 mg/kg; and paralyze with succinylcholine. When initiating mechanical ventilation, the substantial increase in airways resistance will mandate slow rates and moderate tidal volumes with permissive hypercapnia to achieve acceptable oxygenation, minimal barotrauma, and optimum cardiac output, as for asthma (see Chapter 29). Excessive mean intrathoracic pressure is likely to compromise venous return and cardiac output. Manage hypotension and bronchospasm with intravenous epinephrine. Pancuronium, rocuronium or vecuronium are preferred for paralysis after intubation. Benzyl isoquinoline derivatives (e.g., curare, cisatracurium) are to be avoided because of their ability to release histamine.

When and How to Extubate

Extubation in a patient who has been intubated for some time carries significant risk, and a strategy to manage this risk is mandatory. The extubation of patients who were easily intubated and in whom no intervening event has occurred to jeopardize their airways might be regarded as a *routine extubation*. Those who were easily intubated but who are at greater risk of requiring reintubation (due to hypoxemia, hypercapnia, inadequate clearance of secretions, inability to protect their airway or airway obstruction) are *intermediate-risk extubations*. Those in whom airway management is likely to be challenging or complex if reintubation were to be required represent *high-risk extubations*. The last group includes (a) patients with a difficult tracheal intubation (failure to visualize the glottis, requiring multiple attempts or alternative techniques); (b) those with interval complications (airway edema, extrinsic compression, glottic injuries); and (c) those with clinical conditions associated with difficult ventilation or intubation. This latter group would include, for example, patients with paradoxical vocal cord motion, morbid obesity, obstructive sleep apnea, airway surgery, maxillofacial surgery (particularly when it involves intermaxillary fixation), deep neck infections, cervical surgery, or prolonged intubation.

Patients in critical care units often have limited physiological reserve, altered secretions, or an impaired capacity to protect their airways, elevating the risk of reintubation. In these instances, the practitioner may have limited clinical information, equipment, supportive personnel, and preparation time. Furthermore, the patient may be hemodynamically unstable with associated airway obstruction, hypoxemia, and acidosis. There may be a reluctance to administer paralytics when there is uncertainty about the airway. Topical anesthesia may be ineffective due to time constraints or the presence of secretions and edema leading to a struggle between the caregiver and a confused and possibly hypoxic patient. Generally, any urgent reintubation is likely to be more challenging than the original procedure.

Perhaps the most troublesome accompaniment of prolonged intubation in an ICU patient leading to postextubation upper airway obstruction and reintubation is the presence of upper airway edema. In adults, the swelling is generalized involving all glottic and supraglottic structures. In children, subglottic swelling predominates. The degree of edema is increased by positioning (e.g., prone or Trendelenburg), angioedema, thermal injuries, or with conditions associated with generalized swelling such as anaphylaxis and volume overload. In addition, injuries sustained during intubation or ensuing after intubation may exacerbate swelling in the upper airway.

Because of the hazards associated with extubation of the injured or edematous airway, several techniques to assess the degree of injury or swelling have evolved, some better than others. Direct visualization of the glottis with a laryngoscope prior to extubation is of limited value unless the image can be magnified, in which case the assessment of the anatomy is reasonable. Direct examination of the airway using a bronchoscope through an LMA during spontaneous ventilation after extubation provides a good assessment of both form and function.

Tissue swelling may encroach on an ETT at any point along its length. For this reason, a "cuff leak test" has been recommended to determine if air is moving around the ETT. For this test, the oropharynx is suctioned, and the cuff is slowly deflated. The patient is asked to inhale and exhale slowly as the ETT is occluded. An audible leak indicates the flow of air around the ETT. This has been found to be a useful predictor of successful extubation in pediatric trauma and burn victims as well as children with croup. However, its reliability in adults in predicting postextubation stridor and the need for reintubation is poor. Administering the test during controlled mechanical ventilation permits one to quantify the leak volume, and this method has been shown to be a better predictor of postextubation stridor, the need for reintubation, or both.

Airway edema may be reduced by head elevation and the use of racemic epinephrine. Steroids, fluid restriction, and diuretics have been employed with varying results.

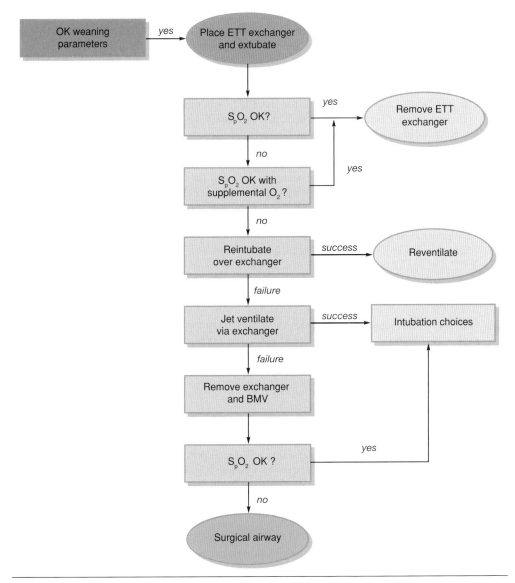

Figure 31-1 ● Extubation algorithm for moderate- and high-risk patients. See text for details.

Patients who meet moderate and high-risk extubation criteria must be treated cautiously. Figure 31-1 is an algorithm designed to guide one through the extubation of such patients. The algorithm is predicated on the following:

• That a pre-extubation evaluation of the airway is performed
• That the patient has adequate weaning parameters
• That an ETT exchange catheter is incorporated into the plan
• That the ability to rapidly perform a cricothyrotomy is assured

Several commercially available ETT exchange catheters are available on the market, including the Cook Airway Exchange Catheter (Cook Critical Care), the Endotracheal Ventilation Catheter (CardioMed Industries), and the Sheridan Tracheal Tube Exchanger

(Hudson Respiratory Care). Substitutes (e.g., gum elastic bougie, nasogastric tube) are not acceptable because they are not sufficiently stiff to guide the replacement tube into position. The dedicated exchange catheters are hollow and are supplied with adapters to permit some degree of gas exchange (insufflation or ventilation). The catheter is inserted through the existing ETT with the distance markings on the tube exchange catheter aligned with those on the ETT to ensure it is positioned correctly in the mid trachea. The tube exchange catheter remains in the airway after the ETT is withdrawn. The patient tolerates the exchange catheter better if lidocaine is instilled down the ETT prior to the insertion of the exchange catheter.

Once the decision to extubate has been made, Figure 31-1 guides subsequent decisions. An exchange catheter is inserted, and the ETT removed. The exchange catheter is taped to the cheek and the forehead to prevent movement of the device. If all is well after a period of time, the exchange catheter is removed. The period of time the exchange catheter ought to be maintained in situ after the ETT is removed remains uncertain and is a matter for clinical judgment. If the patient becomes hypoxic while the exchange catheter is in place, supplemental oxygen by face mask is administered. If this fails to rectify the problem and reintubation is required, an ETT is inserted over the exchange catheter. It is crucial that the ETT size approximate that of the exchange catheter to the extent possible to prevent the leading edge of the ETT from impinging on airway structures and preventing passage. It is also imperative that a laryngoscope be used to move oral tissue out of the way and minimize the angle of approach to the glottis (in much the same fashion as intubation over an Eschmann introducer, see Chapter 6). If this maneuver fails, oxygenation through the exchange catheter should be attempted while one prepares another approach to the airway. If oxygenation via the exchange catheter is unsuccessful, it must be removed and bag-mask ventilation attempted while a cricothyrotomy or intubation is performed.

ICU Airway Equipment

Just as in the operating room (OR) and the emergency department, the ICU ought to have adequate airway management equipment to meet its needs, and there ought to be policies overseeing its management (responsibility, checking, restocking, etc). Routine airway management equipment, as well as devices to manage a difficult or a failed airway, must be immediately available. Moreover, all staff must be familiar with how to use and support the use of these devices.

EVIDENCE

1. **Is there evidence to suggest that managing the adverse physiological effects of intubation improves outcome?** There is substantial evidence that orotracheal intubation produces adverse responses and that those responses lead to adverse patient outcomes (1–7). It is also clear from the literature that obtunding those adverse responses results in an improved outcome (5–7). The critically ill patient has the most to lose and the most to gain from obtunding the responses. The mainstays of controlling the responses are the technique chosen (8–10) and medications. Less stimulating techniques, such as the lighted stylet and nontracheal devices (e.g., LMA), produce less response than traditional laryngoscopic intubation. Opioids, such as fentanyl, alfentanil, sufentanil, and recently, remifentanil, are the mainstays of the pharmacological strategy. However, induction agents, nitrates, beta-blockers (e.g., esmolol), and others have also been used successfully (4,5,7,11–18).

2. **How common is it to have to manage an airway in an ICU patient?** It is not uncommon for airway management to be performed outside the controlled OR environ-

ment. A recent review of cardiac arrest associated with emergency airway management outside the OR in 3,035 patients confirms that the many of these occur in the ICUs (19). Furthermore, we know that the incidence of cardiac arrest in the ICU setting is as high as 2%, much higher than the 0.068% rate in the OR (20). Interestingly, the authors of these two cited studies note that hypoxemia is a prearrest factor and comment that improvements have been seen since the introduction of more experienced staff and the use of ancillary airway devices in ICU. In addition, non-intubated patients with cardiorespiratory decompensation are admitted to the ICU for monitoring. Some of these patients will deteriorate, as with the patient described previously, and require tracheal intubation and mechanical ventilation.

3. **How are most ICUs equipped when it comes to airway management?** A recent survey of ICUs revealed that most maintain an airway cart, but only about 50% maintain a "difficult" airway cart, and less than 5% conform to the suggested list of equipment offered by American Society of Anesthesiologists guidelines (21). Devices used to confirm tracheal intubation and detect esophageal intubation are present in 93% of ICUs, but they are only routinely used in 68% of cases. Only 4% of ICUs had both a bulb syringe and end-tidal carbon dioxide detectors, as suggested by the American Heart Association (22). A fiberoptic bronchoscope (FOB) is the most popular device selected for use in a difficult airway situation, even though it is immediately available less than one-third of the time. Fifty-one percent of respondents believed that the FOB was the primary backup when conventional intubation fails. In a "can't intubate, can't ventilate" situation, 20% believed that the FOB was the method of choice, an LMA (which was in only 50% of the airway kits) was only chosen 36% of the time, and a cricothyrotomy was the first choice for 32% of respondents. The authors commented on the underutilization of the LMA and the need for "continued efforts to educate medical personnel on airway management in the ICU setting" (22).

REFERENCES

1. Schwab TM, Greaves TH. Cardiac arrest as a possible sequela of critical airway management and intubation. *Am J Emerg Med* 1998;16:609–612.

2. Bishop MJ, Bedford RF, Kil HK. Physiologic and pathophysiologic responses to intubation. In: Benumof JL, ed. *Airway Management: Principles and Practice.* St. Louis, MO: Mosby; 1996:102–115.

3. Fox EJ, Sklar GS, Hill CH, et al. Complications related to the pressor response to endotracheal intubation. *Anaesthesiology* 1977;47:524–525.

4. Horak J, Weiss S. Emergent management of the airway: new pharmacology and the control of comorbidities in cardiac disease, ischemia, and valvular heart disease. *Crit Care Clin* 2000;16:411–427.

5. Bruder N, Ortega D, Granthil C. Consequences and prevention methods of hemodynamic changes during laryngoscopy and intratracheal intubation. *Ann Fr Anesth Reanim* 1992;11:57–71.

6. Rodricks MB, Deutschman CS. Emergent airway management: indications and methods in the face of confounding conditions. *Crit Care Clin* 2000;16:389–409.

7. Kovac AL. Controlling the hemodynamic response to laryngoscopy and endotracheal intubation. *J Clin Anesth* 1996;8:63–79.

8. Habib MP. Physiologic implications of artificial airways. *Chest* 1989;96:180.

9. Nishikawa K, Kawamata M, Namiki A. Lightwand intubation is associated with less hemodynamic changes than fibreoptic intubation in normotensive, but not in hypertensive patients over the age of 60. *Can J Anaesth* 2001;48:1148–1154.

10. Kitamura T, Yamada Y, Chinzei M, et al. Attenuation of haemodynamic responses to tracheal intubation by the styletscope. *Br J Anaesth* 2001;86:275–277.

11. Adachi YU, Satomoto M, Higuchi H, et al. Fentanyl attenuates the hemodynamic response to endotracheal intubation more than the response to laryngoscopy. *Anesth Analg* 2002;95:233–237.

12. Habib AS, Parker JL, Maguire AM, et al. Effects of remifentanil and alfentanil on the cardiovascular responses to induction of anaesthesia and tracheal intubation in the elderly. *Br J Anaesth* 2000;88:430–433.

13. Maguire AM, Kumar N, Parker JL, et al. Comparison of effects of remifentanil and alfentanil on cardiovascular response to tracheal intubation in hypertensive patients. *Br J Anaesth* 2001;86:90–93.

14. Casati A, Fanelli G, Albertin A, et al. Small doses of remifentanil or sufentanil for blunting cardiovascular changes induced by tracheal intubation: a double-blind comparison. *Eur J Anaesthesiol* 2001;18:108–112.

15. Albertin A, Casati A, Deni F, et al. Clinical comparison of either small doses of fentanyl or remifentanil for blunting cardiovascular changes induced by tracheal intubation. *Minerva Anestesiol* 2000;66:691–696.

16. Salihoglu Z, Demiroluk S, Demirkiran O, et al. Comparison of effects of remifentanil, alfentanil and fentanyl on cardiovascular responses to tracheal intubation in morbidly obese patients. *Eur J Anaesthesiol* 2002;19:125–128.

17. Bensky KP, Donahue-Spencer L, Hertz GE, et al. The dose-related effects of bolus esmolol on heart rate and blood pressure following laryngoscopy and intubation. *AANA J* 2000;68:437–442.

18. Figueredo E, Garcia-Fuentes EM. Assessment of the efficacy of esmolol on the haemodynamic changes induced by laryngoscopy and tracheal intubation: a meta-analysis. *Acta Anaesthesiol Scand* 2001;45:1011–1022.

19. Mort TC. The incidence and risk factors for cardiac arrest during emergency tracheal intubation: justification for incorporating the ASA guidelines in the remote location. *J Clin Anesth* 2004;16:508–516.

20. Olssen GL, Hallen B. Cardiac arrest during anesthesia: a computer aided study in 250,542 anesthetics. *Acta Anesthesthesiol Scand* 1988;32:653–654.

21. Practice guidelines for management of the difficult airway: an updated report by the American Society of Anesthesiologists Task Force on Management of the Difficult Airway. *Anesthesiology* 2003;98:1269–1277.

22. Oliwas N, Mort T. National ICU difficult airway survey: preliminary results. *Anesthesiology* 2003;99:A403.

32

The Pregnant Patient

Holly Ann Muir and Richard D. Zane

THE CLINICAL CHALLENGE

Along with many other physiological changes, late-term pregnancy also presents unique difficulties related to the airway. In fact, complications related to airway management in the parturient patient are the most significant cause of anesthetic-related maternal mortality. Despite advances in difficult airway management, the incidence of airway management failure in the parturient patient at term remains *ten times higher* than in the age-matched, non-pregnant population. Pregnancy causes an approximately 20% reduction in expiratory reserve volume, residual volume, and functional residual capacity (FRC), which, along with an increased maternal basal metabolic rate and oxygen demand by the fetal unit, leads to rapid desaturation of pregnant women when rendered apneic. Maternal minute ventilation increases early in pregnancy largely due to an increase in tidal volume. This results in alteration of "normal" blood gas parameters, which must be taken into account when managing mechanical ventilation. Maternal $PaCO_2$ falls to approximately 32 mm Hg, which is associated with a compensatory decrease in bicarbonate from 26 to 22 mEq/L in order to maintain a normal maternal pH. Mechanical ventilation must provide some degree of hyperventilation in order to maintain maternal pH, and it is reasonable to increase minute ventilation by approximately 20% for the pregnant woman in first trimester, progressing to 40% by term. During the late stages of pregnancy when the patient is placed supine, the effects of the gravid uterus on the diaphragm and, occasionally, increased breast size on the chest wall, further decrease the FRC. In addition to decreasing FRC, supine positioning in the late second and third trimester of pregnancy can result in aortocaval compression by the gravid uterus. This significantly reduces blood return to the heart, thus impairing maternal and fetal perfusion. This can be mitigated to a certain degree by placing the patient in the left lateral decubitus position.

Pregnancy also can affect laryngoscopy and bag-mask ventilation (BMV). Weight gain and increased breast size may make direct laryngoscopy difficult, while mucosal venous engorgement of the nasal passages and pharynx cause airway tissues to become friable and prone to bleeding. This mucosal edema can also lead to distortion of the airway structures, leading to difficulty both in identifying structures and in passing the endotracheal tube through the larynx and trachea. This upper airway distortion can be worsened by pre-eclampsia, active labor with pushing, and the infusion of large volumes of crystalloid fluids. Vascular engorgement also leads to a decrease in luminal size in the trachea requiring a smaller than expected endotracheal tube (6.5–7.0 on average). BMV can be difficult because of redundant and engorged upper airway tissues and limitations of chest wall and diaphragmatic excursion by the breasts and abdominal contents, respectively.

As pregnancy progresses, gastric acid secretion increases, causing a decrease in maternal gastric pH as well as an increase in gastrin levels, a reduction in gastric activity, and an increase in gastric emptying time that can result as an increase in resting gastric volume. Gastroesophageal sphincter tone is also reduced in pregnancy. With enlargement of the uterus, increasing pressure is exerted on the stomach, combined with a reduction in gastroesophageal sphincter tone, so the risk of reflux is especially high. Administration of neuromuscular blockade will exacerbate this further by causing a loss of supporting abdominal muscle tone. These normal changes in gastrointestinal physiology start early in the second trimester but become most problematic in the mid to late second and third trimesters.

Maternal plasma cholinesterase activity is reduced by 25%; however, this does not result in any significant effects on elimination half-life or duration of effect of succinylcholine. Pregnancy, however, does result in enhanced sensitivity to the aminosteroid muscle relaxants such as vecuronium and rocuronium, while the pharmacodynamics and pharmacokinetics of atracurium, a bis-quaternary ammonium benzylisoquinoline compound, are not changed.

APPROACH TO THE AIRWAY

In early pregnancy, fluid and FRC changes predominate, but the airway itself is unchanged. As pregnancy progresses, difficulty in both intubation and BMV can be anticipated, regardless of the absence of difficult airway markers. Nevertheless, the approach to airway management in the pregnant patient is no different from that of any other emergent intubation, except for consideration of the unique features of pregnancy described previously, which may create airway difficulty beyond the sixth month of pregnancy.

1. Use the difficult airway algorithm for patients in the third trimester of pregnancy. If careful assessment indicates that RSI is reasonable, have backup devices readily at hand, and anticipate more rapid oxyhemoglobin desaturation than for the nonpregnant patient. Avoid nasotracheal intubation, if possible. The mucosa may be engorged, edematous, and friable, and nasotracheal intubation is more likely to lead to mucosal damage and bleeding.
2. Preoxygenate carefully, using at least eight vital capacity breaths or 3 minutes of breathing 100% oxygen; as FRC is reduced, oxygen consumption is increased, and apnea leads to desaturation more rapidly.
3. All opioids and induction agents may reduce maternal blood flow to the placenta and, therefore, blood flow to the fetus. These agents also cross the placental barrier. Because muscle relaxants are quaternary ammonium salts and are fully ionized, they do not readily cross the placenta. Antihypertensive agents such as metoprolol, labetalol, and esmolol cross the placenta and carry a risk of inducing fetal bradycardia. In the context of emergent airway management, however, maternal well-being supersedes the potential for fetal exposure. When these agents are administered and delivery of the fetus is imminent, the caregiver charged with the management of the neonate immediately after delivery should be fully briefed regarding the agents administered to the mother.
4. Although there is not hard evidence in support of Sellick's maneuver, it is widely used and recommended in pregnant patients, in particular, because of the gastrointestinal changes described previously. An assistant trained in the application of cricoid pressure may be important in this situation.
5. Although rescue airway devices, such as the LMA, intubating LMA, and the Combitube, can be used in the event of failed intubation as for the nonpregnant patient, the enhanced risk of aspiration in pregnancy creates additional urgency for definitive airway control. The successful placement of one of these extraglottic rescue devices may achieve adequate gas exchange, giving the provider additional time to secure a definitive airway and avoid a surgical airway. Nonetheless, as the term pregnant patient may rapidly desaturate, cricothyroidotomy should not be delayed when intubation fails and BMV is not successful.

Recommended Intubation Sequence

- **Preparation:** A detailed difficult airway examination, including LEMON, MOANS, RODS, and SHORT, should always be performed before making a decision regarding the appropriateness of RSI (see Chapter 7). When the routine difficult airway assessment does not predict difficulty, obesity, enlarged breasts, and physiological airway edema can nevertheless complicate the ability to successfully secure the airway of the pregnant patient. Even if predictors of a difficult airway are not present, the difficult airway algorithm should be employed for late term pregnancy. If, during application of the difficult airway algorithm, the intubator does not have confidence that BMV and intubation will be successful, it may be advisable to consider an awake, sedated, topically anesthetized technique, such as awake flexible or rigid fiberoptic or video laryngoscopy, or awake direct laryngoscopy.

Assemble your airway equipment both for immediate management and potential rescue of a failed airway. Be sure to include a selection of smaller-size endotracheal tubes with stylets loaded; a bougie, short-handle laryngoscope if direct laryngoscopy will be attempted; and, if available, a rescue device with which you are familiar and equipment for a surgical airway.

- **Preoxygenation:** Eight vital capacity breaths or 3 minutes with 100% oxygen. Use left lateral decubitus positioning when in the supine position to avoid aortocaval compression; tilt the abdomen slightly to the left with a wedge or pillow under the right hip to displace the gravid uterus from the inferior vena cava.
- **Pretreatment:** Avoid pretreatment with defasciculating agents. Lidocaine and fentanyl are indicated as for the nonpregnant patient if time allows. Fentanyl should be used in the eclamptic or pre-eclamptic patient to mitigate hypertensive responses. Note the previously mentioned caveats regarding opioids.
- **Paralysis with Sedation:** As for the nonpregnant patient. Unless contraindicated, succinylcholine remains the gold standard for achieving rapid paralysis in a dose of 1 to 1.5 mg/kg. If succinylcholine is contraindicated, a nondepolarizing agent should be administered at the full dose recommended for RSI, despite the risk of prolonged effect after administration. Rocuronium currently offers the most favorable onset time when given in a dose of 1 mg/kg. The choice of induction agent is dictated by maternal hemodynamic condition as in the nonpregnant patient. There is no evidence to support the use of one particular induction agent in pregnancy.
- **Positioning:** Intubation success can be significantly enhanced with proper positioning prior to administration of induction agents. For the obese parturient patient or one with excessive breast tissue placing a roll, a pillow, or a liter bag of IV fluid vertically between the shoulder blades moves the glottic structures forward and assists in displacing the breasts away from the neck. Positioning of the occiput is equally important because too much extension of the neck can move the glottic structures anteriorly and impede visualization. Placing a pad or folded sheet under the patient's head to bring it into a neutral position may eliminate this. A head up position can help with ventilation both in the spontaneously breathing patient and when positive-pressure ventilation is required.

  Cricoid pressure may be more important in the pregnant patient, but evidence supporting its use is scant. If glottic visualization is difficult, cricoid pressure may be released in order to improve the view.
- **Placement with proof:** It is critical to confirm placement of the endotracheal tube using both auscultation and confirmation of end-tidal carbon dioxide before releasing cricoid pressure.

SPECIFIC CLINICAL CONSIDERATIONS

Management of the Failed Intubation

As with any patient where emergent intubation is required expeditiously, unanticipated difficulty can be encountered despite a careful difficult airway assessment. In the pregnant patient, the approach needs to be modified slightly to accommodate the anticipated physiological impairments imposed by pregnancy. Primarily, this is driven by the rapidity with which the mother desaturates and the commonly encountered airway edema and friability. The recommendation for number of attempts at laryngoscopy prior to moving to a rescue device is reduced to two from three in the pregnant patient, unless success on the third attempt is believed to be highly likely. Even though maintaining oxygenation and ventilation is important for all patients, it is paramount in the pregnant patient, who has reduced physiological reserve. In this circumstance, one should always choose a rescue device with which he or she is most facile and has the most experience. Properly performed, two-handed, two-person BMV may buy time to allow an alternative to cricothyrotomy. Nevertheless, one needs to be prepared to move on to a surgical airway if the rescue device is not able to provide adequate ventilation. Keep in mind that upper airway edema is a common cause of inability to both visualize the glottic structures and ventilate with BMV or supraglottic devices. Resistance to diaphragmatic excursion by the uterus and the weight of the gravid breast on the chest will further impede successful ventilation, so the surgical approach may be the only option.

POSTINTUBATION MANAGEMENT

Pregnancy is associated with an increased metabolic rate, which requires progressively increased minute ventilation as the pregnancy progresses. At term, this translates into a 30% to 50% increase in minute ventilation. Arterial blood gases or pulse oximetry and end-tidal carbon dioxide monitoring will aid in adjusting the ventilation parameters. Modest adjustments of both rate (start at 12–14 per minute) and tidal volume (start at 12 mL/kg) will meet the ventilatory need. If ventilation pressures are high, placing the patient in reverse Trendelenburg and left lateral decubitus position to move the abdominal contents down off the diaphragm may bring some improvement.

TIPS AND PEARLS

Taking the time to position the patient slightly head up with a roll between the shoulders and good support under the occiput before induction and attempting intubation may improve success.

Supraglottic airway edema is a common cause for failure in the pregnant patient; therefore, a smaller (6.5–7.0 mm ID) endotracheal tube may be required. In the event of a failed airway when placing an LMA for rescue, briefly decreasing the degree of cricoid pressure may improve success at placement.

When choosing pharmacological agents to facilitate intubation, the general rule of thumb is: "if it benefits the mother in the acute setting, it will ultimately benefit the fetus."

EVIDENCE

1. **Which extraglottic device is best for the pregnant patient?** There are no randomized studies comparing the various rescue airway devices in pregnant patients. There are, however, a number of case reports detailing the use of the LMA Classic, LMA ProSeal, LMA Fastrach, laryngeal tube, and Combitube. Naturally, these case reports largely focus on the positive outcomes when these devices are used so the risks and benefits of each are difficult to discern. None of these devices provide complete protection against aspiration, which remains a significant concern in the airway management of the pregnant patient. The laryngeal tube modification with the second lumen for passing an oral gastric tube and the LMA ProSeal with a similar design may offer at least a conduit for stomach contents to exit if regurgitation occurs. Both the Combitube and the laryngeal tube have a lumen/balloon that can provide some barrier to regurgitation; however, experience with both devices in obstetrics is limited.

Although the LMA ProSeal, laryngeal tube, and Combitube may offer some advantage against the risk of aspiration, they cannot be used to secure definitive endotracheal intubation as can the intubating LMA. Currently, the intubating LMA is probably the best choice as a rescue device in the pregnant patient because it can be used as both a rescue device and an intubation device. Nonetheless, the choice of rescue device should be influenced by operator experience (1–7).

REFERENCES

1. Backus Chang A. Physiologic changes of pregnancy. In: DH Chestnut, ed. *Obstetric Anesthesia: Principles and Practice,* 3rd ed. Philadelphia: Mosby; 2004:15–36.

2. Crosby ET. The difficult airway in obstetric anaesthesia. In: Benumof JL, ed. *Airway Management: Principles and Practice*. St. Louis, MO: Mosby; 1996:638–665.

3. Dennehy KC, Pian-Smith MC. Airway management of the parturient. *Int Anesthesiol Clin* 2000;38:147–159.

4. Lewin SB, Cheek TG, Deutschman CS. Airway management in the obstetric patient. *Crit Care Clin* 2000;16:505–513.

5. Minville V, N'guyen L, Coustet B, et al. Difficult airway in obstetrics using ILMA Fastrach. *Anesth Analg* 2004;99:1873.

6. Munnur U, de Boisblanc B, Suresh M. Airway problems in pregnancy. *Crit Care Med* 2005;33:S259–S268.

7. Zand F, Amini A. Use of the laryngeal tube-S for airway management and prevention of aspiration after a failed tracheal intubation in a parturient. *Anesthesiology* 2005;102:481–483.

33

Prolonged Seizure Activity

Robert J. Vissers

THE CLINICAL CHALLENGE

A general discussion of the diagnosis and treatment of seizure disorder is beyond the scope of this book. This chapter focuses on the considerations of airway management in the seizure patient. In the simple, self-limited, grand mal seizure, airway management is directed at termination of the seizure and prevention of hypoxia from airway obstruction. Paralysis and intubation should be considered when S_pO_2 falls below 90% or when typical first-line measures fail to terminate the seizure in a reasonable time. For the simple seizure, basic airway maneuvers, expectant observation (most seizures end spontaneously), supplemental high-flow oxygen, and vigilance are usually all that is necessary. Airway protection from aspiration is rarely required in the simple, self-limited seizure because the uncoordinated motor activity precludes coordinated expulsion of gastric contents.

Determining when to proceed from supportive measures to intubation is the main clinical challenge in the airway management of the seizing patient. *Status epilepticus* has been defined as continuous seizure activity for 30 minutes or multiple seizures without recovery of consciousness in between. The rationale for 30 minutes was that this is the minimum seizure duration that has been believed to produce neuronal injury. Recent neurology literature questions the practical value of this and suggests that clinicians wait no longer than 10 minutes before initiating aggressive therapy. Some have suggested any seizure lasting longer than 5 minutes is concerning because most single seizures are much shorter in duration than this. The mortality rate for status epilepticus is more than 20% in most series. Therefore, the discussion focuses on when intubation may be indicated in the patient with prolonged seizure activity. The absolute and relative indications for intubation in the seizing patient are listed in Box 33-1.

APPROACH TO THE AIRWAY

Self-limited Seizure

Most seizures terminate rapidly, either spontaneously or in response to medication, and require only supportive measures. Positioning the patient on his or her side, providing oxygen by face mask, suctioning secretions and blood carefully, and occasionally using the jaw thrust to relieve obstruction from the tongue are usually all that is necessary to prevent

---

BOX 33-1 Indications for Endotracheal Intubation for the Seizing Patient

Absolute indications
1. Hypoxemia (S_pO_2 <90%) secondary to hypoventilation or airway obstruction
2. Treatment of underlying etiology (e.g., intracranial bleed with elevated intracranial pressure)
3. Prolonged seizure refractory to anticonvulsants (to prevent accumulating metabolic debt [acidosis, rhabdomyolysis])
4. Generalized status epilepticus

Relative indications
1. Prophylaxis for the respiratory depressant effect of large doses of anticonvulsants (e.g., benzodiazepines, barbiturates)
2. Termination of seizure activity to facilitate diagnostic workup (e.g., CT scanning)
3. Airway protection in prolonged seizures

hypoxia and aspiration. Bite-blocks should not be placed in the mouths of seizing patients. They are not indicated and will only serve to increase the likelihood of injury. Attempts to ventilate during a seizure are usually ineffective and rarely necessary.

Prolonged Seizure Activity

Although most self-limited seizures do not require intubation, there are several indications for intubation in the prolonged seizure. Extensive generalized motor activity will eventually cause hypoxia, significant acidosis, rhabdomyolysis, and hyperthermia. Respiratory depression may result from high doses or combinations of anticonvulsants. Oxygen saturation of <90%, despite supplemental high-flow oxygen, is an indication for immediate intubation.

There is no clear guideline that specifically defines the duration of seizure activity requiring intubation. A good rule of thumb is that seizures lasting more than 10 minutes despite appropriate anticonvulsant therapy should be considered for intubation. Generally, when first-line (benzodiazepine) anticonvulsants fail to terminate grand mal seizure activity, rapid sequence intubation (RSI) is indicated. Phosphenytoin, which has a relatively short loading time, may be initiated as a second-line agent before intubation, if time allows. Other second-line anticonvulsants (phenytoin, phenobarbital) require at least 20 minutes for a loading dose; therefore, at the time of initiation of such a load, intubation is advisable. The initiation of a propofol or phenobarbital infusion is also an indication for intubation because of its respiratory depressant effects. Both agents also act synergistically with benzodiazepines, which increases the likelihood of apnea and the need for airway management.

TECHNIQUE

RSI is the method of choice in the seizing patient. In addition to its technical superiority, RSI ends all motor activity, allowing the body to begin to correct the metabolic debt. However, cessation of motor activity while the patient is paralyzed does not represent termination of the seizure, and effective loading doses of appropriate anticonvulsants (e.g., phenytoin) are required immediately after intubation. The recommended technique for the seizure patient is described in Box 33-2.

BOX 33-2 Rapid Sequence Intubation for Patients with Prolonged Seizure Activity

Time	Action
Time	**Action**
Zero minus 10 minutes	Preparation
Zero minus 5 minutes	Preoxygenation
Zero minus 3 minutes	Pretreatment
Zero	Continue anticonvulsant therapy
	Paralysis with induction
	Sodium thiopental 3 mg/kg *or*
	midazolam 0.3 mg/kg *or*
	propofol 1 mg/kg
	Succinylcholine 1.5 mg/kg
Zero plus 30 seconds	Protection and positioning
Zero plus 45 seconds	Placement with proof
Zero plus 60 seconds	Postintubation management
	Vecuronium 0.1 mg/kg IV
	Lorazepam 0.02 mg/kg IV
	Consider midazolam drip
	Consider propofol drip,
	1–5 mg/kg/hour IV

Standard RSI technique is appropriate in the seizing patient with the following modifications:

1. Preoxygenation may be suboptimal because of uncoordinated respiratory effort; therefore, pulse oximetry is critical. After giving succinylcholine, the patient may desaturate below 90% before complete relaxation and thus may require oxygenation using a bag and mask before attempts at intubation.

2. Sodium thiopental shares anticonvulsant activity with other barbiturates and may be the best choice for induction in the absence of hypotension. Midazolam is an equally efficacious alternative and preferred in the hemodynamically compromised patient. The induction dose of midazolam for an actively seizing patient is 0.3 mg/kg, but it can be reduced to 0.1 to 0.2 mg/kg if the patient is hemodynamically compromised. Etomidate has an unclear effect on seizure activity and therefore should be considered only if associated hypotension precludes the use of sodium thiopentothal or midazolam. Although etomidate may raise the seizure threshold (and therefore inhibit seizure activity) in generalized seizures, it lowers the threshold in focal seizures. Propofol has also been used as an induction agent in this setting at doses of 1 mg/kg. Little data exist on propofol as an induction agent in patients with seizures, however.

3. Prolonged, deep sedation with an agent that suppresses seizures is desirable for the first hour after intubation to facilitate investigations (e.g., CT scan) and to allow acidosis to correct with controlled ventilation. Long-term neuromuscular blockade should be avoided, if at all possible; however, if it is used, it should be accompanied by EEG monitoring, if available (see item 4).

4. Continuous bedside EEG monitoring is necessary in the paralyzed patient to assess for ongoing seizure activity. If this is not immediately available, motor paralysis frequently should be allowed to wear off to evaluate the effectiveness of anticonvulsant therapy.

5. If elevated intracranial pressure (ICP), head injury, known central nervous system pathology, or suspected meningitis is present, ICP intubation technique should be used (see Chapter 28).

Drugs and Dosages

1. Preintubation seizure management
   - Lorazepam 0.02 mg/kg intravenously (IV)
   or
   - Diazepam 0.1 mg/kg IV or 0.5 mg/kg per rectum
   with
   - Phosphenytoin 18 mg/kg (as milligrams of phenytoin equivalent)
2. Induction agents
   - Sodium thiopental 3 mg/kg
   or
   - Midazolam 0.3 mg/kg
3. Postintubation sedation and therapy
   - Midazolam 0.05 to 0.1 mg/kg/hour IV infusion, or
   - Propofol 1–5 mg/kg/hour IV infusion

TIPS AND PEARLS

1. Always ensure that hypoglycemia is not the cause of the seizure. Check glucose or administer IV dextrose solution in all cases. Similarly, check for hyponatremia.
2. Even in the difficult airway, RSI is generally preferred for airway management in the actively seizing patient. If the airway is assessed to be difficult, a double setup may be desirable.

3. The paralyzed patient may continue to seize, possibly causing neurological injury despite the lack of motor activity. Administer effective doses of long-acting anticonvulsants, and use benzodiazepines for long-term sedation. Avoid long-term paralysis, if possible. If a long-acting neuromuscular blocking agent is used, arrange continuous EEG monitoring, if possible, or allow motor recovery frequently (at least every hour) to assess response to therapy.

4. Prolonged seizure activity almost always represents a significant change in seizure pattern for the patient. A careful search for an underlying cause, including head CT scan, is indicated.

EVIDENCE

1. **Which benzodiazepine is best?** The answer depends on the setting in which it is being used. In one multicenter study, 570 patients with status epilepticus were randomized to lorazepam (0.1 mg/kg), phenytoin (18 mg/kg), diazepam (0.15 mg/kg), and phenytoin or phenobarbital (15 mg/kg) (1). Lorazepam alone was most effective in terminating seizures within 20 minutes and maintaining a seizurefree state in the first 60 minutes after treatment. There was no difference in 30-day outcome or adverse events (1). Lorazepam also performed better than diazepam or placebo in a double-blind prehospital study of 205 patients with status epilepticus, where termination of seizures occurred in 59% of patients versus 43% and 21%, respectively (2). Diazepam remains a popular agent in the emergency setting because of its rapid onset (<20 seconds, compared to 1 minute for midazolam and 2 minutes for lorazepam) (3). Diazepam is stable at room temperature in a premixed form and is readily absorbed rectally; therefore, it is often the benzodiazepine of choice stocked on a resuscitation cart.

   There are no data on the ideal benzodiazepine as an induction agent in status epilepticus; however, the relatively rapid onset, familiarity, and effectiveness of midazolam argue that it is the best choice.

2. **Midazolam, propofol, or pentobarbital for postintubation therapy?** For postintubation care, the patient should be sedated using a drug that not only provides amnesia and anxiolysis, but also optimizes antiepileptic therapy. Benzodiazepines have all these properties and are readily available in the acute care setting. Midazolam is preferred over diazepam and lorazepam as a continuous IV infusion because of its shorter half-life, water solubility, hemodynamic stability, and greater clinical experience in refractory status epilepticus (3,4).

   Recent reports suggest midazolam or propofol being preferred as a first-line agent, then pentobarbital as a second-line drug; however, no prospective randomized trial exists comparing these therapies directly (5,6). A systematic review to evaluate the efficacy and outcomes of these three agents in refractory status epilepticus found 28 studies that described a total of 193 patients (5). Pentobarbital was more effective at preventing breakthrough seizures; however, it was also associated with more episodes of hypotension, and there was no difference in outcomes between any of the agents. Pentobarbital is less desirable because it is rarely used in the emergency setting, making it less familiar or available.

   Despite the popularity of propofol for refractory seizure management in the intensive care unit setting, there is little experience in the emergency setting, and the ICU studies are too small to draw any conclusions (7–10). The recommended dosing for propofol is 1 to 2 mg/kg IV bolus (or induction) followed by a 1 to 5 mg/kg/hour infusion (11). Higher sustained doses have been associated with a propofol infusion syndrome.

REFERENCES

1. Abou Khaled KJ, Hirsch LJ. Advances in the management of seizures and status epilepticus in critically ill patients. *Crit Care Clin* 2006;22(4):637–659.

2. Treiman DM, Meyers PD, Walton NY, et al. A comparison of four treatments for generalized convulsive status epilepticus. *N Engl J Med* 1998;339(12):792–798.

3. Alldredge BK, Gelb AM, Isaacs SM, et al. A comparison of lorazepam, diazepam and placebo for the treatment of out-of-hospital status epilepticus. *N Engl J Med* 2001;345(9):631–637.

4. Treiman DM. Pharmacokinetics and clinical use of benzodiazepines in the management of status epilepticus. *Epilepsia* 1989;30:4–15.

5. Kumar A, Bleck TP. Intravenous midazolam for the treatment of refractory status epilepticus. *Crit Care Med* 1992;20:483.

6. Claassen J, Hirsch LJ, Emerson RG, et al. Treatment of refractory status epilepticus with pentobarbital, propofol, or midazolam: a systematic review. *Epilepsia* 2002;43(2):146–153.

7. Claassen J, Hirsch LJ, Emerson RG, et al. Continuous EEG monitoring and midazolam infusion for refractory nonconvulsive status epilepticus. *Neurology* 2001;57:1036–1042.

8. Prassad A, Worrall BB, Bertam EH, et al. Propofol and midazolam in the treatment of refractory status epilepticus. *Epilepsia* 2001;42:380–386.

9. Stecker MM, Kramer TH, Raps EC, et al. Treatment of refractory status epilepticus with propofol: clinical and pharmacokinetic findings. *Epilepsia* 1998;39(1):18–26.

10. Bradford JC, Kyriakedes CG. Evaluation of the patient with seizures: an evidence-based approach. *Emerg Med Clin North Am* 1999;17:203–220.

11. Rossetti AO, Reichhart MD, Schaller MD, et al. Propofol treatment of refractory status epilepticus: a study of 31 episodes. *Epilepsia* 2004;45:757–763.

34

The Geriatric Patient

Patrick A. Nee and Diane M. Birnbaumer

THE CLINICAL CHALLENGE

People age 65 and older now represent about 15% of the population. The number of retirees in the United States will reach 52 million by 2020. Those age 85 years and older will number 7 million by that year and increase to 14 million by 2040. Elderly patients present disproportionately frequently to the emergency services. A recent U.S. study identified increasing numbers of very old patients requiring urgent airway interventions in the emergency department (ED). Chronic obstructive pulmonary disease (COPD), cardiogenic shock, and severe sepsis are predominantly diseases of older age. Table 34-1 shows the ten most frequent diagnoses in ED patients (older than 65 years) who were intubated in a UK general hospital.

Aging is characterised by a progressive, irreversible deterioration in physiological reserve.

Advanced age affects airway management decision making in three primary areas.

A. *Respiratory Reserve*

Age-related changes in the lungs impair gas exchange, reducing oxygen tension at baseline. The normal PaO_2 falls by 4 mm Hg per decade after the age of 20 years and may be calculated by the formula $100 - (age/4)$ mm Hg or $13.3 - (age/30)$ kPa. Reduced sensitivity of central respiratory drive, weakened respiratory muscles, and altered chest wall mechanics reduce the ability of the older adult to respond to hypoxia and hypercarbia. Consequently, oxygen saturation may fall rapidly in the face of a respiratory threat. Impaired airway reflexes, swallowing disorders, drug effects, and delayed gastric emptying may worsen the situation because of increased risk of pulmonary aspiration. Finally, the presence of cardiovascular or cerebrovascular disease reduces the patient's tolerance of hypoxemia.

B. *High incidence of difficult airway*

Elderly patients have a relatively high incidence of difficult airways, necessitating early planning of the approach and contingencies in case of failure to intubate.

C. *Ethical Considerations*

Advanced age should not be a contraindication to advanced airway interventions, but the patient's desires, advance directives, and comorbidities must be considered. Poor outcomes relate to functional limitation and comorbidities rather than chronological age.

Continuous positive airway pressure and bilevel positive airway pressure are often used in elderly patients with respiratory failure, in whom invasive ventilation is deemed inappropriate. Life-sustaining interventions, including intubation, may not be appropri-

TABLE 34-1

Most Common Diagnoses in Patients (older than 65 years) Intubated in the Emergency Department

- Pneumonia
- Ventricular tachycardia or fibrillation
- Spontaneous intracranial hemorrhage
- Status epilepticus
- Cardiogenic shock
- Traumatic brain injury
- Self-poisoning
- Chronic obstructive pulmonary disease
- Anoxic coma
- Left ventricular failure

ate (or desired) in all cases. The principle of autonomy determines that a patient's views on treatment and treatment limitation must be respected. However, communication with sick, elderly patients in the ED setting may be difficult, especially in those with cognitive dysfunction.

APPROACH TO THE AIRWAY

In view of their poor tolerance of hypoxia, elderly patients may be considered for intubation at an earlier point in the course of an airway or respiratory emergency. Rapid sequence intubation (RSI) is the procedure of choice and may be appropriate even in patients with clinical features suggesting difficulty. Advanced age may be attended by poor mouth opening, carious or missing teeth, stiff lungs, and reduced cervical range of motion.

Preoxygenation is critically important; older patients desaturate relatively quickly due to age-associated changes in the lungs and pre-existing heart and lung disease. For the same reasons, preoxygenation may not be completely effective. Oxygen saturation must be monitored meticulously, and bag-mask ventilation (BMV) with high-flow oxygen must be instituted if saturation falls below 90%. Mask seal may be problematic because of facial wasting, and a two-handed, two-person technique, with a nasal or oral airway, may be required. Well-fitting dentures should be left in place during BMV and removed for intubation. Mouth opening may be limited by temporomandibular joint arthrosis, and cervical spondylosis may restrict neck flexion and head extension. Loss of elastic tissues promotes collapse of the upper airways and partial obstruction. Reduced lung compliance and chest wall stiffness may make BMV, and ventilation with an extraglottic device difficult. This situation is made worse by coexisting COPD or heart failure.

Anticipating a difficult intubation, the physician must attempt to optimize all six components of the *best attempt* (see Chapter 6) before proceeding. Alternative airway approaches, such as fiberoptic intubation, may be considered at the outset, or if difficulty is encountered. Blind nasotracheal intubation is a poor choice in older subjects due to increased risk of pharyngeal perforation and bleeding.

Surgical cricothyrotomy is the appropriate choice in a "can't intubate, can't oxygenate" failed airway situation, but abnormal airway anatomy, past radiation therapy or surgery, and relatively inelastic tissues increase the challenge.

Drug Dosage and Administration

A. *Pretreatment*

The pretreatment agents for older adults are the same as for others: lidocaine and fentanyl. These are used according to the "ABC" mnemonic in Chapter 3. Lidocaine is recommended for elderly patients with elevated intracranial pressure or reactive airways disease, and does not require dose adjustment. Fentanyl mitigates catecholamine response to laryngeal manipulation, which can be particularly important in the elderly who have a high incidence of cardiovascular and cerebrovascular disease. Although senescence blunts these autonomic responses to some extent, critically ill hypoxic and acidotic older patients remain at risk of stroke, myocardial infarction, aortic dissection, or rupture of an abdominal aortic aneurysm.

Attenuation of these responses is not without risk. Older patients are more sensitive to the respiratory depressant and hypotensive effects of opioids. Consequently, fentanyl should be given more slowly (over 2–3 minutes) and in smaller doses (1–2 μg/kg) in the elderly.

B. *Paralysis with induction*

Etomidate is the preferred agent in older patients because of its superior hemodynamic stability. Etomidate will not blunt the pressor response to laryngoscopy, and fentanyl pretreatment is indicated. The controversy regarding etomidate in shock and its effects on adrenal function are addressed in Chapter 18.

Thiopental can cause significant hypotension in the elderly, and, if used, the dose should be reduced to 1.5 or 1 mg/kg, even in euvolemic, normotensive patients. Similarly, propofol can be used, with the dose reduced to 1 mg/kg or even lower. Ketamine causes less cardiovascular lability and is useful in reactive airways disease. However, its sympathomimetic properties are a disadvantage in patients with ischemic heart disease, cerebrovascular disease, elevated intracranial pressure, or Parkinson disease.

Succinylcholine is the paralytic agent of choice for RSI in the elderly, but older patients are more likely to have conditions that can predispose to succinylcholine-induced hyperkalemia, especially stroke. Recent denervating stroke (occurring 3 days to 6 months before the succinylcholine is given) is associated with a risk of hyperkalemia. When there is any uncertainty regarding precisely when the stroke occurred, use of an alternative paralytic agent, such as rocuronium or vecuronium, is advised. In chronic renal failure, absent other risk factors, succinylcholine is safe.

POSTINTUBATION MANAGEMENT

The principles of postintubation management set out in Chapter 3 are appropriate to the aging adult. Sedatives (midazolam, propofol) and analgesics (morphine, fentanyl, alfentanil) should be given at reduced doses, and titrated to response, to minimize adverse effects ("start low, go slow"). Neuromuscular blocking agents are rarely necessary and, if used, should also be given in reduced doses and with increased intervals between doses. Ventilator settings are not usually affected by age, but decreased chest wall and pulmonary compliance may elevate ventilation pressures. In COPD, it is advisable to limit peak pressure and allow a prolonged expiratory phase. Positive-pressure ventilation, particularly with high levels of positive end-expiratory pressure, can unmask relative hypovolemia and may exacerbate the hypotensive effects of sedative drugs. Pressure-controlled ventilation is the preferred mode.

TIPS AND PEARLS

RSI is the procedure of choice, but the physician must anticipate difficulty and prepare for alternative approaches. Elderly patients desaturate quickly, and preoxygenation is important. Interposed breaths may be required after induction. Age-related cardiovascular changes, pre-existing disease, and drug interactions enhance the hypotensive response to induction, and reduced doses of sedatives and hypnotics should be used. Reduced cardiac output prolongs the arm-brain circulation time, and a delayed onset of action should be expected for all intravenous drugs. Pretreatment is as for younger patients. Rocuronium may be substituted where there are contraindications to succinylcholine. Finally, where there is incomplete information in respect of the patient's views on treatment limitation, it is advisable to proceed with interventions.

EVIDENCE

1. **Is older age an independent predictor of difficult intubation?** Airway morphology may be adversely affected by age. Turkish investigators found the greatest reduction

in thyromental and sternomental distances, as well as reduced Mallampati class and cervical range of movement, in patients ages 50 to 70 years (1). In contrast, in a Scottish ED-based study of 156 intubations, there was no relationship between mean age and (Cormack-Lehane) grade at intubation (2).

Independent covariates associated with difficulty in intubation were derived in two sizeable prehospital studies. Age was not independently associated with intubation difficulty in either population (3,4).

Injury during tracheal intubation is more common in the elderly. A North American group found an almost threefold increase in the risk of pharyngoesophageal perforation in patients older than 60 years (5). Of 203 dental injuries reported in Israeli hospitals over a 7-year period, the majority were sustained in patients ages 50 to 70 years (6).

2. **Which pretreatment drugs should be used in the elderly?** There is no specific evidence regarding the use of lidocaine in older adults with reactive airways disease or increased intracranial pressure in the emergency setting. Pending confirmatory evidence, we recommend that the elderly be considered for pretreatment agents (lidocaine, fentanyl) as for their younger counterparts. Although fentanyl is most familiar to emergency physicians, theoretically, shorter-acting opioids may offer advantage in the elderly. Alfentanil and remifentanil attenuated the pressor response to laryngoscopy and intubation in 40 elective surgical patients older than 65 years. However, adverse effects were common; in fact, hypotension was noted in three and four patients, respectively (7). Opioids onset more slowly in older subjects, and their effects persist longer, compared with younger age groups. The elderly are more sensitive to the respiratory and cardiovascular effects of these drugs and a 30% to 50% dose reduction is required (8,9).

3. **Which induction agent (and what dose) should be used in the elderly?** Options for intravenous induction in the elderly include etomidate, midazolam, propofol, and thiopental. Observational studies have shown that the plasma concentration required to induce the (desired and undesired) effects of these agents is up to 50% less in older subjects. Clinical effects take longer to become apparent and persist longer. A 40% reduction in dose of propofol, midazolam, or thiopental sodium is recommended in patients older than 65 years (9,10).

Etomidate (0.3 mg/kg) was used as the induction agent in 522 intubations in a Canadian hospital during a 42-month period. Sedation (and paralysis with succinylcholine) was deemed to be excellent in 88% of intubations. There was a high incidence of technical facility and a low rate of complications, with clinically insignificant elevations in heart rate and blood pressure, not related to age. Cardiac arrest occurred within 15 minutes of intubation in 17 patients, 10 of whom were older adults. In these cases, cardiac and cerebrovascular disease predominated as indications for the procedure, and the induction agent was not implicated in the outcome (11).

In a study of 160 cases from Hong Kong, midazolam caused significantly more hypotension than etomidate, particularly in patients with age older than 70 years (12). Similar advantage was found for etomidate compared to propofol when used for procedural sedation in the critically ill ED patients (13). A recent review of the literature on the use of etomidate in the ED setting concluded that the drug was effective and appropriate, even in hypovolemic patients and those with limited cardiac reserve (14). Dose reduction of etomidate in adults undergoing elective procedures has been described without loss of effect. However, evidence is lacking in the emergency situation, and 0.3 mg/kg continues to be recommended (15).

4. **Which muscle relaxant (and what dose) should be used in RSI in the elderly?** The advantages of succinylcholine in RSI are set out in Chapter 19. Many of the adverse effects are germane to the elderly patient and consideration is as for nonelderly adults. A reduced dose of succinylcholine (0.6 mg/kg) produced acceptable intubat-

ing conditions in elective surgical patients, with shortened neuromuscular recovery time (16,17), but data specific to the elderly are lacking, and we recommend that the standard RSI dose of 1.5 mg/kg be used for emergency intubation of all patients, regardless of whether they are elderly (15).

REFERENCES

1. Turkan S, Ate Y, Cuhruk H, et al. Should we re-evaluate the variables for predicting the difficult airway in anesthesiology? *Anesth Analg* 2002;94(5):1340–1344.

2. Reed MJ, Dunn MJG, McKeown DW. Can an airway assessment score predict difficultly at intubation in the emergency department? *Emerg Med J* 2005;22:99–102.

3. Wang HE, Kupa DF, Paris PM, et al. Multivariate predictors of failed pre-hospital endotracheal intubation. *Acad Emerg Med* 2003;10(7):717–724.

4. Combes X, Jabre P, Jbeili C, et al. Prehospital standardization of medical airway management: incidence and risk factors of difficult airway. *Acad Emerg Med* 2006;13(8):828–834.

5. Domino KB, Posner KL, Caplan RA, et al. Airway injury during anesthesia: a closed claims analysis. *Anesthesiology* 1999;91(6):1703–1711.

6. Givol N, Gershtansky Y, Halamish-Shani T, et al. Perianesthetic dental injuries: analysis of incident reports. *J Clin Anesth* 2004;16(3):173–176.

7. Habib AS, Parker JL, Maguire AM, et al. Effects of remifentanil and alfentanil on the cardiovascular responses to induction of anaesthesia and tracheal intubation in the elderly. *Br J Anaesth* 2002;88(3):430–433.

8. Vuyk J. Pharmacodynamics in the elderly. *Best Pract Res Clin Anaesthesiol* 2003;17(2):207–218.

9. Martin G, Glass PSA, Breslin D, et al. A study of anesthetic drug utilization in different age groups. *J Clin Anesth* 2003;(3):194–200.

10. Schnider TW, Minto CF, Shafer SL, et al. The influence of age on propofol pharmacodynamics. *Anesthesiology* 1999;90:1502–1516.

11. Zed PJ, Abu-Laban RB, Harrison DW. Intubating conditions and hemodynamic effects of etomidate for rapid sequence intubation in the emergency department: an observational cohort study. *Acad Emerg Med* 2006;13(4):378–383.

12. Choi YF, Wong TW, Lau CC. Midazolam is more likely to cause hypotension than etomidate in emergency department rapid sequence intubation. *Emerg Med J* 2004;21:700–702.

13. Miner JR, Martel ML, Meyer M, et al. Procedural sedation of critically ill patients in the emergency department. *Acad Emerg Med* 2005;12(2):124–128.

14. Oglesby AJ. Should etomidate be the induction agent of choice for rapid sequence intubation in the emergency department? *Emerg Med J* 2004;21:655–659.

15. Reynolds SF, Heffner JH. Airway management of the critically ill patient: rapid sequence intubation. *Chest* 2005;127:1397–1412.

16. Mohammad I, El-Orbany M, Ninos JJ, et al. The neuromuscular effects and tracheal intubation conditions after small doses of succinylcholine. *Anesth Analg* 2004;98:1680–1685.

17. Naguib M, Samarkandi A, Riad W, et al. Optimal dose of succinylcholine revisited. *Anesthesiology* 2003;99(5):1045–1049.

35

The Morbidly Obese Patient

Sarah H. Wiser and Richard D. Zane

THE CLINICAL CHALLENGE

The World Health Organization defines obesity by using body bass index (BMI), with "normal" defined as a BMI of 18.5 to 24.9 kg/m^2. Obesity is present when BMI is 30 or higher, morbid or severe obesity when BMI is 40 or higher, and superobesity is a BMI in excess of 50. The 1999–2002 National Health and Nutrition Examination Survey estimates that one-third of U.S. adults are obese, representing a dramatic increase from the prior survey in 1994 and underscoring the epidemic of obesity within the United States.

APPROACH TO THE AIRWAY

As for all patients, the approach to managing the airway of obese patients requires a structured, methodical assessment to identify the specific predictors of difficult bag-mask ventilation (BMV), cricothyrotomy, extraglottic device use, and tracheal intubation. Patient attributes differ, and some obese patients may have multiple anatomical risk factors for difficulty in addition to obesity, whereas others may not. Nevertheless, morbidly obese patients develop both physiological and anatomical changes that can make airway management all the more challenging.

The degree of physiological and anatomical changes correlates with the extent of obesity, and dictates the level of airway difficulty. The physiological and anatomical changes associated with morbid obesity are listed in Box 35-1. The main effects of obesity on airway management are (a) rapid arterial desaturation, secondary to a decreased functional residual capacity (FRC) and increased oxygen consumption; (b) difficult BMV, due to increased risk of obstruction from excess pharyngeal adipose tissue and increased resistance due to the weight of the chest wall and the mass of abdominal contents limiting diaphragmatic excursion; and (c) difficult laryngoscopy, intubation, and cricothyrotomy.

Obesity affects almost every aspect of normal physiological function, most notably the respiratory and cardiovascular systems. Obese patients often have baseline hypoxemia with a widened alveolar–arterial oxygen gradient, which is primarily due to ventilation-perfusion (V/Q) mismatching. Lung volumes develop a restrictive pattern with multiple disturbances, the most important of which is decreased FRC. Notably, these indices change exponentially with the degree of obesity. The fall in FRC has been ascribed to "mass loading" of the abdomen and splinting of the diaphragm. FRC may be reduced to the extent that it falls within the range of closing capacity, thus leading to small airway closure and V/Q mismatch. The FRC declines further when the individual assumes the supine position, resulting in worsening of the V/Q mismatch, right-to-left shunt, and arterial hypoxemia. Although the vital capacity, total lung capacity, and FRC may be maintained in mild obesity, they can be reduced by up to 30% in morbidly obese patients and up to 50% in severe or superobese patients. The decreased FRC causes rapid oxyhemoglobin desaturation during the apneic phase of rapid sequence intubation (RSI), even in the setting of adequate preoxygenation (see Chapter 3).

The work of breathing is increased 30% to 400% in morbidly obese patients because of decreased chest wall compliance, increased airway resistance, and an abnormal diaphragmatic position. These changes limit the maximum ventilatory capacity. The obese patient has elevated oxygen consumption and carbon dioxide production due to the metabolic activity of the excess body mass.

Cardiovascular changes in obesity include increased extracellular volume, cardiac output, left ventricular end diastolic pressure, and left ventricular hypertrophy. The absolute total blood volume is increased, but it is relatively less on a volume/weight basis when compared to lean patients (50 mL/kg vs. 75 mL/kg). Cardiac morbidity, including hypertension, ischemic heart disease, and cardiomyopathy, correlates with progressive obesity.

BOX 35-1 Physiological and Anatomical Changes Associated with Obesity

Physiological changes associated with obesity according to system

Pulmonary:
- Increased intrathoracic pressure with a respiratory restrictive pattern: ↓FRC, ↓ERV, ↓TLC
- Increased WOB, decreased MVC
- V/Q mismatching (predisposes to hypoxemia)
- Risk of pulmonary HTN
- Obesity hypoventilation syndrome

Cardiac:
- Increased cardiac output
- Increased BV, SV
- HTN, LVH
- Increased metabolic rate: ↑ VO_2, ↑ CO_2 production

Renal:
- Increased RBF and GRF

Hepatic/Gastrointestinal:
- Fatty infiltration of the liver
- Increased intra-abdominal pressure
- Risk for hiatal hernia, GERD

Endocrine:
- Increased risk of diabetes
- Hyperlipidemia

Hematologic:
- Increased risk of DVT
- Polycythemia (with chronic hypoxemia)

Musculoskeletal:
- Degenerative joint disease
- Decubital changes

Anatomical changes associated with obesity

- Increased facial girth
- Increased tongue size
- Smaller pharyngeal area
- Redundant pharyngeal tissue (risk of OSA)
- Increased neck circumference
- Increased chest girth
- Increased breast size
- Increased abdominal girth

FRC, functional residual capacity; ERV, expiratory reserve volume; TLC, total lung capacity; WOB, work of breathing; MVC, maximum ventilatory capacity; V/Q, ventilation to perfusion; HTN, hypertension; BV, blood volume; SV, stroke volume; LVH, left ventricular hypertrophy; VO_2, oxygen consumption; CO_2, carbon dioxide; RBF, renal blood flow; GFR, glomerular filtration rate; GERD, gastroesophageal reflux; DVT, deep venous thrombosis; OSA, obstructive sleep apnea.

Other changes include an increase in renal blood flow and glomerular filtration rate (GFR), fatty infiltration of the liver, and a propensity for diabetes mellitus and obstructive sleep apnea (Box 35-1).

Increased chest wall weight, increased facial girth, and redundant pharyngeal tissue all contribute to defining obesity as an independent risk factor for difficult BMV (see Chapter 7). Obese patients tend to have a smaller pharyngeal space because of deposition of adipose tissue into the tongue, tonsillar pillars, and aryepiglottic folds. Patients with obesity have an increased risk of having obstructive sleep apnea and facial hair (in men), which are also independent risk factors for difficult BMV. Difficult BMV should be anticipated in the obese patient, often requiring a two-person technique with both oral and nasopharyngeal airways in place. In severe or superobese patients, BMV may simply be impossible as the mask seal pressure required to overcome the increased weight and resistance may be far in excess of that possible with a bag and mask. In addition, challenging BMV is associated with difficult intubation in 30% of the cases. Intubation difficulty is also associated with increased neck circumference and high Mallampati scores. Cricothyrotomy is more difficult because of the increase in neck circumference, the thickness of the subcutaneous tissues, anatomical distortions, and adipose tissue obscuring landmarks, often requiring deeper and longer incisions. Extraglottic devices may not be able to overcome the high resistance of the weighted chest wall and restricted diaphragms.

TECHNIQUE

Morbidly obese patients vary with respect to airway difficulty, and a methodical LEMON assessment is essential to anticipate and plan appropriately for intubation (see Chapter 7). When the airway appears particularly difficult, the difficult airway algorithm advocates careful preparation and often an awake laryngoscopy or a fiberoptic approach with topical anesthesia and systemic sedation.

Proper positioning is essential in obese patients in order to ensure the best attempt at direct laryngoscopy and tracheal intubation. Ideally, the patient should to be propped up on linens, or on a commercially available pillow, from the midpoint of the back to the shoulders and head for proper positioning, as shown in Figure 35-1A and B. To confirm proper positioning, the patient should be viewed from the side, and an imaginary horizontal line should be able to be drawn from the external auditory meatus to the angle of Louis. This position facilitates intubation and both spontaneous and BMV, thus improving preoxygenation and prolonging the duration of time before arterial desaturation with apnea.

To determine the best technique, the risks and benefits of managing the airway with the patient awake versus unconscious are weighed. No matter which route chosen, the proper airway equipment must be available and checked for proper functioning, and help needs to be readily available in the event intubation proves to be difficult. When performing direct laryngoscopy, a short-handled laryngoscope can be easier to insert because the chest prevents the longer handle from gaining blade access to the mouth. The laryngeal mask airway (LMA) has been shown to be an effective, temporary ventilatory device in morbidly obese patients, but in the superobese patient, the pressure required to overcome the weight of the chest will likely exceed the seal pressure of the LMA, making ventilation difficult or impossible. The intubating laryngeal mask airway (ILMA) has been shown to be effective in providing both ventilation and serving as a conduit to tracheal intubation. Rigid fiberoptic intubating devices and the lighted stylet have been shown to be successful in managing the obese airway as well. The insertion technique for the lighted stylet is the same as in the nonobese patient, although one may encounter a greater diffusion of light depending on the degree of obesity, and room lighting may need to be dimmed. During direct laryngoscopy, the bougie may be helpful when only the posterior arytenoids or the tip of the epiglottis are visible.

BMV often requires two providers using two-handed bilateral jaw thrust and mask seal, with oropharyngeal and nasopharyngeal airways in place and the airway pressure relief valve and mask seal set so that continuous positive airway pressure (5–15 cm H_2O) is delivered to the pharynx. Relaxation of the upper airway muscles during RSI will often cause collapse of the adipose-laden, soft-walled pharynx between the uvula and epiglottis, making BMV and tracheal intubation more difficult, and greatly reinforcing the need to use oral and nasal airways.

Cricothyrotomy may be extremely challenging in the severely obese patient because the chin may be directly contiguous with the chest wall, making identification of and

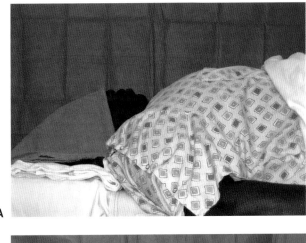

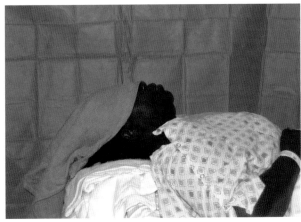

Figure 35-1 ● **A:** Patient is supine with the weight of the breast/chest obstructing access to the airway. **B:** Patient is propped on linens to establish better anatomical landmarks and remove the weight of the breasts/chest off of the airway. Here it is possible to draw an imaginary horizontal line from the external auditory meatus to the angle of Louis.

access to anatomical landmarks difficult. In the moderately obese patient, care must be taken to ensure that landmarks are found. This step may require one or two assistants whose sole role is to hold or retract neck, facial, and chest fat folds. As in all patients, cricothyrotomy is a tactile procedure. In the obese patient, direct visualization will likely be impossible.

Drug Dosage and Administration

Obesity, along with any associated comorbidities, affect all aspects of the pharmacodynamic and pharmacokinetic properties of medications, including absorption, onset, volume of distribution (Vd), protein binding, metabolism, and clearance. In the obese patient, there is not only an increase in the adipose tissue, but also an increase in lean body mass of about 30% of the total excess weight. The ratio of fat to lean mass increases, however, causing a relative decrease in the percentage of lean mass and water in obese patients compared to lean patients. In addition, there is an increase in blood volume and cardiac output. The Vd for a particular agent is affected by the combination of these obesity-associated factors, along with the specific lipophilicity of the drug. Protein binding is affected by an increased concentration of triglycerides, lipoproteins, cholesterol, and free fatty acids. These lipids limit the binding of some drugs, thus increasing the free plasma concentration. In contrast, increased alpha-one glycoprotein may increase protein binding of other drugs, thus decreasing the free plasma concentration. For most agents that undergo hepatic metabolism, there is minimal change despite the high incidence of fatty infiltration of the liver. Agents handled by the kidney, however, have accelerated clearance due to increased GFR. Furthermore, obese patients may be more sensitive to the effects of sedative drugs, opioids, and anesthetic agents. These pharmacokinetic and pharmacodynamic changes can make the net effect of these agents unpredictable. Thus, monitoring of clinical end points is important in addition to empirical drug dosing based on published data.

In general, the lipophilicity of the agent can indicate the dosage requirement. Most anesthetic agents are lipophilic, thus an increase in Vd and dose of the drug is expected, but this is not consistently demonstrated in pharmacological studies because of factors such as end-organ clearance or protein binding. Less lipophilic agents have little or no change in Vd and, therefore, should be dosed according to ideal body weight (IBW) or lean body weight (LBW). Unfortunately, few studies have investigated the effects of obesity on the disposition of anesthetic agents, so for many drugs it is unclear if weight-related dosage adjustments should be made and whether these should be based on actual weight, ideal weight, or a percentage of the actual body weight. See Table 35-1 for specific recommendations.

POSTINTUBATION MANAGEMENT

The changes in the anatomy and physiology of obese patients have important implications for ventilator management. The initial tidal volume should be calculated based on IBW and then adjusted according to airway pressures, with the success of oxygenation and ventilation indicated by pulse oximetry and capnography, or arterial blood gas monitoring. Generally, the use of positive end-expiratory pressure is recommended to prevent end-expiratory airway closure and atelectasis, particularly in the posterior lung regions. In severe or superobesity, it may be necessary to ventilate the patient in the semi-erect position to move the weight of the breasts, abdominal fat, or pannus off the chest wall.

Portable bedside radiographs are usually of poor quality in the obese patient, limiting their clinical value, although one can usually determine if the endotracheal tube (ETT) is in a mainstem bronchus.

When considering extubation of the obese patient, a conservative approach should be taken. Review documentation regarding the difficulty of BMV and tracheal intubation, and consider the possibility of the patient requiring emergent reintubation.

TIPS AND PEARLS

- The predicted difficulty in intubation combined with the decreased physiological reserve in obese patients makes timely airway management important, and the decision to intubate cannot be delayed.
- Most tracheostomy tubes will not be long enough for the morbidly obese patient; a 6-mm inner diameter ETT may be advanced through the cricothyrotomy incision.

TABLE 35-1

Dosing Recommendations for Drugs Commonly Used in Airway Management

Drug	Dosing	Comments
Propofol	LBW	Lipophilic, systemic clearance and Vd at steady-state correlate well with TBW. High affinity for excess fat and other well-perfused organs. High hepatic extraction and conjugation relates to TBW. Cardiovascular depression limits dosage to LBW
Thiopental	LBW	Lipophilic, increased Vd, prolonged duration of action, cardiovascular depression limits dosage to LBW
Midazolam	TBW	Lipophilic, increased Vd, prolonged sedative effect as it accumulates in adipose tissue and inhibition of cytochrome P450 3A4 by other drugs or obesity itself
Succinylcholine	TBW	Hydrophilic, increased plasma cholinesterase activity increases in proportion to body weight
Atracurium	TBW	Hydrophilic, clearance, Vd, and elimination half-life is unchanged. No prolongation of recovery
Vecuronium	IBW	Hydrophilic, Vd increased and clearance decreased, significant delay in recovery if given according to TBW
Rocuronium	IBW	Hydrophilic, similar to vecuronium, prolonged duration of action if used with TBW
Fentanyl	LBW	Lipophilic, increased Vd and elimination half-life, distributes extensively in excess body mass. TBW may cause overdosing
Remifentanil	IBW	Lipophilic, decreased Vd and clearance
Lidocaine	TBW	Increased Vd, no change in clearance and elimination half-life prolonged
Etomidate	TBW	Increased Vd, dose may need to be decreased with liver disease

LBW, lean body weight; Vd, volume of distribution; TBW, total body weight; IBW, ideal body weight.
LBW = IBW + 30% IBW.
See Refs. 3, 10, 12, 13, 14, and 15.

EVIDENCE

1. **Is obesity an independent risk factor for difficult intubation?** Classically, obesity has been considered an independent risk factor for difficult intubation; however, with increasing clinical airway experience with these patients, this has become debatable. Brodsky et al. (1) looked at 100 obese patients and characterized whether they were difficult to intubate. They found that the obese population encounters a frequency of difficult intubations comparable to the general surgical population (1). Conversely, a study by Juvin et al. (2) in obese versus lean patients showed that obesity was asso-

ciated to an increased risk of difficult intubation. Further analysis of these studies demonstrated that the level of BMI above that defined as obesity was not an independent risk factor for intubation difficulties, whereas Mallampati scores of 3 and 4 were risk factors. Brodsky et al. (1) additionally found that increasing neck circumference was the most important independent risk factor for difficult intubation in this patient population, with a 5% risk at 40 cm and a 35% risk at 60 cm. Despite finding similar risk factors, these two groups disagree as to whether obesity should be considered an independent risk factor for difficult intubation. Notably, the different outcome between the two reports may be accounted for by different definition of "difficult airway." In fact, Brodsky et al. had a 12% incidence of "problematic" intubations, although this was not further defined.

In conclusion, it is likely that obesity, by itself, is a marker for difficult airway management, and that the obese patient, like the lean patient, may, in addition, have numerous other markers of difficult airway management.

2. **What is the best position for preoxygenation and intubation of the obese patient?** Positioning is essential to airway management of the obese airway. In the supine position, obesity results in a relative neck extension, leading to a more anterior placement of the larynx. In addition, in the supine position the FRC approaches closing capacity, creating a V/Q mismatch, shunting, and consequent hypoxemia (3). Moreover, it may be difficult to obtain adequate preoxygenation of the patient. Altermatt et al. (4) studied the effect of supine versus sitting position on preoxygenation of obese patients. Patients preoxygenated in the sitting position had 216 seconds of safe apnea time versus 124 seconds in the supine group. Schurmann et al. (5) also showed a significant extension of the "safe apnea period" by employing a 30-degree reverse Trendelenburg position prior to induction of anesthesia. Because the weight of the chest and abdomen is displaced off the airway in this position, BMV is facilitated with lower peak inspiratory pressures (6).

As shown in Figure 35-1B, when the patient is propped on linens or a commercially manufactured device, the airway becomes well defined and removes the weight of the chest, facilitating intubation. To obtain this position, the planking of the patient needs to start at the midpoint of the back and extend to the head (7). When in doubt about the position, take a lateral view of the patient to assess if an imaginary horizontal line can be drawn from the external auditory meatus to the angle of Louis (7). See Figure 35-1A and B.

3. **What is known about the ILMA in obese patients?** The ILMA was designed based on MRI studies of normal weight subjects, but efficacy has been demonstrated in morbidly obese patients (8). Combes et al. (8) compared a group of lean patients to a group of obese patients using the ILMA as the primary airway tool. All patients were successfully intubated with the ILMA, but obese patients required fewer manipulations of the ILMA than lean patients and had fewer failed blind passes of the endotracheal tube and fewer esophageal intubations. Frappier et al. (9) found similar results in their study comparing standard direct laryngoscopy versus ILMA in morbidly obese patients. The ILMA not only provided adequate ventilation, but also achieved intubation in 96.7% of their patients.

The theory behind the efficacy of the ILMA is based on MRIs of obese patients. MRI has shown that decreased pharyngeal area and volume are caused by deposition of adipose tissue, predominately in the lateral pharyngeal walls (8). This information may serve to guide the ILMA into place and stabilize its position with cuff inflation. Furthermore, the ILMA provides for adequate ventilation, whereas BMV may prove to be difficult when collapse of the pharynx occurs with induction. Thus, the ILMA should be considered a valuable and complementary tool to conventional laryngoscopy.

4. **What is the dose of succinylcholine to achieve the best intubating conditions?** In the morbidly obese patient, increased extracellular volume is often associated with

increased levels of plasma pseudocholinesterase, both factors playing a role in the duration of action of succinlycholine. Lemmen and Brodsky (10) found that obese patients receiving IBW and LBW doses of succinylcholine had significantly less blockade, with 33% and 27% having poor intubating conditions, respectively. All patients receiving total body weight (TBW) dosing displayed adequate intubating conditions, although recovery time was prolonged. Of note, even the IBW had a recovery time of 5 minutes, which is still inadequate for resuming spontaneous ventilation before hypoxemia develops in the obese patient (typically 2–3 minutes) (10). Despite the relatively long recovery time with succinylcholine, even with IBW dosing, it is wise to achieve the best intubating conditions possible, hence the recommendation for TBW dosing.

5. **Are obese patients at greater risk for aspiration?** It has been traditionally believed that obesity poses a relatively high risk of aspiration. However, this evidence has been challenged by a report from Tasch et al. (11) that showed lack of association between the degree of obesity and gastric volume or pH. Furthermore, Verdich (12) reported no difference in rates of gastric emptying or lower esophageal sphincter tone.

6. **What is the evidence for drug dosing based on IBW versus LBW versus TBW?** Obesity affects all aspects of pharmacokinetics and pharmacodynamics; thus, it is difficult to predict how an individual patient will respond to a particular agent. Further complicating the issue, there are few studies that have investigated the effects of obesity on the disposition of anesthetic agents. As a result, it is unclear whether weight-related dosage adjustments should be made and whether these should be based on actual weight, ideal weight, or a percentage of the actual body weight. Many drugs may necessitate a higher dosage because of the lipophilicity of the agent, but the dose is limited by cardiovascular depression, hence a LBW dosing method (13). Because others (e.g., vecuronium) have shown to have increased effect even with LBW dosing, despite the increase in Vd from the extra lean body mass, an IBW method is recommended (14). In essence, the best method for dosing an agent is by careful titration to effect (3). In some instances, titration may not be possible, thus empiric drug dosing must be performed in order to achieve a certain goal, whether it be induction or paralysis for intubation (15,16). Refer to Table 13.1 for specific recommendations.

REFERENCES

1. Brodsky JB, Lemmens HJM, Brock-Utne JG, et al. Morbid obesity and tracheal intubation. *Anesth Analg* 2002;94:732–776.

2. Juvin P, Lavaut E, Dupont H, et al. Difficult tracheal intubation is more common in the obese than lean patients. *Anesth Analg* 2003;97:595–600.

3. Adams JP, Murphy PG. Obesity in anaesthesia and intensive care. *Br J Anaesth* 2000;85(1):91–108.

4. Altermatt FR, Munoz HR, Delfino AE, et al. Pre-oxygenation in the obese patient: effects of position on tolerance to apnea. *Br J Anaesth* 2005;95(5):706–709.

5. Schumann R, Jones SB, Ortiz VE, et al. Best practice recommendations for anesthetic perioperative care and pain management in weight loss surgery. *Obesity Res* 2005;13(2):254–266.

6. Leykin Y Pellis T, Lucca M, et al. The effects of cisatracurium on morbidly obese women. *Anesth Analg* 2004;99:1090–1094.

7. Brodsky JB, Lemmens HJM, Brock-Utne JG, et al. Anesthetic considerations for bariatric surgery: proper positioning is important for laryngoscopy. *Anesth Analg* 2003;96:1841–1842.

8. Combes X, Saurat S, Leroux B, et al. Intubating laryngeal mask airway in morbid obese and lean patients. *Anesthesiology* 2005;102(6):1106–1109.

9. Frappier J, Guenoun T, Journois D, et al. Airway management using the intubating laryngeal mask airway for the morbidly obese patient. *Anesth Analg* 2003;96:1510–1515.

10. Lemmen HJM, Brodsky JB. The dose of succinlycholine in morbidly obesity. *Anesth Analg* 2006;102:438–442.

11. Tasch MD, Stoelting RK. Aspiration prevention and prophylaxis: pre-op considerations. In Hagerg C, ed. *Benumof's Airway Management*. Philadelphia: Mosby; 2007:281–302.

12. Verdich C, Madsen JL, Toubro S, et al. Effects of obesity and major weight reduction on gastric emptying. *Int J Obes Relat Metab Disord* 2000;24:899–905.

13. Casati A, Putu M. Anesthesia in the obese patient: pharmacokinetic considerations. *J Clin Anesth* 2005;17:134–145.

14. Cheymol G. Effects of obesity on pharmacokinetics: implications for drug therapy. *Clin Pharmacokinet* 2000;39(3):215–231.

15. Ogunnaike BO, Jones SB, Jones DB, et al. Anesthetic considerations for bariatric surgery. *Anesth Analg* 2002;95:1793–1805.

16. Lemmens HJM, Brodsky JB. Anesthetic drugs and bariatric surgery. *Expert Rev Neurotherapeut* 2006;6(7):1107–1113.

36

Foreign Body in the Adult Airway

Ron M. Walls

THE CLINICAL CHALLENGE

Airway obstruction caused by a foreign body presents a unique series of challenges to the provider. First, when incomplete obstruction is present, there exists the distinct possibility that a particular action, or the failure to take specific action, could drastically worsen the situation by converting a partial obstruction to a complete obstruction. Second, when complete obstruction is present, instinctive and habitual interventions, such as bag-mask ventilation, have the potential to make the situation worse, for example, by causing a supraglottic obstruction to move below the cords, making retrieval more difficult (or impossible). Third, a common maneuver, like endotracheal intubation with bag ventilation, may meet with an unexpected result, such as the complete inability to move any air, defying the provider's attempts to find a solution to a problem perhaps never before encountered. Finally, the completely or partially obstructed airway is a unique clinical situation, requiring a specific set of evaluations and interventions, often in a very compressed period of time.

The patient with a foreign body in the airway may present with signs of upper airway obstruction or may present comatose and apneic, with only the history of onset to provide clues as to the cause of the crisis. The obstruction may be complete, as in the patient who typically has been eating, aspirates a food bolus, and is unable to move sufficient air to phonate. Although these situations usually arise in the prehospital setting, they may occasionally present to the emergency department (ED) or in-hospital. A partially obstructing foreign body will cause symptoms and signs of incomplete upper airway obstruction, specifically stridor, subjective difficulty breathing, and often a sense of fear, panic, or impending doom on the part of the patient. In many cases, there will be a preceding condition that has increased the risk of aspiration. Many patients who aspirate food are physically or mentally impaired, elderly, or intoxicated with drugs or alcohol.

Management of the suspected or known foreign body in the adult airway follows similar rationale to that used in the pediatric patient. The path chosen will depend on the patient's presentation, especially whether the foreign body is causing complete or only partial obstruction.

APPROACH TO THE AIRWAY

Management of the foreign body in the adult airway depends on the location of the foreign body and whether the obstruction is incomplete or complete. Location may be supraglottic, infraglottic, or distal to the carina. Obstruction may be complete or incomplete. Because the precise location of the foreign body is usually not known, the following discussion focuses on the approach to the foreign body whose location is uncertain.

Incomplete Obstruction by a Foreign Body

When the patient presents with an incompletely obstructing foreign body, the most important step is to prevent the conversion of a partial obstruction to a complete obstruction. If the patient is breathing spontaneously and oxygen saturation is adequate (possibly with supplemental oxygen), then the best approach is usually to observe the patient closely for signs of complete obstruction while mobilizing the necessary providers for prompt removal in the operating room (OR). Some foreign bodies are obviously accessible and can be removed in the ED. There is risk, however, with an incompletely obstructing foreign body just proximal to the glottis, that attempts at removal in the ED might result in displacement of the foreign body into the trachea, where it is no longer amenable to removal with common ED instruments. If transfer to the OR is not an option, for example, because it would require transfer to another hospital, a decision must be made as to whether the foreign body should be removed in the ED. If so, the best approach is to handle the airway much as one would handle awake laryngoscopy for a difficult intubation (see Chapter 8). Appropriate equipment is assembled, the patient is fully preoxygenated, and then following explanation of the procedure to the patient, titrated sedation and topical anesthesia are administered. With the patient sedated, the operator carefully begins to insert the laryngoscope with the left hand, inspecting at each level of insertion before advancing to ensure that the foreign body is not pushed farther down by the tip of the laryngoscope. Either a conventional or video laryngoscope may be used. The technique is one of "lift and look" followed by a small advance (perhaps 1 cm), then another lift and look, and so on. It may be necessary to take a break to allow the patient to reoxygenate or to administer more sedation or anesthesia. When the foreign body is identified, the best instrument for removal (Magill forceps, tenaculum, towel clip) is selected. Some foreign bodies, such as hard rubber balls, cannot be grasped well with the Magill forceps. After the object is grasped and successfully removed, laryngoscopy should again be performed to ensure that no additional foreign body remains in the airway. The patient should then be observed for several hours (depending on patient condition) to ensure that there are no further complications and that no foreign body moved distally in the airway.

Upper airway foreign body without complete obstruction should be considered a genuine emergency, and an early decision must be made regarding the appropriateness of attempted removal in the ED versus expedited transfer to the OR. If, at any point, the airway becomes completely obstructed, then the patient will be managed in a manner identical with that described in the following section.

Complete Obstruction of the Airway

When airway obstruction is complete, the patient will be unable to breathe or to phonate and may hold his or her entire neck with one or both hands in the "universal choking sign." The patient will appear terrified and will be making attempts at inspiration. In general, after complete obstruction of the airway with ensuing apnea, oxygen saturation will rapidly fall to levels incompatible with consciousness within seconds to a minute.

Initial management is dictated by whether the patient is conscious or unconscious. If the patient is conscious, the Heimlich maneuver should immediately and repeatedly be applied until either the foreign body is expelled or the patient loses consciousness. (See algorithm, Fig. 36-1.) There is no point in attempting instrumented removal of an upper airway foreign body while the patient is still conscious. If the Heimlich maneuver is successful in removing the foreign body, and the patient can phonate and breathe normally, then observation for a few hours is sufficient, and it is not mandatory to visualize the airway if the patient remains asymptomatic. If the Heimlich maneuver is unsuccessful in removing the foreign body and the patient loses consciousness, or if the patient presents unconscious with an upper airway foreign body, then the first step is immediate direct or video laryngoscopy *before any attempts at bag-mask ventilation, which may cause the foreign body to move from a supraglottic to an infraglottic position.* Generally, the patient will be flaccid, and it will not be necessary to administer a neuromuscular blocking agent. Time should not be lost waiting for an intravenous line to be established. Under direct or video laryngoscopy, a foreign body above the glottis should be easily identifiable. Again, Magill forceps, a tenaculum, a towel clip, or any other suitable device can be used to attempt to remove the foreign body. After removal of the foreign body, the larynx is inspected via laryngoscopy to ensure that there is no residual foreign body in the upper airway. As the foreign body is removed, the patient may begin spontaneous ventilation immediately. If the patient does not begin to breathe spontaneously, immediate intubation and initiation of positive-pressure ventilation is indicated and can be performed during the same laryngoscopy (Fig. 36-1).

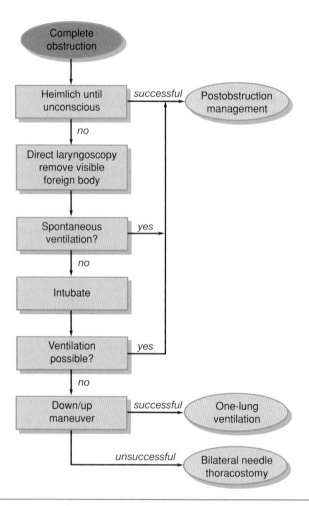

Figure 36-1 ● Management of complete obstruction by a foreign body. See text for explanation.

The laryngoscopy to remove the foreign body should be performed quickly and efficiently. If no foreign body is identified and if the glottis is clearly visualized, then either there is no foreign body or the foreign body is below the vocal cords. In this case, the patient should immediately be intubated and ventilated. If ventilation is successful, then it should be continued and resuscitation proceeds as for any other patient. If bag ventilation via the endotracheal tube meets with total resistance (no air movement, negative end-tidal carbon dioxide detection), then the trachea must be assumed to be completely obstructed. The stylet should immediately be replaced into the endotracheal tube, the cuff deflated, and the tube advanced all the way to its hilt in an attempt to push a tracheal foreign body into the right (or left) mainstem bronchus. The tube is then withdrawn to its normal level, and ventilation is attempted. The strategy here is to try to convert an obstructing tracheal foreign body (which will be lethal) to an obstructing mainstem bronchus foreign body (which can be removed in the OR). Thus, the patient can be kept alive by ventilating one lung while the other lung is obstructed.

If the down-then-up maneuver just described is not successful in establishing one-lung ventilation, there are two clinical possibilities. The only reversible situation is when the patient has one obstructed mainstem bronchus and a tension pneumothorax on the other side. Pneumothorax can occur in foreign body cases because of the abnormally high pressures generated both by the patient, while conscious, and by the rescue maneuvers. Because the operator has no way of knowing into which mainstem bronchus the foreign body was advanced (most commonly the right, but possibly the left), bilateral needle thoracostomy should be performed, in the hope of identifying a tension pneumothorax. If a pneumothorax is not identified, the second clinical possibility is complete bilateral mainstem obstruction, a condition from which survival is not possible, regardless of treatment.

POSTINTUBATION MANAGEMENT

Postintubation management depends on the clinical circumstances. If the foreign body has been successfully removed and the patient remains obtunded, perhaps from posthypoxemic encephalopathy, then ventilation and general management are as for any other postarrest patient. If the foreign body has been pushed down into one mainstem bronchus, the other lung must be ventilated carefully at low rates with markedly reduced tidal volumes to minimize the risk of pneumothorax while waiting for the OR.

TIPS AND PEARLS

1. If the obstruction is incomplete, usually the best approach is to wait for definitive removal in the OR under a double setup. If you are forced to act, move slowly and deliberately to ensure that you do not convert an incomplete obstruction into a complete obstruction.
2. Call for help early.
3. If the obstructing foreign body is above the vocal cords and cannot be removed, immediate cricothyrotomy is indicated.
4. If the obstructed foreign body is distal to the vocal cords and cannot be seen from above by direct laryngoscopy, cricothyrotomy will be of little or no benefit and should not be performed.
5. The Heimlich maneuver is a reasonable first step in any case of complete obstruction and is the only maneuver that can be performed on a patient with a complete obstruction who is awake and responsive.

EVIDENCE

1. **When should I use the Heimlich maneuver versus back blows?** There have been no randomized studies comparing the effectiveness of various methods for expelling an obstructing foreign body. Published reports are almost exclusively case reports and opinion pieces, and most are decades old (1–3). There is no clear evidence to establish the superiority of, for example, the Heimlich maneuver over simple back blows or chest thrusts. The American Heart Association (AHA), in its guidelines for emergency cardiac care, recommends that the Heimlich maneuver be done in the adult patient while conscious (4). If the maneuver is not successful despite repeated attempts, then chest thrusts or back blows can be used. Similarly, for obese patients or women late in pregnancy, chest thrusts are preferred. A cadaver study supports the use of chest thrusts rather than abdominal thrusts when the patient is unconscious, and this evidence is reflected in the AHA recommendations (5).

REFERENCES

1. Penny RW. The Heimlich manoeuvre. *BMJ (Clin Res Ed)* 1983;286:1145–1146.

2. Redding JS. The choking controversy: critique of evidence on the Heimlich maneuver. *Crit Care Med* 1979;7:475–479.

3. Brauner DJ. The Heimlich maneuver: procedure of choice? *J Am Geriatr Soc* 1987;35:78.

4. American Heart Association. 2005 American Heart Association guidelines for cardiopulmonary resuscitation and emergency cardiac care. *Circulation* 2005;112(Suppl 1):IV-19–IV-34.

5. Langhelle A, Sunde K, Wik L, et al. Airway pressure with chest compressions versus Heimlich manoeuvre in recently dead adults with complete airway obstruction. *Resuscitation* 2000;44:105–108.

37

Mechanical Ventilation

Michael F. Murphy and Peter M. C. DeBlieux

INTRODUCTION

Initiating mechanical ventilation is a common task and required skill set for all emergency physicians. The etiologies for respiratory failure are expansive, and the choice between invasive and noninvasive mechanical ventilation can be a challenging clinical decision. This chapter focuses on those patients requiring invasive mechanical ventilation following endotracheal intubation and introduces the concepts essential for the initiation of invasive mechanical ventilation. Chapter 38 focuses on respiratory distress and the institution of noninvasive mechanical ventilation.

Spontaneous ventilation draws air into the lungs (negative pressure), whereas mechanical ventilation pushes it in (positive pressure). In either case, the amount of negative or positive pressure required to deliver the breath (tidal volume) must overcome resistance to airflow. Positive-pressure ventilation alters normal pulmonary physiology by decreasing venous return to the thorax, changing ventilation-perfusion matching in the lung, and increasing airway pressures.

TERMINOLOGY OF MECHANICAL VENTILATION

The following terms are used in mechanical ventilation:

- *Tidal volume (V_t)*. The tidal volume is the volume of a single breath. It is usually in the range of 7 to 8 mL/kg ideal body weight (IBW). Smaller tidal volumes 6 mL/kg IBW with more rapid rates are used in those patients with diffuse infiltrates to prevent excessive airway pressures and to avoid ventilator-induced lung injury (VILI). Such patients with multilobar disease, severe congestive heart failure, adult respiratory distress syndrome (ARDS), or limited healthy lung units should receive these smaller tidal volumes. In reactive lung diseases, the use of permissive hypercapnia and low respiratory rates (RRs; 8–10 breaths per minute) combined with low tidal volumes (6–7 mL/kg IBW) promotes a prolonged expiratory time and diminishes the risk of hyperinflation.
- *RR or frequency (f)*. The usual starting RR is 12 to 20 breaths per minute in the adult. It is much higher in neonates, infants, and small children, and in those conditions where carbon dioxide production is accelerated (e.g., fever, acidosis, other hypermetabolic conditions). The non–gas-exchanging parts of the respiratory system (dead space) constitute a fixed volume of each tidal breath. The remainder of the volume in each breath participates in gas exchange and constitutes alveolar ventilation. Rapid RRs and small tidal volumes risk ventilating little more than dead space, a particular risk in infants and small children. The tradeoff here is rate versus volume (alveolar ventilation).
- *Fractional concentration of inspired oxygen (F_iO_2)*. This ranges from the concentration of oxygen in room air (0.21 or 21%) to that of pure oxygen (1.0 or 100%). When initiating mechanical ventilation, start with a F_iO_2 of 100% and wean the oxygen based on pulse oximetry.
- *Inspiratory flow rate (IFR)*. The IFR is the speed that a tidal volume breath is delivered during inspiration. In an adult, this is typically set at 60 L/minute. During cases of reactive airways disease, the peak IFR may be increased to 90 to 120 L/minute to enhance expiratory time and diminish dynamic hyperinflation.
- *Positive end-expiratory pressure (PEEP)*. PEEP offers a static pressure to the airways during inspiratory and expiratory efforts, and is typically set at 5 cm H_2O. PEEP increases functional residual capacity, total lung volumes, and total lung pressures. When a patient is unable to meet oxygenation goals using a F_iO_2 of 100% then PEEP can be progressively increased to reach oxygenation goals. Excessive PEEP can cause

VILI and alter hemodynamics in patients with limited cardiopulmonary reserve. After a short time, air hunger and fatigue become appreciable. The same thing happens to a patient breathing spontaneously through an endotracheal tube (ETT), especially a small one.

- *Ventilation mode.* There are a variety of modes applicable in invasive mechanical ventilation, and the key to understanding the differences between these modes centers on three variables: the trigger, the limit, and the cycle. The trigger is the event that initiates inspiration: either patient effort or machine-initiated positive pressure. The limit refers to the airflow parameter that is regulated during inspiration, either airflow rate or airway pressure. The cycle terminates inspiration: either a set volume is delivered (volume cycled ventilation), a pressure is delivered over a set time period (pressure cycled ventilation [PCV]), or the patient ceases inspiratory efforts (pressure support [PS] ventilation). The best mode in a given circumstance depends on the needs of the patient.
  - ○ Control mode ventilation (CMV)
  - ○ Assist control (AC)
  - ○ PCV
  - ○ Synchronized intermittent mandatory ventilation (SIMV) and PS
  - ○ Continuous positive airway pressure (CPAP)

Ventilation Modes

- *CMV.* CMV is almost exclusively relegated to the operating room in sedated and paralyzed patients, but an understanding of this mode's limits helps in appreciating the support level of the other modes. In CMV, all breaths are triggered, limited, and cycled by the ventilator. The clinician sets the tidal volume, RR, IFR, PEEP, and F_iO_2. The ventilator then delivers the prescribed V_t (the cycle) at the set IFR (the limit). Even if the patient wanted to initiate an additional breath, the machine would not respond. The analogy is sucking on an empty bottle. In addition, if the patient has not completely exhaled before initiation of the next breath, the machine would generate the required pressure to deliver the full V_t breath. For these reasons, CMV is only employed in those patients who are sedated and paralyzed.
- *AC.* AC mode is the preferred mode for patients in respiratory distress. The clinician sets the V_t, RR, IFR, PEEP, and F_iO_2. In contrast to all other modes, the trigger that initiates inspiration can be either the patient's effort or elapsed time interval. When either occurs, the ventilator delivers the prescribed tidal volume. The ventilator synchronizes set RRs with patient efforts, and if the patient is breathing at or above the set RR, then all breaths are patient initiated. The work of breathing (WOB) is primarily limited to the patient's effort in triggering the ventilator, and altering the sensitivity sets this threshold.
- *SIMV and PS.* SIMV is commonly misunderstood and can lead to excessive WOB on the patient's part. The physician sets the V_t, RR, IFR, PEEP, and F_iO_2. The trigger that initiates inspiration depends on the patient's RR relative to the set RR. When the patient is breathing at or below the set RR, the trigger can be the patient's effort or elapsed time. In these cases, the WOB is similar to an AC mode. If the patient is breathing above the set RR, the ventilator does not assist the patient's efforts. In these instances, the patient's WOB can be excessive due to resistance of the ETT, ventilator circuit, and inherent lung disease. In these additional breaths over the set RR, the patient's effort dictates the size of the tidal volume.

  The WOB detailed previously can be limited through the addition of PS to the SIMV mode. PS is positive inspiratory pressure applied during patient-initiated breaths that exceed the set RR. The WOB and tidal volume in this mode depend on the degree of PS; patient effort; and resistance of the ETT, ventilator circuit, and inherent lung disease. Insufficient PS is associated with high RR and low V_t, also known as rapid, shallow breathing. Typically, RR is the best marker for the appropriate level of PS. RR should be maintained at <30 breaths per minute and ideally below 24 breaths per minute.

- *CPAP.* CPAP is not a true mode of assisted mechanical ventilation. It is equivalent to PEEP and facilitates inhalation by reducing pressure thresholds to initiate airflow. It provides positive airway pressure throughout the respiratory cycle. This static, positive pressure is maintained constant during inhalation and exhalation. In a fashion similar to SIMV, PS can be added to CPAP to function as an assisted form of ventilation. In the CPAP-PS mode, the patient initiates and terminates each breath, dictating the RR with the WOB and tidal volume dependent on the degree of PS; patient effort; and resistance of the ETT, ventilator circuit, and inherent lung disease. This mode should never be used in patients that may have apneic episodes because of the lack of a backup rate.

VENTILATOR TIDAL VOLUME DELIVERY

Volume Cycled Ventilation

In this method of delivering a breath, the operator sets the tidal volume of each breath. The pressure required to deliver this volume varies, depending on the compliance and resistance of the lungs, the flow rate selected, the size and length of the ETT, and other minor factors as discussed previously. In adults, the initial peak flow is usually set to 60 L/minute.

With volume cycled ventilation (VCV), one is also able to determine the flow characteristics of the delivered breaths. The waveform may be square or decelerating (Fig. 37-1). Choosing a square wave results in the tidal volume being delivered at the constant peak flow selected throughout inspiration. This waveform usually generates a higher peak pressure than the decelerating waveform, but has the advantage of a shorter inspiratory time and more time for expiration. A decelerating flow wave causes inspiration to be initiated at the selected peak flow and then decelerates linearly as the breath is delivered. Because resistance to flow normally increases as the breath is delivered, the decelerating waveform generally results in lower peak inspiratory pressures (PIPs). However, this approach

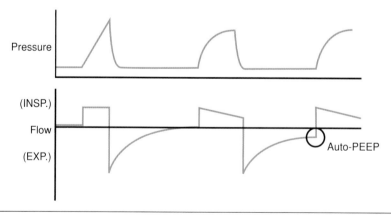

Figure 37-1 ● **Volume-Control Ventilation (VCV).** The lower trace demonstrates a square flow waveform first. The next waveform is a decelerating waveform. Note that the peak pressure generated by the square waveform exceeds that of the decelerating waveform. The third waveform demonstrates inspiration being initiated before expiratory flow has reached zero. This is how breath stacking and auto–positive end-expiratory pressure (auto-PEEP) occur.

increases the inspiratory time, at the expense of expiratory time, potentially trapping gas in the lung (stacking breaths) and leading to a continuous buildup of pressure called *auto-PEEP*. For this reason, the peak flow setting for decelerating flow wave is usually higher than that used in a square wave flow pattern. Auto-PEEP may lead to overdistension and rupture of alveoli (VILI), as well as decreased venous return and cardiac output. Most mechanical ventilators measure auto-PEEP. When setting up the ventilator, one can switch back and forth from one waveform to another in attempting to determine which offers better synchrony for the patient.

Pressure Cycled Ventilation

PCV should not be confused with PS ventilation, described previously. The limit during PCV is a set airway pressure. Instead of V_t, the cycle during PCV is a set inspiratory time (Ti). Some other PCV ventilator models require a RR and inspiratory to expiratory (I:E) ratio to be set. Ti is then calculated by the ventilator based on these settings. The clinician specifies an inspiratory pressure and an inspiratory-expiratory (I/E) ratio predicted to give a reasonable rate and tidal volume, based on the patient's expected resistance and compliance. Tidal volume varies breath to breath based on lung compliance, patient effort, and airways resistance.

In this method of delivering a breath, the peak flow of the administered tidal breath and the flow waveform vary according to the patient's resistance and compliance. Early in inspiration the ventilator generates a flow rate that is sufficiently rapid to reach the preset pressure, automatically alters the flow rate to stay at that pressure, and cycles off at the end of the predetermined inspiratory time. The flow waveform created by this method is a decelerating pattern (Fig. 37-2). A normal I/E ratio is 1:2. If the RR is 10 breaths per minute evenly distributed over the minute, each cycle of inspiration and expiration is 6 seconds. With an I/E ratio of 1:2, inspiration is 2 seconds, and expiration is 4 seconds.

The I/E ratio is usually determined by simply observing the pressure and flow waveforms on the ventilator monitor, especially the termination of flow at the end of expiration to avoid generating auto-PEEP (Fig. 37-3). The inspiratory pressure is selected, and then the inspiratory time is adjusted by watching the monitor so that when the end inspiratory

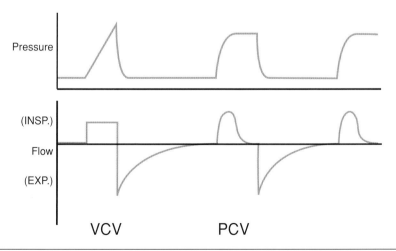

Figure 37-2 ● Pressure-Control Ventilation (PCV). These waveforms demonstrate the differing waveform characteristics between volume-control ventilation (VCV) and PCV. Note that PCV generates lower peak pressures than VCV.

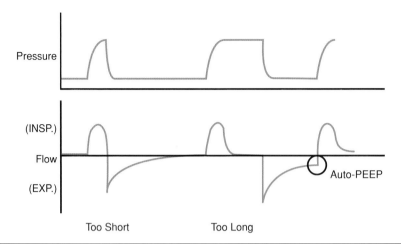

Pressure

(INSP.)

Flow

Auto-PEEP

(EXP.)

Too Short   Too Long

Figure 37-3 ● Pressure-Control Ventilation and Inspiratory-Expiratory Ratio. The first waveform set demonstrates an inspiratory time that is so short that the tidal volume is likely insufficient. The second and third waveform sets demonstrate how an inspiratory time that is too long may lead to breath stacking and auto–positive end-expiratory pressure (auto-PEEP), as illustrated in Figure 37-1.

flow approaches zero, inspiration is terminated and expiration begins. Short inspiratory times lead to low tidal volumes and hypoventilation; long ones may increase mean intrathoracic pressure and compromise hemodynamic function. PCV has been used in reactive airways disease patients, infants, and neonates, and in some transport ventilators.

INITIATING MECHANICAL VENTILATION

The patient who is spontaneously breathing possesses a complex series of physiological feedback loops that control the volume of gas moved into and out of the lungs each minute (minute ventilation). They automatically determine the RR and the volume of each breath necessary to effect gas exchange and maintain homeostasis. The patient who is entirely dependent on a ventilator has no such "servocontrol" mechanism and must rely on the individuals setting the ventilatory parameters to meet their needs adequately. In the past, this meant frequent blood gas determinations. Now we rely on noninvasive techniques such as pulse oximetry and end-tidal carbon dioxide monitoring.

A certain amount of ventilation is required each minute (minute ventilation or minute volume) to remove the carbon dioxide produced by metabolism and delivered to the lungs by the circulatory system each minute. This minute volume approximates 100 mL/kg, provided the metabolic rate is normal. Febrile patients, for instance, produce 25% more carbon dioxide each minute than the same patients when they are afebrile. Minute ventilation would need to increase by 25% to accommodate for this increase, guided by arterial blood gases or end-tidal carbon dioxide monitoring.

In general, we recommend the following settings in an adult:

- Mode—AC
- V_t—7 to 8 mL/kg
- f—12 to 20 breaths per minute
- F_iO_2—1.0
- PEEP—5.0 cm
- IFR—60 L/minute

The vast majority of patients are easily ventilated, and this formula produces reasonable arterial blood gas tensions. Larger tidal volumes and lower rates delivering the same minute ventilation are acceptable, provided the volume/pressure tradeoff is adequate. Similarly, faster rates and smaller tidal volumes are acceptable, provided the rate/dead space ventilation tradeoff is accounted for.

High airway pressures and volumes are real risks to lung injury in mechanical ventilation. The many faces of VILI (pneumothorax, pneumomediastinum, etc.) are visible outcomes of high airway pressures and excessive volumes. This airway pressure is also transmitted directly to the intrathoracic compartment compressing the great veins and the right atrium, and when averaged over the respiratory cycle, is known as the *mean intrathoracic pressure*. This pressure compromises cardiac output and may in severe situations, such as that with the ventilated asthmatic, produce a pulseless electrical activity rhythm. Mean airway pressure exceeding 30 cm of water pressure places patients at risk for VILI. The same applies to mean intrathoracic pressure and venous return.

For some patients, the most perplexing task in establishing adequate mechanical ventilation is trading off rate, volume, and pressure. Ventilating the asthmatic is a good example. The tidal volume has to be sufficient, at a given rate, to provide reasonable minute ventilation, preventing severe acidosis pH <7.2 in permissive hypercapnia. One wants the inspiratory part of the cycle to be short (i.e., high IFR) to allow maximum time for expiration and avoid starting the next inspiration before expiration is complete (stacking breaths). Meanwhile, the rate has to be slow enough to allow reasonable time for expiration and appropriate emptying of trapped volume. The dilemma is how to give a big enough tidal volume 6 to 7 cc/kg IBW, quickly, and without developing excessive pressure. Deliberate hypoventilation (permissive hypercapnia) is one strategy used to attenuate the risks of high airway pressures and dynamic hyperinflation. However, this is one case where attention to detail can make a material difference:

- Use as large an ETT as possible.
- Cut the ETT to minimize the length.
- RR of 8 to 10 breaths per minute.
- V_t of 6 to 7 cc/kg IBW.
- Adjust the peak flow (90 to 120 L/minute) in an attempt to prolong the expiratory phase.

For details and discussion on specific disorders and initiating mechanical ventilation for those conditions, refer to Section 6 of this book.

TIPS AND PEARLS

- Have a respiratory therapist (RT) review the features of ventilators available for use in your particular emergency department. Make sure that your RT is familiar with the ARDSnet protocol, plateau pressure measurements, and the concept of permissive hypercapnia.
- When a ventilator alarms, know how to take a patient off the ventilator and resume bag ventilation until an RT can return. To do this, you must be able to turn the ventilator on and off and know how to silence the alarms. These minimal steps will preserve calm until the RT can respond. Bag ventilation can be used to deal with temporary problems and provides the additional feedback of "feel."
- Understand the typical resistance and compliance characteristics of the various respiratory disorders. This information may help predict specific tidal volumes and rates for your patients.

- Use AC mode in totally apneic patients and in those patients displaying respiratory distress to diminish the WOB. Use SIMV-PS for patients without evidence of respiratory distress.
- Always disconnect the patient from the breathing circuit and bag-mask ventilation during transport. The circuit is heavy and may drag the ETT out, especially in infants and children.

EVIDENCE

1. **Does PIP correlate with lung injury?** The PIP is a function of the ventilator circuitry, ETT, peak flow, and the patient's lung compliance, and does not accurately reflect the risk of VILI. The risk for VILI is best represented by the plateau pressure, measured at the end of inspiration when an inspiratory pause is set. This pause allows for equilibration of pressures between the ventilator and the individual lung units, creating the plateau pressure. The plateau pressure correlates best with the risk of VILI and the current recommendation is to maintain the plateau pressure <30 cm H_2O. Plateau pressures >30 cm H_2O are best managed by reducing either tidal volumes or PEEP.

2. **What is permissive hypercapnia, and is there evidence that it is safe?** Permissive hypercapnia is the technique of ventilating patients with reactive airways disease that manifest dynamic hyperinflation, also known as auto-PEEP or intrinsic PEEP. The concept is based on prolonging expiratory time in hopes of promoting improved lung emptying and reduced pressures. The technique requires low RRs in the 8 to 10 breaths-per-minute range, coupled with a reduced tidal volume of 6 cc/kg/IBW and an elevated peak IFR of 80 to 120 L/minute. This intentional hypoventilation will promote a longer expiratory time and reduce dynamic hyperinflation. Patients will often require significant sedation and possible paralysis to maintain sufficient bradypnea. The consequence of this technique is an elevation in P_{CO_2} and a reduction in pH, with the goal of maintaining the pH >7.2 (1–3).

3. **What is the current ventilator management strategy to limit lung injury in ARDS?** ARDSnet protocol strives for using reduced tidal volume breaths in patients with diffuse lung injury or ARDS. In such clinical scenarios, tidal volume breaths travel predominantly to healthy, nondiseased lung units. The goal in limiting tidal volumes to 6 cc/kg/IBW is to prevent overdistension of the remaining functional lung units, preventing further VILI and an escalation of the inflammatory cascade within the lungs. The initial ARDSnet protocol compared 6 cc/kg to 12 cc/kg, and subsequent studies have compared 6 cc/kg to 10 cc/kg with similar dramatic results in mortality reduction and fewer ventilator days (4–8).

REFERENCES

1. Moore BB, Wagner R, Weis KB. A community based study of near fatal asthma. *Ann All Asthma Immunol* 2001;86(2):190–195.

2. Williams TJ, Tuxen DV, Scheinkestel CD, et al. Risk factors for morbidity in mechanically ventilated patients with acute severe asthma. *Am Rev Respir Dis* 1992;146:607–615.

3. Leatherman JW, McArthur C, Shapiro RS. Effect of prolongation of expiratory time on dynamic hyperinflation in mechanically ventilated patients with severe asthma. *Crit Care Med* 2004;32:1542–1545.

4. Bower RG, Shanholtz CB, Fessler HE, et al. Prospective, randomized, controlled clinical trial comparing traditional versus reduced tidal volume ventilation in acute respiratory distress syndrome. *Crit Care Med* 1999;27:1492–1498.

5. Stewart TE, Meade MO, Cook DJ, et al. Evaluation of a ventilatory strategy to prevent barotrauma in patients at high risk for acute respiratory distress syndrome. *N Engl J Med* 1998;338:355–361.

6. Donahoe M. Basic ventilator management: lung protective strategies. *Surg Clin North Am* 2006;86:1389–1408.

7. The Acute Respiratory Distress Syndrome Network Authors. Ventilation with lower tidal volumes as compared with traditional tidal volumes for acute lung injury and the acute respiratory distress syndrome. *N Engl J Med* 2000;342:1301–1308.

8. Girard TD, Bernard GR. Mechanical ventilation in ARDS: a state-of-the-art review. *Chest* 2007;131(3):921–929.

38

Noninvasive Mechanical Ventilation

Peter M. C. DeBlieux and Kerry B. Broderick

INTRODUCTION

Patients with severe respiratory complaints frequently present to the emergency department (ED) and comprise more than 10% of all presentations. Over the past decade, ED presentations of asthma, pneumonia, and chest pain have increased. A thorough knowledge of mechanical ventilatory support, both invasive and noninvasive is essential for practicing emergency medicine clinicians. Chapter 37 focuses on the institution of invasive mechanical ventilation, and this chapter covers noninvasive positive-pressure ventilation (NPPV or NIVS). Recently, the use of NPPV has grown steadily due to evidence-based research, cost effectiveness, and consideration of patient comfort and complications.

The advantages of NPPV over mechanical ventilation include preservation of speech, swallowing, and physiological airway defense mechanisms; reduced risk of airway injury; reduced risk of nosocomial infection; and probably a decreased length of stay in the intensive care unit (ICU).

TECHNOLOGY OF NONINVASIVE MECHANICAL VENTILATION

Noninvasive mechanical ventilators have several characteristics that are distinct from standard critical care ventilators. NPPV offers a more portable technology due to the reduced size of the air compressor. Because of this reduction in size, these noninvasive ventilators do not develop pressures as high as their critical care ventilator counterparts. Noninvasive ventilators have a single-limb tubing circuit that delivers oxygen to the patient and allows for exhalation. To prevent an accumulation of carbon dioxide, this tubing is continuously flushed with supplemental oxygen delivered during the expiratory phase. Exhaled gases are released through a small exhalation port near the patient's mask. During the respiratory cycle, the machine continuously monitors the degree of air leak and compensates for this loss of volume. NPPV is designed to tolerate air leak and compensates by maintaining airway pressures. This is in sharp contrast to the closed system found in critical care ventilators comprised of a dual, inspiratory and expiratory tubing system that does not tolerate air leak or compensate for lost volume. The device that makes physical contact between the patient and the ventilator is termed the interface. Interfaces for NPPV come in a variety of shapes and sizes designed to cover the individual nares, the nose only, the nose and mouth, the entire face, or the helmet. Ideally, interfaces should be comfortable, offer a good seal, minimize leak, and limit dead space.

MODES OF NONINVASIVE MECHANICAL VENTILATION

In a manner analogous to invasive mechanical ventilation, understanding the modes of NPPV is based on knowledge of three essential variables: the *trigger*, the *limit*, and the *cycle*. The *trigger* is the event that initiates inspiration: either patient effort or machine-initiated positive pressure. The *limit* refers to the airflow parameter that is regulated during inspiration, either airflow rate or airway pressure. The *cycle* terminates inspiration: either a pressure is delivered over a set time period or the patient ceases inspiratory efforts.

Continuous Positive Airway Pressure

Continuous positive airway pressure (CPAP) is a mode for invasive and noninvasive mechanical ventilation. As mentioned in Chapter 37, CPAP is not a stand-alone mode of assisted mechanical ventilation. It is equivalent to positive end-expiratory pressure (PEEP) and facilitates inhalation by reducing pressure thresholds to initiate airflow. It provides positive airway pressure throughout the respiratory cycle. This static, positive pressure is maintained constantly during inhalation and exhalation. This mode should never be used in patients who may have apneic episodes because of the lack of a backup rate.

Spontaneous and Spontaneous/Timed Modes

In spontaneous mode, the airway pressure cycles between an inspiratory positive airway pressure (IPAP) and an expiratory positive airway pressure (EPAP). This is commonly referred to as bilevel or biphasic positive airway pressure (BL-PAP or BiPAP). The patient's inspiratory effort triggers the switch from EPAP to IPAP. The limit during inspiration is the set level of IPAP. The inspiratory phase cycles off, and the machine switches back to IPAP when it detects a cessation of patient effort, indicated by a decrease in inspiratory flow rate, or a maximum inspiratory time is reached, typically 3 seconds. Tidal volume (V_t) varies breath to breath and is determined by degree of IPAP, patient effort, and lung compliance. Work of breathing (WOB) is primarily dictated by initiation and maintenance of inspiratory airflow, with additional WOB linked to active contraction of the expiratory muscles.

Spontaneous mode depends on patient effort to trigger inhalation. A patient breathing at a low rate can develop a respiratory acidosis. The spontaneous/timed (ST) mode prevents this clinical consequence. The trigger in the ST mode can be the patient's effort or an elapsed time interval, predetermined by a set respiratory backup rate. If the patient does not initiate a breath in the prescribed interval, then IPAP is triggered. For machine-generated breaths, the ventilator cycles back to EPAP based on a set inspiratory time. For patient-initiated breaths, the ventilator cycles as it would in the spontaneous mode.

Conceptually, one can consider BiPAP as CPAP with pressure support (PS). The pressure during the inspiratory phase is termed IPAP and is analogous to PS, a pressure boost during inspiratory efforts. The pressure during the expiratory phase is termed EPAP and is analogous to CPAP, or PEEP, positive pressure during the entire respiratory cycle. The IPAP is necessarily set higher than EPAP by a minimum of 5 cm H_2O, and the difference between the two settings is equivalent to the amount of PS provided.

The keys to successfully using NPPV on an emergency basis are patient selection and appropriate aggressiveness of therapy—that is, before resorting to endotracheal intubation and mechanical ventilation.

INDICATIONS AND CONTRAINDICATIONS

The indications for NPPV in the emergency setting are straightforward. The eligible patient must have a patent, nonthreatened airway; be conscious and cooperative; and have an existing, although insufficient, ventilatory drive. Patients who may benefit from NPPV may be hypercarbic, hypoxemic, or both. Patients with an acute exacerbation of chronic obstructive pulmonary disease (COPD), congestive heart failure exacerbation, severe pneumonia, status asthmaticus, or mild postextubation stridor might all be considered for NPPV. NPPV is *contraindicated* if the patient has a threat to his or her airway, is unable to cooperate, or is apneic. If the patient is in extremis, with very poor oxygen tensions and severe and worsening ventilatory inadequacy, immediate intubation is usually indicated, and it is not appropriate to delay intubation for a trial of NPPV. This is a relative contraindication, though, and clinical judgment is required.

The objectives of NPPV are the same as those for invasive mechanical ventilation: to improve pulmonary gas exchange, alleviate respiratory distress, alter adverse pressure/volume relationships in the lungs, permit lung healing, and avoid complications. Patients on NPPV must be monitored closely, using familiar parameters such as vital signs, oximetry, capnography, chest radiograph, bedside spirometry, and arterial blood gases (ABGs).

INITIATING NONINVASIVE MECHANICAL VENTILATION

Either a face mask or a nasal mask can be used, but a nasal mask is generally better tolerated. There are varying mask sizes and styles, and a respiratory therapist must measure the patient to ensure a good fit and seal. First, explain the process to the patient prior to applying the mask. Initially supply 3 to 5 cm H_2O of CPAP with supplemental oxygen. Acceptance on the patient's part may improve if the patient is allowed to hold the mask against his or her face. The mask is secured with straps once the patient demonstrates acceptance. Next, explain to the patient that the pressure will change and either sequentially increase the CPAP pressure by 2 to 3 cm H_2O increments every 5 to 10 minutes, or initiate BiPAP to support the patient's respiratory effort. Recommended initial settings for BiPAP machines in the non-invasive support of patients in respiratory distress or failure are IPAP of 8 cm H_2O and EPAP of 3 cm H_2O, for a pressure support (IPAP minus EPAP) of 5 cm H_2O. The level of supplemental oxygen flowing into the circuit should be governed by goal pulse oximetry and corroborated by ABG results as necessary; it is appropriate to initiate therapy with 2 to 5 L/minute, but this amount should be adjusted with each titration of IPAP or EPAP.

As the patient's response to ventilatory and other therapy is monitored (using cardiac, respiratory, and blood pressure monitors; oximetry; capnography; ABGs as indicated; and the patient's voiced assessment of tolerance and progress), support pressures are titrated. One approach that has been used successfully in hypoxemic patients in impending respiratory failure is to titrate by raising EPAP and IPAP in tandem in 2 cm H_2O steps, allowing a reasonable trial period (e.g., 5 minutes) at each level before increasing further. If the patient is hypercapnic, it may be better to raise the IPAP in 2 cm H_2O steps, with the EPAP being increased in a ratio to IPAP of approximately 1:2.5. The intrinsic positive end-expiratory pressure ($PEEP_i$), or auto-PEEP, cannot be measured by a noninvasive ventilator; therefore, EPAP should generally be maintained below 8 to 10 cm H_2O to be certain that it does not exceed $PEEP_i$ in patients with obstructive lung disease. The IPAP must always be set higher than EPAP. The goals are to reduce the patient's WOB, meet oxygen saturation goals, improve gas exchange, foster patient cooperativity, and maintain a respiratory rate of <30 breaths per minute. If the patient is not approaching these goals after the first hour of NPPV, then strong consideration should be made for rapid sequence intubation and institution of invasive mechanical ventilation.

TIPS AND PEARLS

- Patients who need airway protection must be differentiated from those who need intensive ventilatory support. None of the modes of NPPV provide airway protection.
- Patients with both a patent airway and some preserved respiratory drive—even if that drive is clearly insufficient—may be candidates for NPPV.
- Patients most likely to respond to NPPV in the ED (and therefore avoid intubation) are those with more readily reversible etiologies of distress, such as COPD exacerbation with fatigue, pneumonia with hypoxemia-induced fatigue, or cardiogenic pulmonary edema.
- The ventilatory management of patients in frank or impending respiratory failure with NPPV is a *minute-to-minute*, ongoing strategic decision. Virtually every modern ventilator is capable of delivering noninvasive ventilation (BiPAP, CPAP) and should be readily accessible to the ED or other areas in the hospital where respiratory emergencies arise. Physicians, nurses, and respiratory care personnel must be comfortable with ventilator use and knowledgeable of the limitations.
- Patient selection must take into account the overall condition of the patient, the patient's tolerance of mask support versus intubation, and the anticipated degree of reversal of the underlying insult with ventilatory and pharmacological support.

- One must be prepared for prompt intubation (i.e., difficult airway assessment done, drugs and equipment readily at hand) if therapeutic failure occurs.
- NPPV should be accompanied by aggressive medical therapy of the underlying condition (e.g., angiotensin-converting enzyme inhibitors, diuretics and nitrates for pulmonary edema, beta-adrenergic agonist and anticholinergic aerosols and corticosteroids for reactive airways disease).
- Finally, the patient should be carefully monitored for progress of therapy, tolerance of the mode of support, and any signs of clinical deterioration that indicate a need for intubation with mechanical ventilation.
- Patients treated in the ED with NPPV may require judicious sedation for anxiety in order to tolerate the mask, but doses used, if any, are small because preservation of respiratory drive is essential to the use of these modes.

EVIDENCE

In some published series, patients successfully supported in the ED with NPPV were frequently able to be admitted to telemetry units instead of ICUs, thereby incurring a significant cost savings. Uncontrolled studies without definitive inclusion criteria have found NPPV successful in avoiding intubation and mechanical ventilation in a large variety of patients on whom it has been clinically tested. Most of the studies done with NPPV compare NPPV to standard medical care (SMC) with outcome measures of intubation, ICU length of stay, and mortality. Unfortunately, most of the studies are quite small and have either enrollment criteria or end points that are somewhat subjective. Nonetheless, there is a considerable body of literature analyzing the use of NPPV.

1. **NPPV and COPD.** Two meta-analysis studies have been performed analyzing the use of NPPV in COPD. The most recent meta-analysis was by Peters (1) in 2002 of 15 randomized control trials of NPPV versus SMC. Eight trials enrolled patients with COPD, and seven enrolled patients characterized as a mixed-disease group. NPPV wass associated with an overall 8% reduction in mortality ($p = .03$), 19% reduced need for intubation ($p = .001$), and 2.74 days shorter hospital stay ($p = .004$). The COPD group had more significant reductions with 13% decrease in mortality ($p = .001$), 18% decreased need for MV ($p = .02$), and decrease in hospital stay by 5.66 days ($p = .01$). In 1997, Keenan et al. (2) published a meta-analysis of such trials and identified only 7 out of 212 that met rigorous inclusion criteria for analysis. The analysis showed NPPV to have a decreased mortality (odds ratio, 0.29; 95% confidence interval [CI], 0.15–0.59), and a decreased need for intubation (odds ratio, 0.20; 95% CI, 0.11–0.36) (2).

2. **NPPV and asthma.** Shivaram et al. (3,4) demonstrated both a decreased WOB and an increased patient comfort level during CPAP support of acute asthma exacerbations. Meduri (5) studied NIVS in 17 patients with asthma and acute respiratory failure over a 3-year period and demonstrated marked improvements in pH, $PaCO_2$, and respiratory rates, even at lower pressures of support (2.5 cm H_2O). These small studies should not be considered to constitute evidence that NPPV is of benefit in acute asthma, and NIVS should be used in asthma only with extreme caution.

3. **NPPV and pulmonary edema (PE).** In small studies, there appears to be a benefit to NPPV in the PE patients; however, larger prospective trials are needed before firm conclusions can be drawn. A randomized prospective study of 39 patients with PE compared CPAP to SMC and found a significant decrease in need for intubation ($p = .005$) in the CPAP group. Bersten (6) reported no significant difference in mortality and hospital length of stay. An open nonrandomized study on 29 patients with NPPV found oxygen saturation increased from 73.8 ± 11% to 93 ± 5%, mean pH

increased from 7.22 ± 0.1 to 7.31 ±.07 (p <.01), and $PaCO_2$ decreased from 62 ± 18.5 mm Hg to 48.4 ± 11.5 mm Hg (7). A randomized, controlled, prospective clinical trial on 27 patients comparing nasal CPAP to nasal BiPAP against historical controls for intubation rates and myocardial infarction (MI) found that BiPAP improved ventilation and vital signs more rapidly than CPAP. However, intubation rates, hospital stay, and overall mortality between the two modes of NPPV showed no significant differences in this study. Mehta (8) also reported a higher rate of MI in patients with BiPAP (71%) as compared to CPAP (31%) and usual medical care from historical controls (38%). A randomized prospective study of 40 patients comparing BiPAP to high-dose isosorbide (HDI) reported that 80% of patients in the BiPAP group required intubation as compared with 20% in the HDI group, MI rates of 55% and 10%, and death in two and zero patients, respectively (9). A meta-analysis of NPPV studies in pulmonary edema from 1983 through 1997 found that only 3 of 497 studies were sufficiently rigorous to fulfill their study criteria. These three randomized control trials showed NPPV patients to have a decreased need for intubation (−26%; 95% CI, −13% to −38%), but the decrease in hospital mortality was not significant (−6.6%; 95% CI, +3% to −16%) as compared to standard therapy alone (10). A more recent study compared BiPAP to standard medical therapy in a mixed population of COPD and acute respiratory failure patients. The study ended prematurely after interim analysis of the first 20 patients because the data showed clear benefit in the BiPAP group (11).

REFERENCES

1. Peters JV. Noninvasive ventilation in acute respiratory failure—a meta-analysis update. *Crit Care Med* 2002;30:555–562.

2. Keenan SP, Kernerman PD, Cook DJ, et al. Effect of noninvasive positive pressure ventilation on mortality in patients admitted with acute respiratory failure: a meta-analysis. *Crit Care Med* 1997;25:1685.

3. Shivaram U, Donath J, Khan FA, et al. Effects of CPAP in acute asthma. *Respiration* 1987;52:157.

4. Shivaram U, Miro AM, Cash ME, et al. Cardiopulmonary responses to CPAP in acute asthma. *J Crit Care* 1993;8:87.

5. Meduri GM. Noninvasive positive-pressure ventilation in patients with acute respiratory failure. *Clin Chest Med* 1996;17:513.

6. Bersten AD. Treatment of severe cardiogenic pulmonary edema with continuous positive airway pressure delivered by face mask. *N Engl J Med* 1991;325:1825–1830.

7. Hoffman B. The use of noninvasive pressure support ventilation for severe respiratory insufficiency due to pulmonary oedema. *Intensive Care Med* 1999;25:15–20.

8. Mehta S. Randomized, prospective trial of bilevel versus continuous positive airway pressure in acute pulmonary edema. *Crit Care Med* 1997;25:620–628.

9. Sharon A. High-dose intravenous isosorbide-dinitrate is safer and better than BI-PAP ventilation combined with conventional treatment for severe pulmonary edema. *J Am Coll Cardiol* 2000;36:832–837.

10. Pang D. The effect of positive pressure airway support on mortality and the need for intubation in cardiogenic pulmonary edema: a systematic review. *Chest* 1998;114:1185–1192.

11. Thys F. Noninvasive ventilation for acute respiratory failure: a prospective randomised placebo-controlled trial. *Eur Respir J* 2002;20:545–555.

39

Pulse Oximetry and Capnography/ Capnometry

Michael F. Murphy and Baruch Krauss

PULSE OXIMETRY

Pulse oximetry provides a noninvasive and continuous means of rapidly determining arterial oxygen saturation and its changes. The devices are easy to use and interpret, pose no risk to the patient, and are relatively inexpensive. However, reliable interpretation of the information provided by these devices requires an appreciation of their limitations in certain situations.

Principles of Measurement

There are two kinds of oximetry used in clinical practice: transmission and reflectance. Both transmission and reflectance oximeters consist of light sources, typically red and infrared (IR), and a photodetector ("photodiodes"). The transmission pulse oximeter is the most common type of oximetry employed in clinical practice. It positions light-emitting diodes on one side of a tissue bed (e.g., finger or ear lobe) and a photo detector on the opposite side of the tissue bed. Reflectance oximeters position the emission source and the detector side by side or at least in close proximity to each other. Transmission oximeters have to deal with other absorbers in the light path, including skin, soft tissue, and venous and capillary blood, whereas reflectance oximeters do not.

The principle of "oximetry" is based on oxyhemoglobin (OxyHb) and deoxyhemoglobin having different absorption spectra at the two commonly used sensor wavelengths of 660 nm (red) and 940 nm (IR). At the wavelength of red light (660 nm), reduced hemoglobin absorbs about ten times as much light as OxyHb.

Pulse oximeters assess the pulsatile variation of red and IR light transmitted through (transmission) or absorbed by (reflectance) a tissue bed. These factors are divided into a pulsatile (AC) component due to the pulsatile flow of arterial blood and a nonpulsatile (DC) component of the tissue bed that includes venous blood, capillary blood, and nonpulsatile arterial blood. Data averaged over several arterial pulse cycles are then presented as saturation (S_pO_2). Studies have shown an excellent correlation between arterial hemoglobin (Hb) oxygen saturation and pulse oximeter saturation.

Indications

Pulse oximetry is particularly useful in the emergency department (ED) evaluation of patients with acute cardiopulmonary disorders such as chest trauma, bronchiolitis, asthma, heart failure, and chronic obstructive pulmonary disease. It is a standard monitoring parameter for patients undergoing sedation and in patients with a decreased level of consciousness, such as intoxication, overdose, and head injury. Its ability to decrease the frequency with which arterial blood gases are done has also been demonstrated, particularly when used in conjunction with end-tidal carbon dioxide ($ETCO_2$) determination. Continuous monitoring may indicate the insidious development of shock as vasoconstriction develops. Continuous oximetry is mandatory in patients requiring definitive airway management.

Limitations and Precautions

Limitations to the accuracy of pulse oximetry exist with severe vasoconstriction (e.g., shock, hypothermia), excessive movement, synthetic fingernails and nail polish, severe anemia, or the presence of abnormal hemoglobins. Reflectance oximetry has been demonstrated to reflect oxygen saturations more accurately in the setting of hypothermia and vasoconstriction. Carboxyhemoglobin (COHb) and methemoglobin (MetHb) contribute to light absorption and cause errors in the pulse oximetry readings. The pulse oximeter sees COHb as though it was mostly OxyHb and gives a falsely high reading. MetHb produces a large pulsatile absorbance signal at both the red and IR wavelengths. This effect forces the absorbance ratio toward unity, which corresponds to a S_pO_2 of 85%. Thus, in the presence of high levels of MetHb, the S_pO_2 is erroneously low when the arterial saturation is above 85% and erroneously high when the arterial saturation is below 85%. In dark-skinned patients, erroneously high readings (about 3%–5%) and a higher incidence of failure to detect signal have been reported.

Pulse oximetry has been shown to be of limited accuracy and reliability during cardiopulmonary resuscitation (CPR) and may be misleading. Nevertheless, its use is indicated during resuscitation because information useful to patient management may be gleaned.

In general, transmission oximetry signals are weaker from ears than from fingers, except in the face of hypotension or peripheral vasoconstriction, but ear responses are faster. Nasal bridge probes have been reported to read falsely high in some circumstances. When compared to reflectance sensors, there are fewer potential sensor sites, the response time can be lengthy, and its performance is more adversely affected by ambient light, motion, and poor perfusion.

Reflectance oximeters have emitting and sensing diodes on a single surface. Therefore, they can be placed in anatomical locations that do not require two surfaces in close proximity with a vascular bed in between. In fact, "oximetric Swan-Ganz" catheters employ this technology to monitor venous oxygen saturation. Placement on the forehead implies that there is better correlation with "core" arterial oxygen saturation. The big disadvantage of reflectance sensors lies in their propensity to be subject to contaminating sources of tissue (e.g., arteries, pigmentation).

In general, the reflectance sensor is more sophisticated in design, requires more user skill (to correctly apply the sensor and interpret the results, including waveform morphology), can provide more parameters, and has greater versatility than transillumination methods.

The pulse oximeter measures oxygen saturation, not the partial pressure of oxygen. This means that it is possible for the partial pressure of oxygen to fall substantially before the oxygen saturation starts to fall. The explanation lies in the sigmoid shape of the OxyHb dissociation curve. If a healthy adult patient is given 100% oxygen to breathe for a few minutes and then ventilation ceases for any reason, several minutes may elapse before the oxygen saturation starts to fall (see Chapter 3). The pulse oximeter in these circumstances therefore warns of a potentially fatal complication several minutes after it has begun. This is sometimes referred to as *monitor lag*.

Finally, adequate oxygen saturation does not indicate that the patient is *ventilating* adequately. This is particularly important in patients with decreased levels of consciousness, such as during procedural sedation. Routine carbon dioxide (CO_2) monitoring during procedural sedation is a better means of assessing the adequacy of minute ventilation (see the next section).

END-TIDAL CARBON DIOXIDE MONITORING

The concentration of CO_2 in exhaled breath is intrinsically linked to tissue metabolism, pulmonary (central) circulation, and ventilation. *Capnography* is the noninvasive graphic record of instantaneous CO_2 concentrations in the respired gases during a respiratory cycle represented as a waveform or *capnogram*. Although the concentrations of CO_2 can be displayed continuously through the respiratory cycle, it is conventional that only the maximum CO_2 concentration at the end of each tidal exhalation, the $ETCO_2$, is displayed. *Capnometry* is the quantitative measurement of $ETCO_2$ on a visual display without a waveform. *Colorimetric* detectors use color scales to estimate ranges of $ETCO_2$, but are not sufficiently accurate to give quantitative measurements. Their use is therefore limited to confirmation of endotracheal tube (ETT) placement in the trachea and its continuous location in the trachea.

$ETCO_2$ monitoring is becoming increasingly common in the ED and prehospital setting. A 1998 survey of emergency medicine training programs in the United States found that more than 80% use CO_2 monitoring, with colorimetric devices being the most frequently used at that time.

Principles of Measurement

Four spectrographic methods are used to measure $ETCO_2$ concentration in expired gases: IR, mass, Raman, and photoacoustic spectrography with most stand-alone monitors using the IR technique. CO_2 selectively absorbs IR light with a wavelength of 4.26 μm. The concentration of CO_2 in a gas can be determined by passing filtered IR light through the gas and comparing the amount of light that is absorbed to a reference light beam passing through a CO_2-free chamber.

CO$_2$ monitors are configured as either sidestream or mainstream, depending on the location of the photoelectric detector or sensor. *Sidestream* monitors, more likely to be encountered in emergency medical services and the ED, aspirate a sample of gas through a small catheter into a measuring chamber located inside the monitor. They are lightweight, can be used in intubated and nonintubated patients, and have nasal-oral airway interfaces (cannula) that simultaneously sample CO_2 and deliver low-flow oxygen. This allows for preoxygenation and continuous oxygen delivery during procedural sedation and analgesia. High-flow sidestream systems (150 cc/minute) have several disadvantages, including plugging by secretions, 2- or 3-second delays in response time, and air leaks, which can dilute the sample. Newer generation low-flow systems (50 cc/minute) do not have these problems. *Mainstream* monitors, useful only in intubated patients, are bulky and heavy, with the sensor positioned at the hub of the ETT, and because they must be heated to prevent condensation, may burn patients.

Colorimetric CO_2 detectors use pH-sensitive filter paper impregnated with metacresol purple, which changes color from purple (<4 mm Hg CO_2) to tan (4–15 mm Hg CO_2) to yellow (>20 mm Hg CO_2), depending on the concentration of CO_2, although there is some variability in absolute numbers based on the brand of device. The indicator, housed in a plastic casing, is inserted between the ETT and the ventilator bag, and responds quickly enough to detect changes on a breath-by-breath basis. They are inexpensive and easy to use, and should be available in every ED for confirmation of ETT placement if quantitative methods are not available.

In otherwise healthy patients, a close correlation exists between $ETCO_2$ (i.e., the alveolar CO_2 [$PaCO_2$]) and the arterial partial pressure ($PaCO_2$). The $ETCO_2$ is approximately 2 to 5 mm Hg less than the $PaCO_2$ because of the contribution of physiological dead space to the end-expiratory gases. Most conditions that affect ventilation-perfusion ratios can widen the Pa-$ETCO_2$ gradient, including pulmonary embolism, cardiac arrest, hypovolemia, obstructive lung disease, and the lateral decubitus position. Although $ETCO_2$ may not always accurately reflect the absolute $PaCO_2$ in critically ill patients, it is still valuable in detecting ventilatory trends and identifying sudden airway events (e.g., apnea, extubation, pulmonary embolism).

Phases of the Capnogram

Analysis of the waveform by the measurement of expired CO_2 concentration over time can yield valuable clinical information. A normal capnogram has four phases (Fig. 39-1). Phase A-B represents the CO_2-free portion of the respiratory cycle. Most often, this occurs at the end of the inspiratory phase, although it may represent apnea or a disconnection of the device from the patient. An elevation of this baseline above zero implies CO_2 rebreathing, as might be the case with increased dead space in the circuit, hypoventilation (high-flow sidestream sensors only), or contamination of the sensor.

Phase B-C, the *rapid upstroke* of the curve, represents the transition from inspiration to expiration and the mixing of dead space and alveolar gas. Prolongation of phase B-C (Fig. 39-1) occurs with obstruction to expiratory gas flow (e.g., obstructive lung disease, bronchospasm, kinked ETT) or leaks in the breathing system.

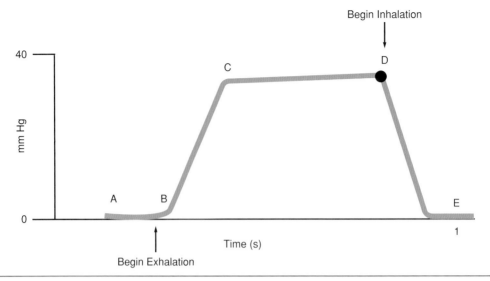

Figure 39-1 ● Normal capnogram.

Phase C-D, the *alveolar plateau,* represents the predominance of alveolar gas rich in CO_2 and tends to slope gently upward with the uneven emptying of alveoli. The maximum CO_2 concentration in each breath (i.e., $ETCO_2$) represents *point D* and is the number that appears on the monitor. The slope of this phase can be increased by the same obstructive factors that increase the slope of phase B-C, as well as a normal physiological variation in pregnancy. A dip in the plateau indicates a spontaneous respiratory effort during mechanical ventilation, as might occur in patients with hypoxia, hypercarbia, or emerging from anesthesia.

Phase D-E, the *inspiratory downstroke,* is a nearly vertical drop to baseline. This slope can be prolonged and blend in with the beginning of the expiratory phase in endotracheal cuff leaks. Abnormal respiratory patterns that are chaotic limit the usefulness of $ETCO_2$ monitoring because characteristic patterns are difficult to discern.

Clinical Uses of Capnography

Capnography can be used in the ED for many clinical scenarios in both intubated and non-intubated patients. These include confirmation of ETT placement in the trachea, continuous monitoring of tube position, providing qualitative and quantitative methods of assessing cardiac output, gauging effectiveness of CPR during cardiac arrest (Fig. 39-2), determining prognosis in CPR and in trauma, maintaining appropriate $ETCO_2$ levels in patients with suspected increases in intracranial pressure, aiding in the detection and diagnosis of pulmonary embolism (air and clot), assessing response to treatment in patients with acute respiratory distress, determining adequacy of ventilation in patients with altered mental status (including drug-induced alterations in consciousness during procedural sedation and analgesia; Fig. 39-3), assessment of ventilatory status of actively seizing patients, and detection of metabolic acidosis in diabetes and gastroenteritis.

Along with visualizing an ETT going through the vocal cords and seeing tracheal rings on bronchoscopy, CO_2 monitoring is another "gold standard" used to confirm intubation of the trachea (see Chapter 3). Misleading $ETCO_2$ readings can occur with erroneous esophageal intubation after bag-mask ventilation and ingestion of carbonated beverages or antacids. These tracings are abnormal in appearance and resolve after six breaths. $ETCO_2$ is also falsely elevated for about 5 minutes after injection of sodium bicarbonate. In nonarrest

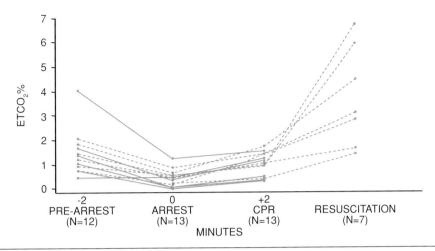

Figure 39-2 ● End-tidal carbon dioxide ($ETCO_2$) pattern during cardiac arrest.

settings, the $ETCO_2$ approaches 100% sensitivity and specificity in confirming correct ETT placement; conversely, it is also useful in detecting accidental extubation.

$ETCO_2$ can estimate $PaCO_2$ in hemodynamically stable patients with normal lung function. Although the normal Pa-$ETCO_2$ gradient is approximately 2 to 5 mm Hg, this may increase in patients with hemodynamic instability and pulmonary disorders, with the width of the gradient dependent on the severity of the lung disease or decrease in perfusion. Characteristic capnographic patterns associated with restrictive and obstructive lung disease are shown in Figure 39-4. Initially, it may be helpful to compare the $PaCO_2$ with the $ETCO_2$ to determine whether a difference is present and to quantify the difference, particularly in ventilated patients with obstructive lung disease (where the ventilator inspiratory cycle ordinarily interrupts the plateau phase before it becomes flat, underestimating the true end-tidal concentration of CO_2) or in unstable patients. With correction for this gradient, $ETCO_2$ trends can generally be used as a substitute for serial $PaCO_2$ measurements.

The airway, breathing, and circulation of critically ill or injured patients can be rapidly assessed using $ETCO_2$ values and the capnogram. The presence of a normal waveform denotes a patent airway and spontaneous breathing, and normal $ETCO_2$ levels indicate adequate perfusion. Therefore, capnography can be used to assess critically ill patients

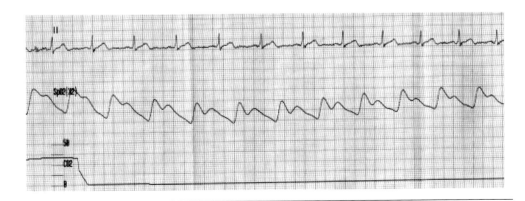

Figure 39-3 ● Capnographic detection of apnea.

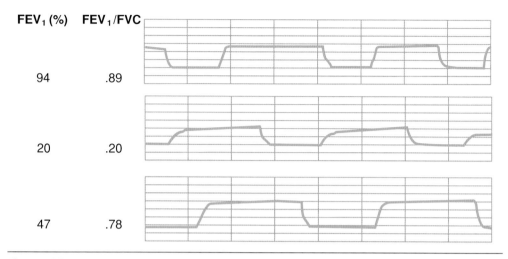

Figure 39-4 ● Capnogram shape in normal subjects and patients with obstructive and restrictive lung disease.

(including victims of chemical terrorism with nerve gas exposure) and actively seizing patients. Unlike pulse oximetry, capnography does not misinterpret motion artifact and provides reliable readings in low perfusion states.

Animal and human studies have shown that $ETCO_2$ is a noninvasive measurement that is highly correlated with cardiac output and is the earliest indicator of return of spontaneous circulation (ROSC) in CPR. ROSC is heralded by an almost immediate increase in $ETCO_2$ from baseline. Multiple studies have shown that $ETCO_2$ has prognostic value in terms of mortality during CPR. No patient with a mean $ETCO_2$ level <10 mm Hg after 20 minutes of CPR survived, giving $ETCO_2$ measurement a high negative predictive value for failure of resuscitation. Despite these promising findings, capnography requires further prospective validation to confirm its utility as a prognostic tool in cardiac arrest.

The measurement of cardiac output ordinarily requires the placement of pulmonary arterial catheters and is rarely done in the ED, although noninvasive methods are continually being identified, including the use of $ETCO_2$. Using modified forms of the direct Fick equation, animal and human studies have shown excellent correlation between $ETCO_2$ measurements and cardiac output over a wide range of values. These measurements seem independent of changes in dead space (hypovolemia) or shunt (pulmonary edema) and may be adaptable to nonintubated patients.

Capnography is the only monitoring modality that is accurate and reliable in actively seizing patients. Capnographic data (respiratory rate, $ETCO_2$, and capnogram) can be used to distinguish among actively seizing patients with apnea (flatline waveform, no $ETCO_2$ readings, and no chest wall movement), with ineffective ventilation and low tidal volume breathing (small waveforms, low $ETCO_2$ values), and with effective ventilation (normal waveform, normal $ETCO_2$ values).

Capnography can also rapidly detect the common airway, respiratory, and central nervous system adverse events associated with the nerve agents in chemical terrorism, including apnea, upper airway obstruction, laryngospasm, bronchospasm, and respiratory failure.

Capnography provides dynamic monitoring of ventilatory status in patients with acute respiratory distress, including asthma, bronchiolitis, chronic obstructive pulmonary disease, congestive heart failure, croup, and cystic fibrosis. By measuring $ETCO_2$ and respiratory rate with each breath, capnography provides instantaneous feedback on the clinical status of the patient. Respiratory rate is measured directly from the airway by nasal-oral cannula, providing a more reliable reading than impedance respiratory monitoring. In upper airway obstruction and laryngospasm, impedance monitoring detects chest wall movement, interprets this as a valid breath, and displays a respiratory rate, even though the patient is not ventilating. In contrast, capnography will detect no ventilation and shows a flatline waveform.

$ETCO_2$ trends can be rapidly assessed in tachypneic patients. A patient with a respiratory rate of 30 will generate 150 $ETCO_2$ readings in 5 minutes. This provides sufficient information to determine the vector of the patient's ventilatory status: worsening despite treatment (increasing $ETCO_2$), stabilizing (stable $ETCO_2$), or improving (decreasing $ETCO_2$).

Bronchospasm in obstructive lung disease leads to upward slanting of the expiratory plateau of the capnogram (Fig. 39-4). Changes in $ETCO_2$ over time and the slope of this phase of the capnogram have been shown to correlate well with spirometric measurements (FEV_1 and PEFR). Capnography has the advantage of being independent of effort, gender, age, and height, and is a useful objective measure in asthmatic patients who are unwilling or unable to cooperate with spirometry (e.g., young children, ventilated patients, patients in acute respiratory distress).

Capnography can also detect the common adverse airway and respiratory events associated with procedural sedation and analgesia. Capnography is the earliest indicator of airway or respiratory compromise and will manifest an abnormally high or low $ETCO_2$ before pulse oximetry detects falling OxyHb saturation, especially in patients receiving supplemental oxygen. Both central and obstructive apnea can be almost instantaneously detected by capnography. Loss of the capnogram, in conjunction with no chest wall movement and no breath sounds on auscultation, confirms the diagnosis of central apnea. Obstructive apnea is characterized by loss of the capnogram, chest wall movement, and absent breath sounds. The absence of the capnogram in association with the presence or absence of chest wall movement distinguishes apnea from upper airway obstruction and laryngospasm. Response to airway alignment maneuvers can further distinguish upper airway obstruction from laryngospasm.

Capnography may be more sensitive than clinical assessment of ventilation in detection of apnea. In a recent study, 10 of 39 (26%) patients experienced 20-second periods of apnea during procedural sedation and analgesia. All ten episodes of apnea were detected by capnography, but not by the anesthesia providers.

Obtunded or unconscious patients, including those with alcohol intoxication, intentional or unintentional drug overdose, and postictal patients (especially those treated with benzodiazepines), may have impaired ventilation. Capnography can differentiate between postictal patients with effective ventilation and those with ineffective ventilation, as well as provide continuous monitoring of ventilatory trends over time to identify those patients at risk for respiratory depression and respiratory failure.

In addition to its established uses for assessment of ventilation and perfusion, capnography is a valuable tool for assessing metabolic status. Recent studies have shown that $ETCO_2$ and serum bicarbonate (HCO_3) are linearly correlated in diabetes and in gastroenteritis, and $ETCO_2$ can be used as an indicator of metabolic acidosis in these patients (Figs. 39-5 and 39-6, respectively). As a patient becomes acidotic, HCO_3 decreases, and a compensatory respiratory alkalosis develops with an increase in minute ventilation and a resultant decrease in $ETCO_2$. The more acidotic the patient, the lower is the HCO_3, the higher the respiratory rate, and the lower the $ETCO_2$. Furthermore, $ETCO_2$ can be used to distinguish diabetics in ketoacidosis (metabolic acidosis, compensatory tachypnea, low $ETCO_2$) from those who are not (nonacidotic, normal respiratory rate, normal $ETCO_2$). In a study of diabetic children presenting to the ED, $ETCO_2$ <29 mm Hg identified 95% of the patients with ketoacidosis, with 83% sensitivity and 100% specificity. No ketoacidosis was detected in patients with $ETCO_2$ >36 mm Hg (Fig. 39-5).

A similar association between $ETCO_2$ and HCO_3 was demonstrated in children with gastroenteritis, with maximal sensitivity occurring at $ETCO_2$ ≤34 mm Hg (sensitivity 100%,

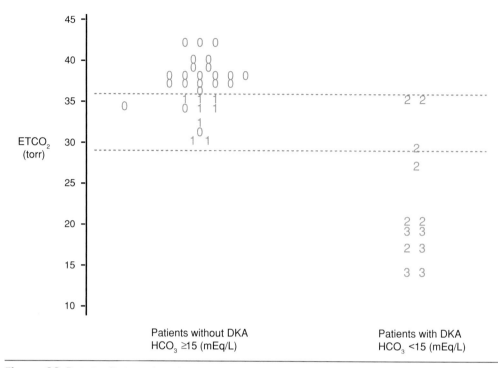

Figure 39-5 ● Predictive value of end-tidal carbon dioxide (ETCO$_2$) in detecting metabolic acidosis in diabetics.

specificity 60%) and optimal specificity without compromise of sensitivity occurring at ETCO$_2$ ≤31 mm Hg (sensitivity 76%, specificity 96%) (Fig. 39-6). As a potential triage tool for determining the need for oral versus intravenous rehydration, ETCO$_2$ could identify patients with a clinically significant acidosis, with an ETCO$_2$ ≤31 mm Hg giving a positive likelihood ratio of 20.4 in detecting HCO$_3$ ≤15 mmol/L and a ratio of 14.1 for HCO$_3$

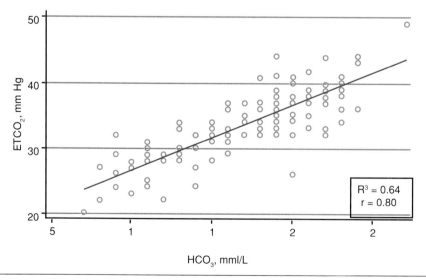

Figure 39-6 ● End-tidal carbon dioxide (ETCO$_2$)-serum bicarbonate (HCO$_3$) correlation in gastroenteritis.

≤ 13 mmol/L. These $ETCO_2$ values are 14 or 20 times more likely to occur in an acidotic patient than in a patient with an HCO_3 >13 mmol/L or >15 mmol/L.

Sublingual Capnography

Studies in the mid-1990s showed that increases in esophageal and gastric PCO_2 ("gastric tonometry") are associated with tissue dysoxia, most commonly found in low perfusion states, occurring early in the course of shock before more conventional measures of tissue oxygenation, such as heart rate, blood pressure, serum lactate, and arterial blood gases. Sublingual capnometry ($P_{SL}CO_2$) correlates with gastric tonometry and is a useful, noninvasive alternative to visceral PCO_2 monitoring.

Sublingual capnometry is relatively simple to monitor. A noninvasive microelectrode CO_2 probe is placed under the tongue. A handheld device similar in appearance to a digital thermometer provides a continuous $P_{SL}CO_2$ reading. The device consists of three major components: a disposable CO_2 sensor, a fiberoptic cable that connects the disposable sensor to a blood gas analyzer, and a blood gas monitoring instrument.

Studies currently underway to determine what absolute measures of $P_{SL}CO_2$ or trends in $P_{SL}CO_2$ will be useful in diagnosing early tissue dysoxia. One study of patients with penetrating torso trauma found that a $P_{SL}CO_2$ <45 mm Hg accurately predicted hemodynamic stability. With further study, this technology may prove useful in emergency medicine and prehospital care, where the early detection of tissue dysoxia is important and currently imprecise. Unfortunately, the discovery of contamination of the sublingual probe with *Burkholderia cepacia* has led to a voluntary recall of the product.

CONCLUSION

Capnography is a versatile noninvasive diagnostic monitoring modality that provides real-time information on the ventilatory, perfusion, and metabolic status of both intubated and nonintubated patients.

EVIDENCE

1. **What are some of the key issues that the emergency airway manager needs to be aware of when it comes to pulse oximetry in the ED?** Monitor lag (the time taken for OxyHb saturation to reflect falling oxygen partial pressure) and response delay (the time taken to equilibrate because of intermittent sampling) are well described by Hill and Stoneham (1). Kellerman et al. (2) demonstrated that ready availability of pulse oximetry in the ED reduces arterial blood gas sampling. Reflectance oximetry has been demonstrated to more accurately reflect oxygen saturations in the setting of hypothermia and vasoconstriction (3,4). The limitations of pulse oximetry in reflecting the adequacy of oxygenation during CPR are well documented (5–7).

2. **What are the key indications for $ETCO_2$ monitoring in the ED?** The most common indications in the ED are to evaluate the adequacy of ventilation in intubated patients, for verification of ETT placement, for nonintubated patients with acute respiratory distress and during procedural sedation and analgesia (8,9). CO_2 monitoring is also commonly used to evaluate perfusion status during cardiac arrest and shock states, having long been known to be an indicator of pulmonary blood flow (10–15).

DISCLOSURE

Baruch Krauss, MD, EdM, is a consultant for Oridion Medical, a capnography company, and holds two patents in the area of capnography.

REFERENCES

1. Hill E, Stoneham MD. Practical applications of pulse oximetry. *Update in anaesthesia* 2000;11:1–2. Available at: http://www.nda.ox.ac.uk/wfsa/html/u11/u1104_01.htm.

2. Kellerman AL, Cofer CA, Joseph S, et al. Impact of portable oximetry on arterial blood gas test ordering in an urban emergency department. *Ann Emerg Med* 1991;20:130–134.

3. Bebout DE, Mannheimer PD, Wun CCW. Site-dependent differences in the time to detect changes in saturation during low perfusion [abstract]. *Crit Care Med* 2001;29:115a.

4. Keogh BF, Kopotic RJ. Recent findings in the use of reflectance oximetry: a critical review. *Curr Opin Anesthesiol* 2005;18:649–654.

5. Griffin M, Cooney C. Pulse oximetry during cardiopulmonary resuscitation. *Anaesthesia* 1995;50:1008.

6. Spittal MJ. Evaluation of pulse oximetry during cardiopulmonary resuscitation. *Anaesthesia* 1993;48:701–703.

7. Moorthy SS, Didorff SF, Schmidt SI. Erroneous pulse oximeter data during CPR. *Anesth Analg* 1990;70:339.

8. Krauss B, Hess DR. Capnography for procedural sedation and analgesia in the emergency department. *Ann Emerg Med* 2007;50:172–181.

9. Soto RG, Fu ES, Vila H, et al. Capnography accurately detects apnea during monitored anesthesia care. *Anesth Analg* 2004;99:379–382.

10. Levine RL, Wayne MA, Miller CC. End-tidal carbon dioxide and outcome of out-of-hospital cardiac arrest. *N Engl J Med* 1997;337:301.

11. Falk JL, Rackow EC, Weil MH. End-tidal carbon dioxide concentration during cardiopulmonary resuscitation. *N Engl J Med* 1988;318:607.

12. Garnett AR, Ornato JP, Gonzalez ER, et al. End-tidal carbon dioxide monitoring during cardiopulmonary resuscitation. *JAMA* 1987;257:512.

13. Deakin CD, Sado DM, Coats TJ, et al. Prehospital end-tidal carbon dioxide concentration and outcome in major trauma. *J Trauma* 2004;57:65.

14. Cantineau JP, Lambert Y, Merckx P, et al. End-tidal carbon dioxide during cardiopulmonary resuscitation in humans presenting mostly with asystole: a predictor of outcome. *Crit Care Med* 1996;24:791–796.

15. Ahrens T, Schallom L, Bettorf K, et al. End-tidal carbon dioxide measurements as a prognostic indicator of outcome in cardiac arrest. *Am J Crit Care* 2001;10:391–398.

INDEX

439

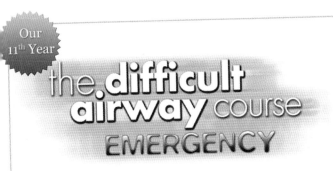
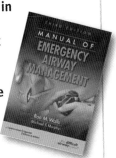

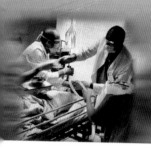
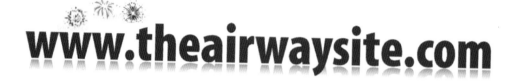
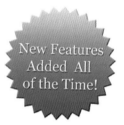
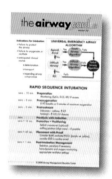
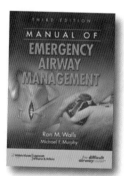
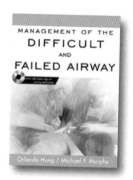